Understanding and treating fear of pain

Understanding and treating fear of pain

Edited by

Gordon J.G. Asmundson
Professor and Research Director
Faculty of Kinesiology and Health Studies
University of Regina
Canada

Johan W.S. Vlaeyen
Associate Professor
Department of Medical, Clinical, and
Experimental Psychology
Maastricht University
Netherlands

Geert Crombez
Professor of Health Psychology
Faculty of Psychology and Educational Sciences
Ghent University
Belgium

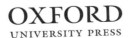

OXFORD
UNIVERSITY PRESS

OXFORD

UNIVERSITY PRESS

Great Clarendon Street, Oxford OX2 6DP

Oxford University Press is a department of the University of Oxford.
It furthers the University's objective of excellence in research, scholarship,
and education by publishing worldwide in

Oxford New York

Auckland Bangkok Buenos Aires Cape Town Chennai
Dar es Salaam Delhi Hong Kong Istanbul Karachi Kolkata
Kuala Lumpur Madrid Melbourne Mexico City Mumbai Nairobi
São Paulo Shanghai Taipei Tokyo Toronto

Oxford is a registered trade mark of Oxford University Press
in the UK and in certain other countries

Published in the United States
by Oxford University Press Inc., New York

A catalogue record for this title is available from the British Library

ISBN 0 19 8525141 (Hbk)

10 9 8 7 6 5 4 3 2 1

Typeset by Newgen Imaging Systems (P) Ltd., Chennai, India
Printed in Great Britain
on acid-free paper by
Biddles Ltd, King's Lynn

Dedications

To Karen and Graham, for being such vibrant and colourful siblings—
G.J.G.A.

To Nicole, Yana, and Jolinde, most precious people in my life—J.W.S.V.

To Lien, Jana, and Ewout, as evidence that thinking can lead to something
you can see and touch—G.C.

Foreword

Kenneth D. Craig
Professor of Psychology
Senior Investigator
Canadian Institutes of Health Research
University of British Columbia

Bottom line: Embracing the innovative understanding of pain and the related healthcare interventions carefully described in this volume would lead to dramatic improvement in care provided to people suffering or disabled by pain. Put in less scholarly terms: "Warning! Failure to heed the messages in this volume leads to unnecessary suffering."

This outburst of intemperate, non-academic language is provoked by the gravity of the problem. Acute pain is virtually inevitable and universal; while it almost always can be controlled through pharmacological and psychological interventions, under-management of pain is commonplace and anxiety, fears of pain, avoidance behavior and related psychological states can render an individual's stress unmanageable. Another serious problem is pain that persists beyond when healing would be expected if the pain had a basis solely in tissue damage or disease. Chronic pain of this type is the focus of this book. At least one in five persons suffers some form of chronic pain requiring health care or leading to personal or social distress and impairment. While many suffer from injuries or diseases adequate to explain the suffering, explanations grounded in physical pathology are inadequate for the majority of people suffering from chronic pain. The best medical interventions will have failed for these people and there is likely to be mounting biological, psychological, and social damage. These commonplace challenges of acute and chronic pain confront all of us, including our loved ones, and many members of our communities. Thus, a sense of urgency to improve pain control reasonably reflects self-interest, altruistic concern for others, and an appreciation of the enormous health care system costs of this major public health problem. Innovative approaches to pain and pain management must be taken seriously.

One could ask, does the volume represent a novel perspective on pain capable of satisfying the needs of many of these unhappy people? The answer is decidedly yes if the question refers to a remarkably well developed, original synthesis of research and theory incorporating both clinical and basic science issues as well as evidence-based assessment and treatment strategies and tools. The answer perhaps would be no if one were asking whether recognition of the role fear plays in pain were novel. Emotions were recognized as powerful features of pain in ancient writings. However, only in recent decades, culminating in the current surge of interest, have resources been devoted to understanding their important role or have methodologies been developed for clinicians concerned about controlling destructive fear and anxiety that commonly is the root of pain related disability. Fortunately, the concepts have captured the attention of clinical investigators long enough for controlled trials demonstrating the effectiveness of interventions focusing specifically upon fear-avoidance and related psychological processes. These are well described in this volume.

A deliberate focus on understanding and controlling emotional processes rather than sensory features of pain stands in contrast to widespread conventional approaches to pain. Definitions typically characterize pain as a subjective experience with sensory and affective features, but there is a widespread tendency to focus upon sensory qualities. This resonates with most peoples' personal experiences of pain, as they are commonly perceived as sensations arising from injury or disease, although even cursory discussions with people about pain rapidly lead to an examination of feelings, thoughts, and personal and social consequences. Reinforcing the focus on pain as a specific sensation was the major surge of enthusiasm for biomedical research discoveries in the 19th and 20th Centuries. Studies of anatomy, physiology, and chemistry were remarkably successful in helping us understand peripheral mechanisms of pain, with these leading to an appreciation of spinal cord processes. The neuroscience approach became progressively more reductionistic, with molecular biology and biopharmacological sciences enjoying great strength at present. Unquestionably, there have been tremendous breakthroughs in the understanding of basic mechanisms responsible for nociception in the past several decades. One also can have confidence that the genome project, protein mapping, molecular structure calculations and the like will continue to yield extremely important information about how pain works.

Surprisingly however, neuroscience advances in understanding pain have not justified the considerable optimism that the discoveries would lead to novel classes of analgesic drugs. They have not translated into dramatic improvements in pharmacological control of pain—opioids and drugs related to salicylic acid (aspirin, etc.) have remained the mainstay analgesic drugs and their properties have provided the basis for practically every pain reliever available. Unfortunately, these are insufficient, as the legion of chronic pain sufferers attests. The current armamentarium of pain drugs does not provide wholly adequate analgesia. There are substantial individual differences in how people respond to specific analgesics, certain forms of pain are not responsive to the usual analgesics, for example, neuropathic pain, and side effects are often unpleasant, if not dangerous, e.g., gastric lesions arising from salicylates. As well, many people suffer from unrecognized, poorly assessed, under-estimated, and inadequately controlled pain because the complex social structures designed to provide care are often unduly preoccupied with biomedical management. Advances in care will arise from attending to psychological and social features of pain, including those related to the concerns delineated at the beginning of the previous sentence.

Models of pain that include consideration of the social contexts of pain, cognition, and emotional processes, particularly fear and anxiety, improve control by introducing novel interventions that focus upon these features of pain. They reflect an appreciation of central and higher order, divergent and interactive brain mechanisms that for long remained elusive, in part because research methodologies did not lend themselves to investigation of brain systems. Brain imaging technologies are now beginning to provide insights into the brain mechanisms responsible for the complexities of the biological systems that regulate the multiple cognitive, affective and sensory features of pain experience. Of course, it is no surprise to the health care practitioner already familiar with the complexities of pain that both distributed and sequential brain activities are engaged or that the substantial individual differences in the experience of pain are associated with variations in brain activity. It would have been surprising if this were not the case. There clearly is a lot to be learned about the biological systems that subserve fear of pain, pain-related anxiety, catastrophic thinking, attentional mechanisms related to pain, etc., but studies focusing upon behavioral outcomes have provided a good understanding of the functions biological systems must serve.

In part, the advances in understanding and controlling pain described in this volume reflect a willingness to address uniquely human capabilities. There is great merit in a detailed understanding of evolved nociceptive systems in progenitor nonhuman animal species that are well-conserved in humans. But, evolution produced a different animal in *Homo sapiens* and the unique features of human biology and its expression in experience and behavior must be considered. Innate mechanisms acquired in *hominid* ancestral environments included the remarkable human capabilities for social learning and the martialing of resources available through the use of complex social systems. "Medically unexplained pain", a concept that applies to most chronic pain, is less "unexplainable" when cognitive, emotional, and social constructs are used in explanatory models. Contextualizing the symptoms and complaints through the use of constructs that have distinctive human features adds explanatory power.

I am aware that the assertions made here do not have the usual references to sources or databases. The reader will find more than adequate documentation in the engaging writings of the outstanding authors in this volume. For the most part, they are the investigators responsible for the remarkable advances described. The individual chapters provide fresh and vital perspective and they are well edited so the entire volume is integrated and coherent. There is much critical analysis that will inspire further excellent research.

In conclusion, I note the irony in my use of a fear-inspiring message to alert readers to the health hazards of failing to pay attention to fear of pain and other psychosocial factors contributing to pain and related disability, so well articulated in this volume. The warning that restrictive use of biological concepts of pain puts people at risk was directed not only at those responsible for the delivery of health care but also to people at risk of pain or suffering from pain. Inclusive models of pain and treatment strategies directly addressing fear of pain and other psychological parameters, as well the social contexts that promote either debilitating invalidism or effective coping, return control of pain to those most likely to suffer.

Preface

Pain has been conceptualized both as an affective experience and as pure sensation arising from noxious simulation. Current theory holds that pain comprises sensory as well as cognitive, affective, and behavioral components. Thus, pain can be viewed as both a sensory and emotional experience. Pain typically occurs in response to actual or potential tissue damage to motivate (when possible) escape from the source of pain and promote recuperative behavior. Although there is some evidence to suggest that the affective, cognitive, and behavioral experiences of those with acute pain are similar to those with chronic pain, the latter will be the primary focus of this volume. For our purposes, chronic pain is defined in accordance with the International Association for the Study of Pain as pain that persists over a period of at least 3 months.

Relative to the emotional context of pain, people with chronic pain tend to be more fearful and anxious than the general population. This fear and anxiety may be related to a variety of factors, including, but not limited to, worries of not regaining lost functional abilities, financial difficulties, feelings of social inadequacy, and uncertainty about the physical consequences of persistent pain. Recently there has been an increase in theoretical and empirical efforts to delineate the precise nature of the relationship between fear, anxiety, and chronic pain. Indeed, based on the proposition that fear of pain and, in the case of chronic musculoskeletal pain, fear of (re)injury, serves as a mechanism through which pain is maintained over time, considerable strides in assessment, treatment, and research have been made. This progress is encouraging but, as will become apparent, there is considerably more work to be done.

How do pain-related fear and anxiety serve to maintain and exacerbate pain? Do they predispose some people to develop pain of a chronic nature? What exactly is it that they fear? How do we best assess and treat patients with fear and anxiety that co-occurs with chronic pain? These are but a few of the questions that will be addressed by the chapters in this volume. The purpose of this volume is to provide you with a resource that comprehensively covers the important issues and developments in theory, research, and treatment of pain-related fear and anxiety. In a general sense, then, this volume will provide a roadmap of where we have been and where we are heading in our attempts to understand and treat fear and anxiety in the context of chronic pain. Theoretical positions will be outlined, research advances in delineating basic mechanisms will be described and evaluated, new and emerging treatment approaches will be detailed, and suggestions for future directions of investigation will be provided. The chapters make ample use of tables and figures and, in the assessment and treatment sections, clinical vignettes, in order to help illustrate important concepts and points.

This volume is organized into four parts. In Part I, you are introduced to current theoretical positions regarding pain-related fear and anxiety. Relevant empirical findings are also covered in Part I. Part II provides a comprehensive coverage of assessment issues, ranging from determining what it is that your patient fears to selecting appropriate assessment instruments. Part III delineates important advances in treatment strategies that can be employed when dealing with patients with significant pain-related fear and anxiety, whether in a primary care or specialty treatment setting. Finally, Part IV summarizes what we believe to be some of the critical points of the previous parts and, further, offers avenues of future investigation.

We hope that this volume will appeal to a wide audience of mental health and medical professionals, including psychologists, psychiatrists, and medical specialists who deal with patients with chronic pain, general practitioners, councilors, physical therapists, occupational therapists, and students in mental health and medical professions (e.g. psychology graduate students, general medicine interns, psychiatry residents). Issues of pain-related fear and anxiety, and their influence on function, are, arguably, amongst the fastest growing areas in pain research and management. So, whether you are a practicing clinician, a researcher, or both, we hope this volume will help guide and shape your efforts to better understand the oft devastating issues that accompany pain-related fear and anxiety.

September 2003

Gordon J.G. Asmundson
Johan W.S. Vlaeyen
Geert Crombez

Acknowledgments

We are very grateful to R. Nicholas Carleton, Kristi D. Wright, and Michael J. Coons for their editorial assistance and to our families for their everlasting support and encouragement.

Contents

About the Editors

Gordon J.G. Asmundson PhD is a Professor and Research Director in the Faculty of Kinesiology and Health Studies at the University of Regina, Canada and an Adjunct Professor of Psychiatry at the University of Saskatchewan. He is currently the North American Editor of *Cognitive Behaviour Therapy* and serves on the editorial boards for the *Journal of Anxiety Disorders*, the *Clinical Journal of Pain*, and the *European Journal of Pain*. He has published over 110 journal articles and book chapters as well as 4 books, including *Clinical Research in Mental Health* (with G. Ron Norton and Murray B. Stein; 2002, Thousand Oaks, CA: Sage), the edited volume *Health Anxiety* (with Steven Taylor and Brian J. Cox; 2001, New York, NY: Wiley), and the co-authored volume *Treating Health Anxiety: A Cognitive–Behavioral Approach* (with Steven Taylor; 2004, New York, NY: Guilford). He served as a member of the *Diagnostic and Statistical Manual of Mental Disorders-IV (DSM-IV)* Text Revision Work Group for the Anxiety Disorders. Dr Asmundson's research contributions have been recognized by early career awards from the Anxiety Disorders Association of America, the Canadian chapter of the International Association for the Study of Pain, and the Canadian Psychological Association. He is actively involved in clinical research and clinical research supervision and has interests in assessment and basic mechanisms of the anxiety disorders, health anxiety, acute and chronic pain, and the association of these with disability and behavior change.

Johan W.S. Vlaeyen PhD is a Clinical Psychologist. He completed an APA-approved Clinical Psychology internship at the University of Washington, Seattle, United States, under supervision of Professor Wilbert Fordyce. He currently is Associate Professor at the Department of Medical, Clinical, and Experimental Psychology of the Maastricht University, member of the Pain Management and Research Center of the University Hospital Maastricht, and affiliated with the Institute for Rehabilitation Research at Hoensbroeck. He also directs the department of pain and somatoform disorders of the Research Institute "Experimental Psychopathology" of the Maastricht University. Dr. Vlaeyen currently serves on the editorial boards of *Cognitive Behaviour Therapy*, the *Clinical Journal of Pain*, and the *European Journal of Pain*. He served as a member of the Pain Curriculum for Psychologists of the International Association for the Study of Pain, and he is recipient of an award from the Belgian chapter of the International Association for the Study of Pain for his contributions in pain research. He is actively involved in clinical research and clinical research supervision, and has interests in assessment and cognitive and behavioral mechanisms of chronic pain and somatoform disorders, the role of pain-related fear and mood in pain disability, and the cognitive–behavioral treatment of pain disorders.

Geert Crombez PhD is Professor of Health Psychology in the Faculty of Psychology and Educational Sciences at the Ghent University, Belgium. He is director of the Research Center "Health and Behavior," and the Research Center "Experimental Psychopathology" at the Ghent University. He has published over 130 journal articles and book chapters. His contributions have been recognized by an early career award from the Belgian chapter of the International Association for the Study of Pain. He is actively involved in experimental and clinical research regarding acute and chronic pain, fatigue, trauma, obesitas, and fear and anxiety disorders, and has interests in the basic processes of learning, attention, and memory.

Contributors

Gordon J.G. Asmundson PhD
Anxiety and Illness Behaviours
Laboratory, Faculty of Kinseiology and
Health Studies,
University of Regina, Regina,
Saskatchewan, Canada S4S 0A2

Benjamin H.K. Balderson PhD
Center for Health Studies,
1730 Minor Avenue, Suite 1600, Seattle,
Washington, USA 98101

Katja Boersma
Section of Behavioral Medicine,
Department of Occupational and
Environmental Medicine, Örebro
University Hospital, Örebro, Sweden

Michael J. Coons MA
Department of Psychology, University
of Waterloo, Waterloo, Ontario,
Canada.

Geert Crombez PhD
Faculty of Psychology and
Educational Sciences, Ghent
University, Belgium

Jeroen de Jong MSc
Department of Medical, Clinical,
and Experimental Psychology,
Maastricht University,
The Netherlands

Peter J. de Jong PhD
Department of Medical, Clinical,
and Experimental Psychology,
Maastricht University,
The Netherlands

Christopher Eccleston PhD
Pain Management Unit,
Royal National Hospital for Rheumatic
Diseases and University of Bath, Bath,
UK BA1 1RL

Els L.M. Gheldof MSc
Vakgroep Gedragswetenschappen—
Psychologie, Limburgs Universitair
Centrum, Universitaire Campus,
Diepenbeek, Belgium

Liesbet Goubert PhD
Faculty of Psychology and Educational
Sciences, Ghent University, Belgium

Heather D. Hadjistavropoulos PhD
Department of Psychology, University
of Regina, Regina, Saskatchewan,
Canada S4S 0A2

Ruud M.A. Houben MSc
Department of Medical,
Clinical, and Experimental Psychology,
Maastricht University, Maastricht,
The Netherlands

Edmund Keogh PhD
Department of Psychology, University
of Bath, Bath, UK BA2 7AY

Kristine M. Kowalyk MA
Department of Psychology, University
of Regina, Regina, Saskatchewan,
Canada S4S 0A2

Maaike Leeuw MSc
Department of Medical, Clinical, and
Experimental Psychology, Maastricht
University, The Netherlands

Elizabeth H.B. Lin MD MPH
Department of Psychiatry and
Behavioral Sciences, University of
Washington, Seattle, Washington, USA
98195-6560

Steven J. Linton PhD
Section of Behavioral Medicine,
Department of Occupational and
Environmental Medicine, Örebro
University Hospital, Örebro,
Sweden

Lance M. McCracken PhD
Pain Management Unit, Royal
National Hospital for Rheumatic
Diseases and University of Bath,
Bath, UK BA1 1RL

Daniel W. McNeil PhD
Department of Psychology, West
Virginia University, Morgantown,
Virginia, USA 26506-6040

Stephen Morley PhD
Academic Unit of Psychiatry
and Behavioural Sciences, School
of Medicine, University of Leeds,
Leeds, UK LS2 9JT

Peter J. Norton PhD
Department of Psychology, University
of Houston,
Houston, Texas, USA 77204-5022

Madelon Peters PhD
Department of Medical, Clinical, and
Experimental Psychology, Maastricht
University, The Netherlands

Jeffrey Roelofs MSc
Department of Medical, Clinical,
and Experimental Psychology,
Maastricht University,
The Netherlands

Henk A. Seelen PhD
Institute for Rehabilitation Research,
Posture and Movement Research
Group, Hoensbroek,
The Netherlands

Stefaan Van Damme PhD
Department of Experimental, Clinical
and Health Psychology Ghent
University, Ghent, Belgium

Jeanine A. Verbunt MD
Rehabilitation Foundation
Limburg, Hoensbroek,
The Netherlands

Jan Vinck
Limburg University Centre,
Department of Human and
Social Sciences, Belgium

Johan W.S. Vlaeyen PhD
Department of Medical, Clinical,
and Experimental Psychology,
Maastricht University,
Maastricht, The Netherlands

Michael Von Korff ScD
Department of Psychiatry and
Behavioral Sciences,
University of Washington,
Seattle, Washington,
USA 98195-6560

Kevin E. Vowles
Department of Psychology, West
Virginia University, Morgantown,
Virginia, USA 26506-6040

Amanda C. de C. Williams PhD
INPUT Pain Management Unit, Guy's
and St. Thomas' Hospital
NHS Trust, London,
UK SE1 7EH

Abbreviations

APP	Affective Priming Paradigm
ASI	Anxiety Sensitivity Index
ASP	Affective Simon Paradigma
BCQ	Body Consciousness Questionnaire
BT	Behavioral Treatment
BVS	Body Vigilance Scale
CBT	Cognitive Behavioral Treatment
CR	Conditioned Response
CS	Conditioned Stimulus
CSQ	Coping Strategies Questionnaire
DSM-IV	*Diagnostic and Statistical Manual of Mental Disorders-IV*
EAST	Extrinsic Affective Simon Task
ERP	Event-Related Management
FABQ	Fear-Avoidance Beliefs Questionnaire
FPQ	Fear of Pain Questionnaire
MPI	Multidimensional Pain Inventory
MSPQ	Modified Somatic Perceptions Questionnaire
NA	Negative Affectivity
PAIRS	Pain and Impairment Relationship Scale
PASS	Pain Anxiety Symptoms Scale
PBQ	Pain Beliefs Questionnaire
PCS	Pain Catastrophizing Scale
PHODA	Photograph Series of Daily Activities
PILL	Pennebaker Inventory of Limbic Languidness
PTSD	Posttraumatic Stress Disorder
PVAQ	Pain Vigilance and Awareness Questionnaire
RCT	Randomized Controlled Trial
SOPA	Survey of Pain Attitudes
TSK	Tampa Scale of Kinesphobia
UCR	Unconditioned Response
UCS	Unconditioned Stimulus

Part I

Theoretical foundations and empirical findings

Chapter 1

Fear-avoidance models of chronic pain: An overview

Gordon J.G. Asmundson, Peter J. Norton, and Johan W.S. Vlaeyen

1 Introduction

Over the past decade there has been a burgeoning of research aimed specifically at better understanding the role that fear, anxiety, and avoidance behavior play in the development and exacerbation of chronic pain following apparently healed acute musculoskeletal injury or benign (harmless) somatic conditions. Although reviewed in recent years (Asmundson *et al.* 1999; Vlaeyen and Linton 2000), this literature has continued to grow, has clarified associations with parallel lines of investigation (e.g. the anxiety disorders), and is now stimulating new and exciting practical applications designed to reduce pain chronicity and associated disability. The primary purpose of this chapter is to outline the general tenets of current fear-avoidance models of chronic pain and to provide some potentially useful updates to these. These models provide a foundation on which the remaining chapters are based. Detailed discussion of the empirical support, strengths, and weaknesses, and applied aspects of the fear-avoidance models will be left to the accomplished scholars who have penned the chapters that follow.

An obvious place to begin our overview is to briefly examine the evolution of the epistemology of pain and chronic pain. Some years ago, a student working with one of us wrote in her thesis something to the effect that "since the dawn of time, the battle against pain has plagued humankind." Melodramatics aside, the intent of her statement is quite clear: Pain and attempts to alleviate it have always been a part of the human experience. And yet, despite our long-standing familiarity with pain, a complete grasp of its causes, facets, functions, and dysfunctions has proven elusive. Why?

One likely reason is that the experience of pain is idiosyncratic. One person may respond vociferously to a physical injury, while another similar person might show minimal response to an identical injury (e.g. Boos *et al.* 1995).

Soldiers in combat have been known to not perceive pain from an injury inflicted during battle, while others with similar injuries report severe pain (Beecher 1956). People have demonstrated extreme pain responses when they incorrectly believed they were injured (see Merskey and Spear 1967) and, in a similar vein, some people report continued pain after an injury or insult has fully healed (Beals and Hickman 1972). Collectively, these sort of observations suggest that the perception of pain can dramatically differ between injuries of similar nature that occur at different times.

Similar individual differences occur with other perceptions. Two people may not perceive the color of a rose to be exactly the same, and they may have a somewhat different perception of the flavor of a glass of chardonnay. But, unless stimuli are very intense or noxious, independent observers are not likely to notice individual differences in perceptions of the rose or the chardonnay. With pain, however, responses to its perception as well as subtle individual differences in these responses are often observable (to both casual and trained observers). These individual differences become particularly important in explaining (1) pain that is decidedly incongruous with the extent of identifiable injury or tissue damage, and (2) pain that occurs in the absence of identifiable injury or organic pathology, or that persists after an injury has apparently healed.

Below we examine elements of various models of pain. We do this in order to demonstrate that, despite their seemingly apparent importance, individual differences and their influence on pain perception have been of theoretical and empirical importance for less than half a century (also see Asmundson and Wright 2004). This historical overview will also set the stage for our consideration of fear, anxiety, and avoidance and the role that they play in chronic pain and the disability often associated with it.

2 Traditional biomedical models of pain and chronic pain

Biomedical models of pain are thousands of years old. Over 2000 years ago Ancient Greek society, largely based on the work of Hippocrates and Galen, provided one of the earliest biomedical models of health, illness, and pain. According to Hippocrates' formulation:

> The human body contains blood, phlegm, yellow bile and black bile. These are the things that make up its constitution and cause its pains and health. Health is primarily that state in which these constituent substances are in the correct proportion to each other, both in strength and quantity, and are well mixed. Pain occurs when one of the substances presents either a deficiency or an excess, or is separated in the body and not mixed with the others. (Lloyd 1978: 262)

Contemporary scholars, while appreciative of Hippocrates' many contributions, consider the humor hypothesis to be a joke. Regardless, this model, and variations thereof, dominated medical thinking for several centuries.

In the mid-seventeenth century, the noted philosopher, René Descartes, presented a model of pain that bears a simplistic resemblance to current neurological formations of pain (Descartes 1664). Descartes postulated that injury or insult is detected by pain receptors in the skin. This information is then transmitted through "animal spirits" and the pulling of threads to the brain and, via the pineal gland, to the mind. Descartes basic model underwent considerable revision (e.g. Müller 1842; von Frey 1894), based on a rapidly improving neuroscience, such that pain came to be viewed as a sensory experience resulting from stimulation of specific noxious receptors (usually as a result of physical damage arising from injury or disease). Again, however, as sophisticated as these biological theories became (for a comprehensive review of the history of pain epistemology, see Bonica 1990), they failed to account for individual differences in pain perception and propensities to develop chronic pain, being reductionistic (i.e. assuming a direct link between disease and physical pathology) and exclusionary (i.e. assuming psychological, social, and behavioral mechanisms are not important in disease) (Engel 1977; Turk and Flor 1999). Chronic pain was generally ignored within the biomedical treatises.

3 Gate control theory

Although scholars of the psychodynamic tradition (e.g. Breuer and Freud 1893–1895/1957; Engel 1959) were the first to propose a central role for psychological factors in pain, particularly chronic pain, it was Melzack and Wall (1965) who first integrated biological and psychological mechanisms in an account of between-person and within-person differences in the experience of pain. The original conceptualization of the Gate Control Theory of Pain, in brief, posited that nociceptive information from the periphery of the body is routed through a hypothetical gating mechanism in the dorsal horn of the spinal cord. The gating mechanism, which modulates the intensity of the ascending (i.e. from periphery to brain) transmission, is influenced by several factors, including descending (i.e. from brain to the gating mechanism) transmission regarding current cognitive and affective states. In essence, the theory suggested that processes mediated by the central nervous system, including cognition and affect, could directly impact the transmission and perception of nociceptive sensory information from the periphery.

The Gate Control Theory and its revisions (Melzack and Casey 1968) are reviewed elsewhere in greater detail (e.g. Wall 1996; Turk and Flor 1999;

Asmundson and Wright 2004). Discussion of recent advances based on the theory, including Price's (2000) parallel-serial model of pain affect and Melzack's neuromatrix theory of pain (Melzack 1999; Melzack and Katz 2004), are also beyond the scope of this chapter. The critical point that we wish to make here is that the Gate Control Theory was the first to provide a cogent explanation for how individuals with the same physical injury could vary widely in their perception of pain and how the same individual could perceive pain from a similar injury differently at two times. However, akin to the biomedical models, the Gate Control Theory was not clear in describing the process by which the experience of pain persists after damaged tissue has apparently healed.

4 Fear and avoidance in chronic pain

In recent years there has been considerable attention devoted to understanding the experience of pain within the context of an approach that integrates its biological, psychological, and social components (for recent reviews, see Turk and Flor 1999; Asmundson and Wright 2004). Relative to earlier explanations, the integrated, or biopsychosocial, approach posits a broader, multi-dimensional perspective on the experience of pain. The basic premises of the approach are as follows:

> Predispositional factors and current biological factors may initiate, maintain, and modulate physical perpetuations; predispositional and current psychological factors influence the appraisal and perception of internal physiological signs; and social factors shape the behavioural responses of patients to the perceptions of their physical perturbations. (Turk and Flor 1999: 20)

Models that fall under the biopsychosocial umbrella have proven particularly useful in advancing the understanding of cases where pain seems to be incongruous with the extent of tissue damage and where it persists in the absence of identifiable tissue damage or organic pathology.

Fear has proven to be a critical element in several biopsychosocial models of pain. The idea of a relationship between these constructs is, however, not a new one. Over 2000 years ago, Aristotle wrote, "Let fear, then, be a kind of pain or disturbance resulting the imagination of impending danger, either destructive or painful." During the first half of the twentieth century a number of investigators observed an association between pain and significant degrees of anxiety (e.g. Rowbotham 1946; Paulett 1947), viewing the latter as a product of intractable forms of the former. That is, people with chronic pain conditions were thought to become anxious as a result of their persistent pain. Beginning in the 1960s, and continuing through to the present, clinical investigators tried to advance their understanding of the association by assessing the prevalence of pain reports in individuals with anxiety disorders. This line of inquiry has shown that pain is more common in people with anxiety disorders relative to those with other psychiatric conditions (e.g. Spear 1967) and that certain anxiety disorders, including social phobia and posttraumatic stress disorder, are more common in people with chronic pain than are others (Asmundson *et al.* 1999; Asmundson *et al.* 2002).

Although avoidance behavior is closely associated with fear responses and anxiety disorders (Marks 1969; Barlow 2002), its role in the field of pain came to the fore in the 1970s with the pioneering work of Fordyce and his colleagues (Fordyce 1976; Fordyce *et al.* 1982). Below we outline Fordyce's early contributions and trace the developments that led from his work to the contemporary fear-avoidance models that form the foundation on which much of the work highlighted in subsequent chapters is based. Other learning mechanisms are described in detail in Chapters 2 and 6.

4.1 Avoidance learning

Fordyce and colleagues (Fordyce 1976; Fordyce *et al.* 1982) described a model that details how reinforcement serves as a mechanism by which behaviors associated with acute injury are maintained over time, become chronic, and promote disability. Operant learning of avoidance behavior was at the heart of this model. They suggested that, following an acute injury, avoidance behavior is negatively reinforced through the reduction of suffering associated with nociception. The avoidance behavior, in turn, serves the short-term benefit of minimizing the likelihood of further injury and affording damaged tissue an opportunity to heal. For the majority of individuals, avoidance behaviors are gradually replaced by approach behaviors, promoting further rehabilitation of the damaged tissue and, ultimately, the return to pre-injury activity levels. However, for a small but significant subset of injured individuals, the negative reinforcement contingencies (e.g. reduction of pain) can shift to other positive (e.g. increased attention) and negative (e.g. reduced work or family responsibilities) reinforcement contingencies that, in turn, serve to maintain avoidance behavior. In essence, these people learn that avoiding activities and situations that they associate with pain reduces the likelihood of experiencing a new episode of pain. Fordyce *et al.* (1982) outlined behavioral interventions designed to modify the learned avoidance behavior and, ultimately, reduce the disability associated with its persistence.

Linton *et al.* (1984) presented a fear-avoidance learning model that included both classical and operant conditioning components. The classical conditioning component refers to the process whereby a neutral stimulus takes on a negative meaning. For example, through direct experience or some other process (e.g. vicarious learning or observation) a previously neutral activity or situation, such as bending to lift an object, becomes associated with pain and elicits sympathetic activation and accompanying fear and anxiety. This response in turn, leads to avoidance behavior. The operant conditioning component, as in the Fordyce model, refers to the process whereby a stimulus—bending to lift an object in our example—comes to *predict* an aversive outcome that activates a fear response on its own. The person learns that avoiding the stimulus reduces pain, fear, anxiety, and the like and, thereby, the avoidance behavior is reinforced. Through this process the person becomes mired in a pattern of avoidance behavior that perpetuates limitations in activity and is difficult to extinguish.

As the behaviorally based models of Fordyce and Linton were stimulating empirical inquiry and guiding treatment interventions, scholars of a cognitive orientation were becoming more active in the field of pain. In a seminal work, Turk *et al.* (1983) provided a cognitive–behavioral perspective on pain that emphasized the notion that people were active processors of both internal and external information and, as such, attribution, expectancies, and feelings of self-efficacy, and the like were also factors of importance to the experience and maintenance of pain. Early fear-avoidance models were a product of this emerging cognitive–behavioral perspective.

4.2 Early fear-avoidance models

The term *fear-avoidance* was first used in the context of pain by Lethem *et al.* (1983) in an article entitled "Outline of a fear-avoidance model of exaggerated pain perception—I" published in *Behaviour Research and Therapy*. Preliminary empirical evidence supporting the model was presented in a second article within the same issue of the journal (Slade *et al.* 1983). Lethem and colleagues were interested in explaining the process by which fear of pain and avoidance behavior become desynchronous from the sensory components of pain; that is, how fear of pain and avoidance behavior contribute to the maintenance of pain in the absence of identifiable organic pathology.

Philips (1987) expanded on the notion that cognitions influence avoidance behavior and, thereby, the maintenance of chronic pain. More specifically, she proposed that avoidance of pain was not only a product of the interplay between current pain levels and negative reinforcement contingencies but also of expectations, based on current feelings of self-efficacy and prior experiences of pain, that encountering certain situations or activities will result in additional pain (see Fig. 1.1). Subtle differences aside, these early models were amongst the first to conceptualize chronic pain behavior as a vicious cycle between behavior and cognition.

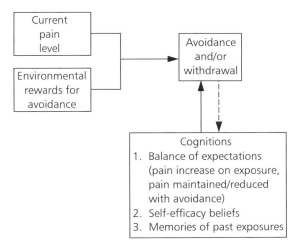

Fig. 1.1 A model of chronic pain avoidance behavior. Reprinted from *Behaviour Research and Therapy*, **25**, H. Philips, "Avoidance behaviour and its role in sustaining chronic pain," p. 277, Copyright 1987, with kind permission from Elsevier Science Ltd., The Boulevard, Langford Lane, Kidlington OX5 1GB, UK.

4.3 Contemporary fear-avoidance model

What we refer to as the contemporary fear-avoidance model of chronic pain is based primarily on the writings of McCracken *et al.* (1992), Waddell *et al.* (1993), Vlaeyen *et al.* (1995), and Asmundson *et al.* (1999). Each of these scholars takes a slightly different perspective on conceptualizing the role of fear and avoidance in perpetuating pain. For example, in addition to fear of pain itself (i.e. of nociception), Waddell *et al.* (1993) focus specifically on fear of pain provoking activities (e.g. work, leisure) whereas Asmundson *et al.* (1999; also see Asmundson and Taylor 1996) suggest that fear of pain may be secondary to fear of anxiety-related sensations associated with pain episodes. Subtle differences aside, the main ideas of each of these scholars are captured in the model proposed by Vlaeyen and Linton (2000) in their state-of-the-art review of the field. This model, illustrated in Fig. 1.2, can be summarized as follows:

1. When pain is perceived, a judgment of the meaning or purpose of the pain is placed on the experience (pain experience).

2. For the majority of individuals, the pain is judged to be undesirable and unpleasant, but not as catastrophic or suggestive of a major calamity (no fear). In this case, the individual engages in appropriate behavioral restriction followed by graduated increases in activity (Confrontation) until healing has occurred (Recovery).

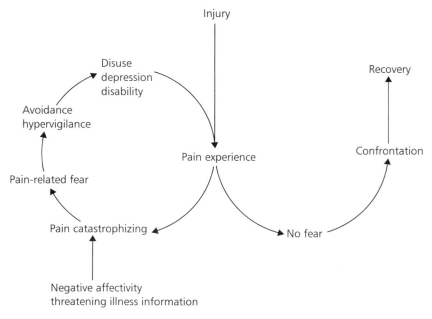

Fig. 1.2 Fear-avoidance model. Reprinted from *Pain*, **85**, J.W.S. Vlaeyen and S.J. Linton, "Fear-avoidance and its consequences in chronic musculoskeletal pain: A state of the art," p. 329, Copyright 2000, with kind permission from the International Association for the Study of Pain, 909 NE 43rd Ave, Suite 306, Seattle, WA, USA.

3. For a significant minority of individuals, a catastrophic meaning is placed on the experience of pain (pain catastrophizing). Catastrophizing, influenced by predispositional and current psychological factors, leads to pain-related fear (i.e. fear of pain, fear of (re)injury) and thereafter spirals into a vicious and self-perpetuating fear-avoidance cycle that promotes and maintains activity limitations, disability, and pain.

This model has served as a useful heuristic upon which considerable amounts of empirical research and related practical applications have been based (for an example of findings current to the beginning of this millennium, see Vlaeyen and Linton 2000). In addition to advances in empirical findings and practical applications to this field of inquiry (as detailed in the remaining chapters of this volume), there has been continuing refinement of the contemporary fear-avoidance model. For example, Norton and Asmundson (2003) proposed an amendment to the model of Vlaeyen and Linton in an effort to clarify the contributions of autonomic nervous system dysregulation and muscular tension on negative expectancies (or anxious anticipation) regarding future pain

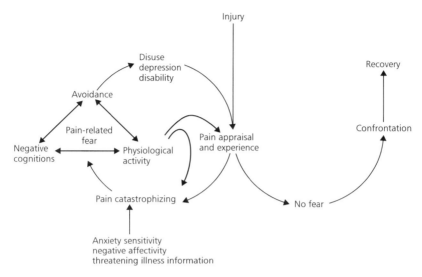

Fig. 1.3 Amended Vlaeyen-Linton fear-avoidance model of chronic pain. Reprinted from *Behavior Therapy*, **34**, P.J. Norton and G.J.G. Asmundson (2003), "Amending the fear-avoidance model of chronic pain: What is the role of physiological arousal?," p. 19, Copyright 2003, with kind permission of the Association for the Advancement of Behavior Therapy.

(see Fig. 1.3). Our efforts at refinement have also been based on the issue of elucidating the distinction between fear and anxiety and the classes of behavior motivated by these states.

5 Fear and anxiety—a closer look

What is, and what is not, considered *fear*? Is it the same as anxiety? How does it relate to behaviors that postpone or prevent exposure to an aversive situation or activity (e.g. avoidance), and behaviors that terminate such exposure (e.g. escape, neutralizing)? Fear and anxiety are highly related constructs. They are, however, distinct (Blanchard and Blanchard 1990) and it is important to recognize and understand their differences. We believe that oversight of the differences may hamper progress in understanding and treating fear of pain.

5.1 Fear

Fear, often described as one of the basic or pure emotions (Izard 1992), is a *present-oriented* state that is designed to protect the individual from a perceived *immediate threat*. It is usually directed toward a concrete stimulus, activity, or situation. Presumably under primarily amygdalar control (Gray and McNaughton 2000), fear is the emotional manifestation of the *fight or flight* response (Cannon 1929). Although the emotional experience is often the most salient aspect, fear is a multifaceted phenomenon. Most notably, Lang (1968) identified three major dimensions along which fear is expressed— cognitive, physiological, and behavioral. These components of fear are loosely coupled and can change at different speeds. This gives rise to desynchronous changes; for example, cognitive changes can precede the behavioral or vice versa.

The cognitive component (previously labeled the verbal component; Lang 1968) is characterized by increases in thoughts of danger, threat, or death (i.e. negative automatic thoughts; see Beck and Emery with Greenberg 1985). These thoughts serve two functions, including increasing attention directed to the threat and away from irrelevant distracters, and motivating action. Activation of fear may also trigger evaluations of one's ability to cope with the perceived threat (Lazarus and Folkman 1984) and this appraisal will largely determine the degree of fear experienced and the response to it.

The physiological component of fear is characterized by activation of the sympathetic nervous system. This activation results in a variety of physiological changes designed to increase the likelihood of survival over the threat. The liver releases surplus sugars to provide increased energy for action. Respiration rate accelerates, increasing the amount of oxygen, which is used to burn the surplus sugars transported into the blood stream. Epinephrine and norepinephrine are released, increasing the heart rate to more quickly transport oxygen to the musculature. Circulatory changes occur, directing increased blood flow to the major musculature and away from the smaller muscles, dermis, cranium, and gastrointestinal tract. The major musculature shows a general increase in tension to better facilitate fighting or fleeing (see Hoehn-Saric and McLeod 1993). In essence, then, arousal is increased and nonessential functions are decreased in order to maximize attempts to escape from or defend against the perceived threat (i.e. the fight-or-flight response).

While Lang (1968) described the third component of fear as behavioral, it might be more appropriate to conceive of it as a motivational response that provides the impetus for engaging in *defensive behavior*. Defensive behaviors typically arise in direct response to the activation of fear and are designed to protect the individual from the perceived threat that prompted activation of the emotional state. Activation of the sympathetic nervous system seems to favor fight-or-flight behaviors, but other defensive behavior patterns commonly arise, particularly when the threat cannot be fought or fled/escaped. Such alternate defensive behaviors include passive coping behaviors (e.g. freezing or immobility) and active coping behaviors (e.g. washing or neutralizing). People often do not engage in overt defensive behaviors for a variety of reasons, such as situational demands or sex role expectations, but still experience fear and the motivation for defensive action. This suggests that the defensive actions are not likely part of the emotion *per se* but a response to it.

5.2 Anxiety

Anxiety, in contrast to fear, is a *future-oriented* cognitive-affective state that appears to arise from the septo-hippocampal system (Gray and McNaughton 2000). It occurs in response to *anticipated* threats that are often vague or uncertain in nature. Like fear, anxiety appears to comprise cognitive, physiological, and motivational (behavioral) components. However, unlike fear, anxiety typically has a greater cognitive component and a more suppressed physiological element (Barlow 2002). The physiological response, described by Barlow (2002) as a "preparatory set" or "over preparedness," appears to place defensive physiological systems in a state of heightened alert. This state serves to facilitate and expedite a fight-or-flight response should the potential threat be encountered. Therefore, when anxious, physiological changes similar to those experienced during fear (e.g. increased heart rate, muscle tension, motility changes) are evident but typically at a less intense level (see Kleinknecht 1986).

Cognitively, shifts occur to enhance threat detection and narrow attention to potential threat cues. This increases the likelihood that a potential threat, if actually present, will be detected (Mathews and MacLeod 1985). Interpretive biases and threat-relevant schemata are also activated to ensure that any perceived evidence of threat is filtered such that incoming data is acted upon based on past experiences (memories) and beliefs about the threat (Beck and Emery with Greenberg 1985).

Differences in motivational/behavioral responses also exist between fear and anxiety. While fear involves motivation to engage in defensive behaviors, anxiety typically involves motivation for engaging in *preventative behaviors* (Blanchard and Blanchard 1990). This latter class of behaviors, which includes avoidance and use of safety cues, serves to protect the individual from an anticipated future threat. The mechanism by which the individual is protected from the perceived threat can, however, vary significantly. Avoidance behavior, for example, serves to minimize the likelihood of encountering the anticipated threat, whereas use of safety cues or other compensatory behaviors serve to minimize the amount of risk or to mitigate the severity of the threat if it is actually encountered.

5.3 Mutually reinforcing dyads

Fear motivates defensive behaviors such as escape. Anxiety motivates preventative behaviors such as avoidance. But, how are the fear-escape and anxiety-avoidance dyads interrelated? It would appear that both of these protective systems may trigger each other in a mutually reinforcing fashion. Anxiety, particularly with increased vigilance for evidence of threat, may increase the likelihood that a threat will be perceived and fear will be experienced. Fear, in turn, forces one to recognize something as a threat that may potentially reoccur. Moreover, stimuli that have been associated (directly or otherwise) with a fear-provoking threat can, in turn, become cues suggesting potential threat and thereby provoke anxiety.

Interestingly, and significant in the context of this volume, this detailed analysis of the fear-escape and anxiety-avoidance dyads may contradict some of the terminology used in describing fear and avoidance behavior in chronic pain. From this perspective, fear provides motivation toward engaging in defensive behaviors such as escape. Anxiety provides motivation toward preventative behaviors such as avoidance. By definition, then, one does not avoid encountering a threat that is already present and one does not escape from something that is not yet present. This creates a problem for the contemporary fear-avoidance model of chronic pain if it presupposes a direct link from fear to avoidance behavior without recognizing anxiety as intervening variable.

6 Fear-anxiety-avoidance model of chronic pain

Based on this formulation of fear, anxiety, and avoidance behavior, an updated model is presented (see Fig. 1.4). As in the Vlaeyen and Linton (2000) model, pain is perceived subsequent to an injury. This model also allows for pain perception following onset of organic pathology. For most, the pain is interpreted as a natural consequence of injury or disease state, and is not viewed as being catastrophic in and of itself (no catastrophizing). The injured or diseased structures are rested and protected, often under appropriate medical supervision, to allow for proper healing. Eventually, the individual begins engaging in graded activity, despite the presence of mild pain and discomfort, and returns to a tolerable level of activity. This may be at levels similar to or, depending on the nature of pathology, somewhat diminished from pre-injury or pre-disease levels.

The perception of pain, for some people, will be imbued with a catastrophic interpretation (pain catastrophizing). Data from the areas of personality theory, developmental psychology, and cognitive theories of psychopathology, as well as preliminary studies of chronic pain, suggest that this tendency to catastrophically interpret pain may arise as a function of predispositional factors such as anxiety sensitivity (Reiss and McNally 1985; Reiss 1991), negative affectivity (Clark and Watson 1991), and attention to and interpretation of threatening illness information (predisposing risk factors; see Chapters 3 and 4).

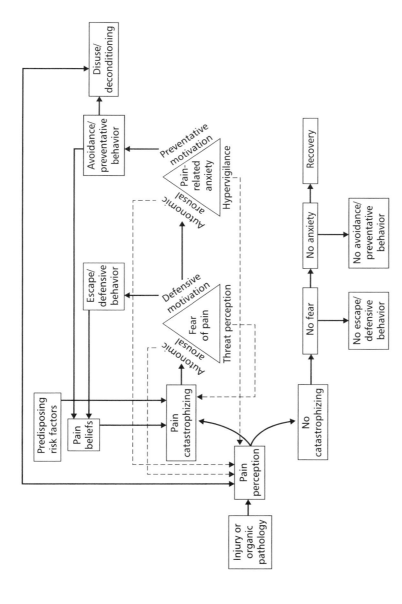

Fig. 1.4 Fear-anxiety-avoidance model of chronic pain. Bold solid lines represent direct links between variables. Dashed lines represent indirect feedback links between variables.

In addition, beliefs that a person holds regarding pain (pain beliefs; see Chapter 6), including beliefs stemming from previous experiences of pain, will influence the extent to which pain is catastrophically interpreted. The catastrophic interpretation produces a fear-based emotional state designed to protect the individual from the perceived catastrophic threat (fear of pain) and this may promote the onset of anxiety (pain-related anxiety). Fear and anxiety pathways are described below. Some of the proposed pathways are more speculative than others and, as such, represent areas in which additional empirical scrutiny is warranted.

6.1 Fear of pain pathways

In the context of our model, fear is directed at pain sensations as well as activities and situations that the person has associated with pain. A detailed discussion of the object of fear in fear of pain is presented in Chapter 9 of this volume and, as shown in the available empirical literature, suggests that this extends beyond the sensory experience of pain itself to include work-, injury-, illness-, and social-context variables (see Asmundson *et al.* 1999).

Consistent with Lang's (1968) description of a three-response system of fear, cognitive, physiological, and motivational shifts occur, which are designed to maximize the likelihood of surviving the perceived threat. As noted before, the various responses of fear do not exist in isolation from each other but, rather, act and interact with each other, often in a mutually reinforcing and exacerbating cycle. In addition, each of the components may promote, directly or indirectly, some of the factors that precipitated the pain-related fear. The direct and indirect paths between the variables are illustrated in Fig. 1.4 with bold solid lines and dashed lines, respectively.

The cognitive shifts that enhance threat perception, as described earlier, may serve to exacerbate, or at least perpetuate, catastrophic interpretations regarding pain, thereby re-effecting the fearful response (path from threat perception to pain catastrophizing). For example, immediately following a moderate ankle sprain a person may catastrophize about having significantly injured the joint (e.g. "It hurts so badly. I must have broken a bone and torn a tendon. I am probably never going to be able to run again.") and thereby becomes fearful. His or her attention narrows to the ankle injury and the accompanying sensations. The point tenderness, weight-bearing pain, and sensations of throbbing or numbness may strengthen the veracity of the catastrophic interpretation. Indeed, the attentional shift may promote additional catastrophic interpretations, such as expectations of developing a permanent limp and being unable to participate in any recreational activities.

As described by Norton and Asmundson (2003), physiological arousal also plays an important role in perpetuating the experience of pain (path from autonomic arousal to pain perception). While the physiological changes associated with fear are designed to help protect the individual, they can have an unintentional negative effect. These effects are akin to those experienced by individuals with other fear- and anxiety-based conditions. In people with panic disorder, for example, an elevated heart rate prompts the fear of impending death from a heart attack which, in turn, prompts increased heart rate and accompanying exacerbation of the fear of dying (see Barlow 1988). In social anxiety disorder an individual giving a speech fears that others will judge their nervousness in a negative way, experiences increased muscular tension and shaking, and, as a consequence, exacerbations of their fear (see McEwan and Devins 1983). For people with pain-related fear, the symptoms of sympathetic arousal may exacerbate the pain-related fear in several ways. First, physiological symptoms of sympathetic arousal may be *misinterpreted* as evidence of pain or injury (Weisenberg *et al.* 1984; Al Absi and Rokke 1991; Nisbett and Schachter 1966). Second, arousal symptoms may impact biomechanical efficiency, which can, in turn, produce movements that damage tissues and create pain (Watson *et al.* 1997). Finally, arousal symptoms such as muscular tension may directly aggravate weakened or injured tissues and thereby increase pain (Flor *et al.* 1985, 1992). These hypothesized mechanisms may act by increasing pain perception and its catastrophic interpretation. However, more empirical evaluation is needed to substantiate these propositions: Most studies, primarily from Herta Flor's group (see also Spense *et al.* 2001), have found stress-related and symptom-specific muscular reactivity but *not* increased muscle tone to be associated with increased pain.

The motivational component of pain-related fear is seen as encouraging the person to escape from or defend against the pain, the fear, or both (path from defensive motivation to escape/defensive behavior; see Chapter 3). This is accomplished through escape from the current pain producing stimuli (e.g. disengaging from a pain-producing activity) or by modifications to behavior that reduce the intensity of pain (e.g. bracing, limping). While effective in the short term for reducing pain and fear, escape and defensive behaviors can serve to strengthen maladaptive pain beliefs (path from escape/defensive behavior to pain beliefs), increase the likelihood that future perceptions of pain will be interpreted catastrophically (path from pain beliefs to pain catastrophizing), and promote additional pain-related fear.

6.2 Pain-related anxiety pathways

Fear of pain and escape/defensive behavior are negative and unpleasant phenomena in their own right. They do not, however, completely explain the experience of chronic pain in the absence of identifiable injury or organic pathology and ongoing pain-related disability. To illustrate, being frightened by an older sibling who leaps up from behind the sofa during a scary movie is certainly fear provoking and unpleasant but likely does not functionally interfere with one's future life. Likewise, while an episode of intense acute pain, perhaps following a low back strain or surgical procedure, can be fear-provoking, it need not necessarily lead to anything more than short-term limitations in function. However, in some cases, fearful responses to a perceived threat may create significant anxiety regarding potential *future encounters* with the same or similar stimuli (pain-related anxiety).

When anxious due to anticipated pain or injury, the cognitive (hypervigilance), physiological (autonomic arousal), and motivational (preventative motivation) components are evoked. Expectancies (Crombez *et al.* 1996) and attentional shifts (for review see Pincus and Morley 2001) promote hypervigilance for evidence of potential pain or injury. Memories and pain-relevant schemata are activated to filter and appraise the evidence of pain. Autonomic activation primes the fight-or-flight system for activation, if necessary, and motivation to avoid or protect against the potential threat increases dramatically. Similar to the three components in pain-related fear, the cognitive, physiological, and motivational components of pain-related anxiety can increase the likelihood, directly or indirectly, of actually experiencing pain and responding fearfully.

Hypervigilance for evidence of threat, by definition, increases the likelihood that the threat, in this case pain, will be detected (path from hypervigilance to pain perception; see Chapter 4 for detailed discussion of hypervigilance). Somatic scanning, for example, may highlight sensations of pain to which the person may not have otherwise given attention. External scanning may highlight potentially pain-producing stimuli or activities that might otherwise have been ignored. Additionally, hypervigilance may interact with memories and pain-relevant schemata such that innocuous stimuli may be *misinterpreted* as evidence of pain. The physiological component can interact with the cognitive component, providing target symptoms to be attended to and possibly misinterpreted, and can influence the perception of pain (path from autonomic arousal to pain perception).

Perhaps most importantly in the development of long-term chronicity, the motivational aspect of anxiety can result in the engagement of avoidance and preventative behaviors (path from preventative motivation to avoidance/preventative behavior). As suggested in earlier avoidance learning and fear-avoidance models, avoidance and preventative behaviors, while effective in the short-term to help avoid pain, have negative long-term sequalea that actually increase the likelihood of experiencing future pain.

First, engaging in avoidance or preventative behaviors can seemingly confirm beliefs about pain (path from avoidance/preventative behavior to pain beliefs). Consider, for example, the case where John anticipates that eating a certain meal will provoke intense gastrointestinal pain. He becomes anxious about this possibility and attempts to prevent it by instead eating a very bland meal. When he does not develop gastrointestinal pain, John reasons that:

(1) I expected the spicy meal to cause pain;

(2) I ate a bland meal instead;

(3) I did not experience pain because I ate the bland meal rather than the spicy meal, and therefore;

(4) The spicy meal would have caused pain.

Although not logically sound, this reasoning often has a powerful effect on strengthening beliefs about potential threat. John might not have experienced any pain had the spicy meal been eaten but, by engaging in avoidance preventative behavior, the belief is not disconfirmed but, rather, strengthened. A similar reasoning process is engaged in by those who anticipate pain related to movement or participation is physical activity and from the effects of other types of stimulation; for example, "If I bend over to pick up that box, my pain will increase" and "If I feel pain, it means that my injury is getting worse." In the case of such dysfunctional assumptions, the search for confirming evidence, and the lack of disconfirming evidence, reinforces the credibility of the false assumptions (also see Smeets *et al.* 2000).

Second, avoidance of activity due to anticipation of pain may lead to muscular atrophy, loss of coordination, loss of ligamentous flexibility, decalcification and weakening of skeletal structures, and degeneration of associated tissue due to lack, or restriction, of use (path from avoidance/preventative behavior to disuse/deconditioning) (Bortz 1984). These effects, while aversive in their own right, can promote further experiences of pain (path from disuse/deconditioning to pain perception), as the compromised tissues and structures become less capable of engaging in mechanical actions, weight bearing, or other activities. This is an area that requires additional empirical inquiry. Indeed, to date, there appears to be little support for the "disuse syndrome," at least as proposed by Bortz (Verbunt *et al.* 2003; also see Chapter 7), and more support for disordered muscular coordination than muscle atrophy (Watson *et al.* 1997; Lamoth *et al.* 2002).

6.3 Model summary

The fear-anxiety-avoidance model of chronic pain is based on current conceptualizations of fear and anxiety. By isolating fear and its associated behaviors from anxiety and its associated behaviors, the model accounts for the puzzle of both (1) pain intensity that is incongruous with actual injury, through feedback from fear of pain to pain perception, and (2) pain that occurs in the absence of identifiable injury or organic pathology or that persists after an injury has apparently healed, via feedback from pain-related anxiety to pain perception. The model also serves to clarify some of the confusion in the field that revolves around the use of the seemingly congruent but distinct constructs of fear and anxiety.

7 **Conclusion**

Models or pain (and chronic pain) have changed considerably over the past several thousand years. Aristotle's early conceptualization was that pain occurred when one of blood, phlegm, yellow bile, or black bile was either deficient or present in excess within the body. Today, pain is viewed as a multi-dimensional phenomenon, comprising biological, psychological, social, and cultural components. Contemporary fear-avoidance models, based largely on the operant model of Fordyce (1976), have developed over the past 15–20 years to the point where they are no longer fledglings. Indeed, the amount of empirical and clinical work stimulated by these models has warranted several reviews (e.g. Asmundson *et al.* 1999; Vlaeyen and Linton 2000). These models have proven heuristic in understanding pain intensity that is incongruous with actual injury and pain that occurs in the absence of identifiable injury or organic pathology or that persists after an injury has apparently healed. In an attempt to draw the oft-overlooked distinction between the constructs of fear and anxiety, an issue that has caused some confusion in this field (as well as others), we have presented a model that clarifies the issue. Our intent in making this clarification is to promote further conceptual, empirical, and practical developments. The remaining chapters in Part I of this volume highlight other important theoretical issues and empirical findings. Practical issues, including those related to assessment and treatment of pain-related fear and anxiety, are detailed respectively in Parts II and III. Challenges and future research directions are highlighted in all chapters and, in closing, are summarized in Part IV.

Acknowledgments

Preparation of this article was supported, in part, by an operating grant and investigator award to the first author from the Canadian Institutes of Health Research (CIHR) and the Saskatchewan-CIHR Regional Partnerships Program.

References

Al Absi, M. and Rokke, P.D. (1991). Can anxiety help us tolerate pain? *Pain*, **46**, 43–51.

Asmundson, G.J.G. and Taylor, S. (1996). Role of anxiety sensitivity in pain-rleated fear and avoidance. *Journal of Behavioral Medicine*, **19**, 577–86.

Asmundson, G.J.G. and Wright, K.D. (2004). The biopsychosocial model of pain. In T. Hadjistavropoulos and K. D. Craig (eds.), *Pain: Psychological Perspectives*, pp. 35–57. New Jersey, NJ: Erlbaum.

Asmundson, G.J.G., Norton, P.J., and Norton, G.R. (1999). Beyond pain: The role of fear and avoidance in chronicity. *Clinical Psychology Review*, **19**, 97–119.

Asmundson, G.J.G., Coons, M.J., Taylor, S., and Katz, J. (2002). Invited article (peer-reviewed). PTSD and the experience of pain: Research and clinical implications of shared vulnerability and mutual maintenance models. *Canadian Journal of Psychiatry*, **47**, 930–7.

Barlow, D.H. (1988). *Anxiety and its Disorders*. New York, NY: Guilford Press.

Barlow, D.H. (2002). *Anxiety and its Disorders*, 2nd ed. New York, NY: Guilford Press.

Beals, R.K. and Hickman, N.W. (1972). Industrial injuries of the back and extremities. *The Journal of Bone and Joint Surgery*, **54-A**, 1593–611.

Beck, A.T., Emery, G., and Greenberg, R.L. (1985). *Anxiety Disorders and Phobias: A Cognitive Perspective*. New York, NY: Basic Books.

Beecher, H.K. (1956). Relationship of significance of wound to pain experienced. *Journal of the American Medical Association*, **161**, 1609–13.

Blanchard, R.J. and Blanchard, D.C. (1990). An ethoexperimental analysis of defense, fear and anxiety. In N. McNaughton and G. Andrews (eds.), *Anxiety*, pp. 124–33. Dunedin, New Zealand: Otago University Press.

Bonica, J.J. (1990). *The Management of Pain*, 2nd edn. Philadelphia, PA: Lea and Febiger.

Boos, N., Rieder, R., Schade, V., Spratt, K.F., Semner, N., and Aebi, M. (1995). The diagnostic accuracy of magnetic resonance imaging, work perception and psychosocial factors in identifying symptomatic disk herniations. *Spine*, **20**, 2613–25.

Bortz, W.M. (1984). The disuse syndrome. *Western Journal of Medicine*, **141**, 691–4.

Breuer, J. and Freud, S. (1957). *Studies on Hysteria*. (J. Strachey, ed. and Trans.) New York, NY: Basic Books. (Original work published 1893–1895).

Cannon, W.B. (1929). *Bodily Changes in Pain, Hunger, Fear and Rage: An Account of Recent Researches into the Functions of Emotional Excitement*, 2nd edn. New York, NY: Appleton-Century-Crofts.

Clark, L.A. and Watson, D. (1991). Tripartite model of anxiety and depression: Psychometric evidence and taxonomic implications. *Journal of Abnormal Psychology*, **100**, 316–36.

Crombez, G., Vervaet, L., Lysens, R., Eelen, P., and Baeyens, F. (1996). Do pain expectancies cause pain in chronic low back patients? A clinical investigation. *Behaviour Research and Therapy*, **34**, 919–26.

Descartes, R. (1664). *L'homme*. Paris: e Angot.

Engel, G.L. (1959). "Psychogenic" pain and pain-prone patient. *American Journal of Medicine*, **26**, 899–918.

Engel, G.L. (1977). The need for a new medical model: A challenge for biomedicine. *Science*, **196**, 129–35.

Flor, H., Turk, D.C., and Birbaumer, N. (1985). Assessment of stress-related responses in chronic back pain patients. *Journal of Consulting and Clinical Psychology*, **53**, 354–64.

Flor, H., Birbaumer, N., Schugens, M.M., and Lutzenberger, W. (1992). Symptom-specific psychophysiological responses in chronic pain patients. *Psychophysiology*, **29**, 452–60.

Fordyce, W.E. (1976). *Behavioral Methods for Chronic Pain and Illness*. St Louis: Mosby.

Fordyce, W.E., Shelton, J.L., and Dundore, D.E. (1982). The modification of avoidance learning in pain behaviors. *Journal of Behavioral Medicine*, **5**, 405–14.

von Frey, M. (1894). Berichte der sachlichen gesellschaft der wissenschaften. *Leipzig*, **46**, 185–283.

Gray, J.A. and McNaughton, N. (2000). *The Neuropsychology of Anxiety: An Enquiry into the Function of the Septo-hippocampal System*, 2nd edn., New York, NY: Oxford University Press.

Hoehn-Saric, R. and McLeod, D.R. (1993). Somatic manifestations of normal and pathological anxiety. In R. Hoehn-Saric and D.R. McLeod (eds.), *Biology of Anxiety Disorders*. Washington, DC: American Psychiatric Press.

Izard, C.E. (1992). Basic emotions, relations among emotions, and emotion-cognition relations. *Psychological Review*, **99**, 561–5.

Kleinknecht, R.A. (1986). *The Anxious Self: Diagnosis and Treatment of Fears and Phobias*. New York, NY: Human Sciences Press.

Lamoth, C.J., Meijer, O.G., Wuisman, P.I., van Dienn, J.H., Levin, M.F., and Beek, B.J. (2002). Pelvis-thorax coordination in the transverse plane during walking in persons with non-specific low back pain. *Spine*, **27**, E92–E99.

Lang, P.J. (1968). Fear reduction and fear behavior: Problems in treating a construct. In J.M. Shlien (ed.), *Research in Psychotherapy*. Washington, DC: American Psychological Association.

Lazarus and Folkman (1984). *Stress, Appraisal, and Coping*. New York, NY: Springer.

Lethem, J., Slade, P.D., Troup, J.D.G., and Bentley, G. (1983). Outline of a fear-avoidance model of exaggerated pain perception—I. *Behaviour Research and Therapy*, **21**, 401–8.

Linton, S.J., Melin, L., and Götestam, K.G. (1984). Behavioral analysis of chronic pain and its management. *Progress in Behavior Modification*, vol. 18. New York, NY: Academic Press.

Lloyd, G.E.R. (ed.) (1978). *Hippocratic Writings*. Harmondsworth, New York: Penguin Classics.

Marks, I.M. (1969). *Fears and Phobias*. London: Heinemann Medical and Academic Press.

Mathews, A. and MacLeod, C. (1985). Selective processing of threat cues in anxiety states. *Behaviour Research and Therapy*, **23**, 563–9.

McCracken, L.M., Zayfert, C., and Gross, R.T. (1992). The pain anxiety symptoms scale: Development and validation of a scale to measure fear of pain. *Pain*, **50**, 67–73.

McEwan, K.L. and Devins, G.M. (1983). Is increased arousal in social anxiety noticed by others? *Journal of Abnormal Psychology*, **92**, 417–21.

Melzack, R. (1999). From the gate to the neuromatrix. *Pain*, **82** (Suppl. 6), S121–S126.

Melzack, R. and Casey, K.L. (1968). Sensory, motivational and central control determinants of pain. In D.R. Kennshalo (ed.), *The Skin Senses* (pp. 423–43). Springfield, IL: Thomas.

Melzack, R. and Katz, J. (in press). The gate control theory: Reaching for the brain. In T. Hadjistavropoulos and K.D. Craig (eds.), *Pain: Psychological Perspectives*. New Jersey, NJ: Erlbaum.

Melzack, R. and Wall, P.D. (1965). Pain mechanisms. *Science*, **150**, 971–9.

Merskey, H. and Spear, F.G. (1967). *Pain: Psychologic and Psychiatric Aspects*. London: Baillière, tindall, and cassell.

Müller, J. (1842). *Elements of Physiology*. London: Taylor and Walton.

Nisbett, R.E. and Schachter, S. (1966). Cognitive manipulation of pain. *Journal of Experimental Social Psychology*, **2**, 227–36.

Norton, P.J. and Asmundson, G.J.G. (2003). Amending the fear-avoidance model of chronic pain: What is the role of physiological arousal? *Behavior Therapy*, **34**, 17–30.

Paulett, J.D. (1947). Low back pain. *Lancet*, **253**, 272–6.

Pincus, T. and Morley, S. (2001). Cognitive-processing bias in chronic pain: A review and integration. *Psychological Bulletin*, **127**, 5999–6617.

Philips, H. (1987). Avoidance behavior and its role in sustaining chronic pain. *Behaviour Research and Therapy*, **25**, 273–9.

Price, D.D. (2000). Psychological and neural mechanisms of the affective dimension of pain. *Science*, **288**, 1769–72.

Reiss, S. (1991). Expectancy theory of fear, anxiety, and panic. *Clinical Psychology Review*, **11**, 141–53.

Reiss, S. and McNally, R.J. (1985). The expectancy model of fear. In S. Reiss and R.R. Bootzin (eds.), *Theoretical Issues in Behavior Therapy* (pp. 107–21). New York: Academic Press.

Rowbotham, G.F. (1946). Pain and its underlying pathology. *Journal of Mental Science*, **92**, 595–604.

Slade, P.D., Troup, J.D.G., Lethem, J., and Bentley, G. (1983). The fear-avoidance model of exaggerated pain perception—II. Preliminary studies of coping strategies for pain. *Behaviour Research and Therapy*, **21**, 409–16.

Smeets, G., de Jong, P.J, and Mayer, B. (2000). If you suffer from a headache, then you have a brain tumour: Domain-specific reasoning "bias" and hypochondriasis. *Behaviour Research and Therapy*, **38**, 763–76.

Spear, F.G. (1967). Pain and psychiatric patients. *Journal of Psychosomatic Research*, **11**, 187–93.

Spence, S.H., Sharpe, L., Newton-John, T., and Champion, D. (2001). An investigation of symptom-specific muscle hyperactivity in upper extremity cumulative trauma disorder. *Clinical Journal of Pain*, **17**, 119–28.

Turk, D.C. and Flor, H. (1999). The Biobehavioral perspective of pain. In R.J. Gatchel and D.C. Turk (eds.), *Psychosocial Factors in Pain. Clinical Perspectives* (pp. 18–34). New York, NY: The Guilford Press.

Turk, D.C., Meichenbaum, D., and Genest, M. (1983). *Pain and Behavioral Medicine: A Cognitive-Behavioral Perspective*. New York, NY: The Guilford Press.

Verbunt, J.A., Seelen, H.A., Vlaeyen, J.W.S., van de Heijden, G.J., Heuts, P.H., Pons, K., and Andre Knottnerous, J. (2003). Disuse and deconditioning in chronic low back pain: concepts and hypotheses on contributing mechanisms. *European Journal of Pain*, **7**, 9–21.

Vlaeyen, J.W.S. and Linton, S.J. (2000). Fear-avoidance and its consequences in chronic musculoskeletal pain: A state of the art. *Pain*, **85**, 317–32.

Vlaeyen, J.W.S., Kole-Snijders, A.M.K., Boeren, R.G.B., and van Eek, H. (1995). Fear of movement/(re)injury in chronic low back pain and its relation to behavioral performance. *Pain*, **62**, 363–72.

Waddell, G., Newton, M., Henderson, I., Sommerville, D., and Main, C.J. (1993). A fear-avoidance beliefs questionnaire (FABQ) and the role of fear-avoidance beliefs in chronic low back pain and disability. *Pain*, **52**, 157–68.

Wall, P.D. (1996). Comments after 30 years of the gate control theory of pain. *Pain Forum*, **5**, 12–22.

Watson, P.J., Booker, C.K., and Main, C.J. (1997). Evidence for the role of psychological factors in abnormal paraspinal activity in patients with chronic low back pain. *Journal of Musculoskeletal Pain*, **5**, 41–56.

Watson, P., Booker, C.K., Main, C.J., and Chen, A.C.N. (1997). Surface electromyography in the identification of chronic low back pain patients: The development of the flexion relaxation ratio. *Clinical Biomechanics*, **12**, 165–71.

Weisenberg, M., Aviram, O., Wolf, Y., and Raphaeli, N. (1984). Relevant and irrelevant anxiety in the reaction to pain. *Pain*, **20**, 371–83.

Chapter 2

Pain-related fear and avoidance: A conditioning perspective

Liesbet Goubert, Geert Crombez, and Madelon Peters

1 Introduction

Pain is more than an unpleasant perceptual and emotional experience. It elicits innate responses and action tendencies that prepare and facilitate escape from pain. Par excellence, pain is an experience that drives learning. We learn about the circumstances of everyday pain. We discover the events or actions that precede the experience of pain, and find out what predicts and causes pain. We learn to fear impending pain, and learn which actions should be undertaken to minimize pain, and to avoid it on future occasions. The same applies for the experience of clinical and chronic pain. The relevance of learning in chronic pain has been recognized early on in the field of pain (Fordyce 1976), and continues to play a role in more recent biopsychosocial accounts of chronic pain. For example, fear-avoidance models have elaborated the role of fear and avoidance behavior in the development of chronic pain problems (for an overview, see Vlaeyen and Linton 2000). At present, the concepts of "pain-related fear" and "avoidance" have become established in the pain literature. However, the precise mechanisms by which learning takes place are often taken for granted or left unspecified.

One reason may be that contemporary learning psychology became associated with outdated and unfashionable paradigms and theories. Pavlov and Skinner are remembered as the godfathers of learning and conditioning from introduction courses of psychology. Often their views of learning are explained within the rise and fall of behaviorism, implicitly making it an unworthy topic of further inquiry. Learning psychology has, however, survived. During the last decades, a revolution in the field of learning has occurred, focusing on the development of new paradigms and new theoretical accounts about the nature of the process of learning. For most of us, this revolution took place unnoticed. Modern learning theorists were not as interested as the founding fathers in the relevance of their findings for understanding psychopathology. The two fields went separate ways with little cross-fertilization of ideas (Bouton *et al.* 2001). This also applies for the field of pain.

The aims of this chapter are to introduce and summarize some of the new ideas about learning, and to discuss the implications of these ideas for both the process of therapeutic change and research. We begin with a historical overview of both classical and instrumental conditioning. Emphasis is on the application of these concepts to pain in the context of empirical evidence and modern accounts of learning psychology. Subsequently, we summarize the basic tenets of a modern learning psychology of fear and avoidance, and illustrate their relevance for current views of clinical and chronic pain.

2 Historical conceptualizations

2.1 Classical conditioning and pain

Being perplexed and observing carefully are often two characteristics of great scientists. This was not different for Pavlov. Initially he investigated the effects of food upon the gastrointestinal system in dogs, work for which he received a Nobel Prize in 1904. During these experiments, he noticed that physiological effects that were assumed to occur only in response to the ingestion of food also occurred when he entered the room, or when a bowl of food was presented to the dog. This phenomenon intrigued Pavlov, and, in a series of experiments, he started to dismantle this phenomenon in search for its essential features. The classical paradigm of conditioning should be understood in that context. It is the result of an attempt to reduce the complex reality of learning into an experimental paradigm that still captured the essence of learning.

The prototype of classical conditioning is well-known. The sound of a bell or of a metronome (the conditioned stimulus, CS) was repeatedly presented before the ingestion of food (the unconditioned stimulus, UCS) in hungry dogs. Where initially salivation could be observed only in response to the food (the unconditioned response, UCR), after a few pairings between the sound and the food, also the sound started to elicit similar responses (conditioned response, CR). The same form of learning has been observed in a wide range of species, motivational systems, and responses (see Turkkan 1989). Taking a rational perspective, one can only be puzzled about the emergence of CRs. After all, the CR seems to have no function: It has no effect upon the probability of the UCS, nor does it help the organism to control the UCS. Nevertheless, evolutionary accounts have stressed the adaptive value of classical conditioning within the natural environment of living organisms. Innate and hardwired responses to biologically significant events are swiftly learned in anticipation of these events, allowing an effective preparation for and efficient response to these events in most natural situations (Hollis 1982).

Classical conditioning has also been applied to pain. It has been argued that the innate and hardwired reflexes to noxious stimuli such as vocalization, sudden withdrawal, and increased pupillary diameter can be conditioned toward previously neutral stimuli or events, such as the doctor's office or a parent's angry face (Sternbach 1978). Two of the most discussed issues in the field of pain are (1) the conditioning of muscle tension and (2) the conditioning of the pain experience. We review both phenomena.

2.1.1 Classical conditioning of muscle tension

One of the innate responses to pain is tensing the muscle surrounding the injured area. Possibly, its evolutionary functions are to limit further damage by the immobilization of the injured site, or to dampen the pain experience by increasing non-nociceptive input that might inhibit the transmission of nociceptive input at the spinal level (Melzack and Wall 1965). However, a chronic tension of the muscle can have a negative and detrimental effect upon the pain experience by stimulating and sensitizing nociceptors via ischemia and hypoxia (Linton *et al.* 1985). A popular view of the maintenance of chronic pain is that patients may become trapped into a vicious pain-tension cycle (Gentry and Bernal 1977). It is further argued that muscle tension may come under the control of classical conditioning processes, further fuelling the vicious circle (Gentry and Bernal 1977).

Although the literature attaches much importance to the phenomenon of conditioned muscle tension, there is almost no experimental evidence showing either its existence or its impact on acute or chronic pain. Most often reported are the findings that chronic pain patients respond with increased levels of muscle tension to physical as well as personally relevant stressors, and that they show slow return to baseline levels subsequent to stress induction (for a review see Flor and Turk 1989). For example, Flor and colleagues (Flor *et al.* 1985, 1992) found localization-specific muscle tension in patients with chronic back pain and temporomandibular joint pain in response to personally relevant stress. During imagery of personal stress situations, patients with pain in the maxillary joint responded with more muscle tension in that area, whereas patients with pain in the back responded with more muscle tension in the erector spinae muscles. These studies, however, illustrate individual response stereotypy; that is, the tendency of groups of individuals to respond to a wide variety of stressors with a similar physiological response. It has not yet been demonstrated (1) that the origins of individual response stereotypy are owing to the classical conditioning, and (2) that the muscle tension moderates the experience of acute and chronic pain (Knost *et al.* 1999). Moreover, even symptom-specific psychophysiological responses have not been consistently found (e.g. Spence *et al.* 2001).

A decade ago Flor and colleagues started to investigate the conditioning of muscle tension using a classical conditioning paradigm (Flor and Birbaumer 1994). They subjected students to moderately aversive electric shock using simple tones or slides of different emotional valence (such as angry or happy faces) as neutral stimuli (CSs). Intracutaneous shock to the finger was used as the UCS, and lead to an increase in muscle tension in the flexor communis digitorum muscle (UCR). After several pairings of the shock and the tone or slide, the tone or slide itself elicited a learnt muscular response (CR), which showed high resistance to extinction. Students who frequently complained about neck and shoulder pain (a sub-chronic pain group) acquired these conditioned muscular responses more rapidly and showed more resistance to extinction. Results suggest that, especially in individuals at risk for chronic pain (e.g. having a parent or a family member with a chronic pain problem), conditioned muscle tension emerges as a CR. These findings await further corroboration.

2.1.2 Classical conditioning of pain sensations

It has been proposed that the pain sensation itself can be brought under control of environmental contingencies. According to Jaynes (1985), for example, conditioning takes place between verbal statements, such as "I hurt," and the experience of pain. In the long term, these verbalizations will produce the conscious pain response by itself. Chapman and Gagliardi (1980) also suggested that pain can be directly conditioned via the association of a previously neutral stimulus with a painful situation. The CS may then become a substitute for the UCS, and activate the sensory and affective attributes of the noxious stimulus in such a vivid way that it is perceived as a perceptual reality. It is clear that this position is an extreme example of the original substitution theory of Pavlov (Konorski 1967; Holland 1990): The CS elicits an experience with the same perceptual quality as pain.

There are few empirical studies that support such an extreme view for perceptual systems in general and for pain in particular (see Crombez *et al.* 1994). There is no systematic evidence that perceptual experiences (e.g. in the visual or auditive modality) can be directly conditioned. There are some early studies indicating that pain sensations can be conditioned (Garvey 1933; Leuba 1940), but these are often based upon methodologically weak procedures. Moreover, the CR often lacks the qualia of a perceptual experience.

In one of the experiments of Leuba (1940), a hypnotized participant was pricked five or six times with a needle on the left hand while a metal waste paper basket was tapped with a metal pencil. After the participant had been awakened he was asked to report anything he experienced while the experimenter did various things: ". . . from the moment the basket was tapped he (the participant) moved his left hand quickly, looked at it, felt the fleshy part, and looked puzzled. When further probed for his experience, he replied 'Feels as though it had been pricked by something small and sharp. It comes when you make that noise and disappears when you stop'" (p. 349). Leuba (1940) also described the conditioning of other sensations, for instance visual stimuli, odours, and auditory signals. However, the experimental procedure can be criticized on several grounds. Aside from the fact that demand characteristics cannot be ruled out, the reported sensations did not have a clear reality status. Even Leuba (1940) mentioned that the images were "fleeting and difficult to examine."

A complete dismissal of the above findings is probably throwing away the baby with the bath water. Surely, a straightforward conditioning of perceptual experiences most often makes no sense. It would result in hallucinations and in a lesser sensitivity to important changes in the environment (Konorski 1967; Crombez *et al.* 1996). In that context, the distinction between the orienting and the defensive system of Sokolov (1963) is useful. According to Sokolov (1963), events that are novel, unexpected, and of low to moderate intensity elicit an orienting response that facilitates an intake and a detailed analysis of incoming information. A defensive response is elicited by painful stimuli and is aimed at facilitating escape and dampening its impact. Sokolov (1963) has documented that, during classical conditioning with painful stimuli, a defensive focus may become conditioned. In these situations, activity of the defensive system overrules an otherwise careful and detailed analysis of the incoming information. Participants then react after a minimal perceptual analysis of the information. This mechanism may be responsible for the finding that, under strong expectancies of intense pain, one may observe extreme psychophysiological reactions to low intense pain, but also a subsequent self-report that indicates that the painful experience is far less than expected (see Epstein 1973).

2.1.3 Conclusions

Classical conditioning may occur whenever an event precedes the occurrence of an aversive painful event. Of importance is that CRs emerge despite the fact that they have no effect upon the probability of the painful experience. Most often, studies have focused upon the putative role of muscle tension as a CR, and upon the possibility that the perceptual experience of pain can be directly conditioned. For both theses, empirical evidence is limited and scarce. Several authors point out that the emergence of conditioned responding is best understood in the context of the adaptability and the flexibility of evolutionary old behavioral systems. It is a misconception that CRs are identical to, or always mimic, the UCRs. Detailed chemical analysis has revealed that even in the classical study of Pavlov with conditioned salivation this was not the case. This line of reasoning has also been applied to pain. Bolles and Fanselow (1980) have convincingly argued that CRs in anticipation of pain are preparatory defensive responses best conceived of as conditioned fear. This is in line with the more recent idea concerning the important role of fear in the expectation and avoidance of pain (see later).

2.2 Operant conditioning and pain

Skinner has made a sharp distinction between classical and operant conditioning. In his view, the critical difference between these forms of learning is the extent of control over the environment. In classical conditioning, there is no control over the occurrence of events in the environment. In operant conditioning, control over the environment is the quintessence of learning. The organism learns to "operate" upon the environment: A pigeon learns that pecking upon an illuminated key brings along grains. A rat learns to have control over the occurrence of food pellets by pressing a lever. The basic principles of operant conditioning are quite simple. Any behavior that is followed by a favorable consequence is more likely to recur: It will show an increase in frequency. Any behavior that is followed by an aversive consequence will be less likely to recur and will show a decrease in frequency.

Fordyce (1976) was the first to apply the principles of operant conditioning to the problems of chronic pain patients. His application was truly a revolutionary way of thinking about chronic pain. His work stemmed from the shortcomings of the attempts of traditional health care to resolve chronic pain problems by focusing upon tissue damage and disease. Central was the idea that "pain behavior" should be the focus of treatment, that is, the whole range of actions a patient undertakes when in pain (Fordyce 1988). In doing so, he shifted the goal of treatment from a reduction in pain intensity toward the diminution of the impact of pain upon life and the restoration of functional behavior. His influence upon theory and treatment of chronic pain was substantial.

Pain behaviors include verbal complaints, nonverbal sounds, taking medication, taking bed rest, avoidance of home and work responsibilities, body postures, and facial expressions of pain. According to Fordyce, all these behaviors should be conceived of as behaviors that are learned and maintained by their consequences. They are displayed because patients receive empathy from solicitous spouses, get access to pain medications, are financially compensated, avoid pain-worsening activities, or escape from distressing events. In sum, pain behavior emerges whenever the benefits outweigh the costs.

In the context of pain-related fear and avoidance, the principles of operant conditioning are of paramount importance. Through operant conditioning, patients may avoid future pain by taking medication or by restricting their activity level. However, the mechanisms underlying avoidance behavior are far less investigated than the impact of the social consequences upon pain behavior. We review both areas of research.

2.2.1 The role of social consequences in pain behavior

The idea that pain behavior can be shaped and maintained by social reinforcement has received considerable attention from researchers. Indeed, attention from significant others is an obvious example of positive reinforcement of pain behaviors. Fordyce has provided several clinical examples of this mechanism (Fordyce 1983). This idea has, however, also led to persistent and popular misunderstandings, such as the pernicious and erroneous idea that pain behavior is a deliberate strategy that occurs whenever the benefits outweigh the costs (Eccleston *et al.* 1997).

There are no experiments in chronic pain patients that have tried to experimentally manipulate the type and extent of social reinforcement of clinically relevant pain behavior. However, there is ample research that has looked at the impact of the presence of the spouse upon self-reports of pain and pain behavior. One of the first studies was of Block *et al.* (1980). They showed that self-reported pain during a taped structured interview depended on whether the patients were observed by their spouses or ward clerks. Patients who reported that their spouses were relatively non-solicitous in responding to pain behavior reported significantly lower pain levels in the spouse-observing condition than in the neutral-observer condition. Patients who reported that their spouses were relatively solicitous in responding to pain behavior reported marginally higher levels of pain in the spouse-observing condition than in the neutral-observer condition. The results of this study have been interpreted as evidence for an operant view upon pain behavior. It is assumed that the solicitous spouse acted as a discriminative stimulus, in whose presence pain behavior would be likely received positively and empathically.

A similar study by Lousberg *et al.* (1992), using the procedure of Block *et al.* (1980), assessed spouse solicitousness from the perspective of the patients and from the perspective of the spouse. Their results partially replicated the findings of Block *et al.* (1980). Only a categorization of spouse solicitousness according to the perspective of the spouse—and not of the patient—was in line with the operant view. More specifically, patients with solicitous spouses reported more pain and walked for a shorter duration in the presence of their spouse than patients with relatively non-solicitous spouses. Further support for an operant view was provided by Romano *et al.* (2000). They found that, after controlling for patient age, gender, and pain intensity, the solicitous behaviors of the partner were significantly associated with higher rates of patient verbal and nonverbal behavior. It was also revealed that negative responses of the partner were associated negatively with patient nonverbal pain behavior. In a study of Flor *et al.* (1995), patients showed reduced pain thresholds and pain tolerance levels during the cold-pressor task in the presence of a solicitous spouse than in the absence of the spouse.

Experimental research in pain-free volunteers has mainly investigated whether the level of pain that is verbally reported during an experimental pain procedure can be shaped by social reinforcement. In the study of Linton and Götestam (1985), healthy volunteers were required to rate the pain intensity during a series of ischemic pain experiences induced by inflating a blood-pressure cuff. In the up-conditioning of pain report, the participant was verbally rewarded each time the pain report was increased in comparison with the previous trial. Down-conditioning of pain report was achieved by rewarding a decrease in reported pain. Both forms of conditioning were successful.

A recent study of Flor *et al.* (2002) further investigated operant conditioning of self-reported pain during painful intracutaneous electric stimulation of the finger. Somatosensory-evoked potentials of pain were measured as well. In an up-training group, participants were given positive reinforcement when their actual pain rating was higher than the average rating during a baseline period. In the down-training group the positive/negative feedback assignment was defined conversely. Both healthy controls and chronic low back pain patients showed the expected learning pattern: Higher pain reports were obtained after up-conditioning and lower pain reports after down-conditioning. However, the cortical pain response (N150) of the chronic pain patients was generally elevated. This may reflect an enhanced reactivity to painful stimuli in chronic back pain patients. Moreover, the back pain patients displayed slower extinction of both the verbal and the cortical (N150) pain response. In addition, the back pain group displayed prolonged elevated electromyogram levels to the task. According to the authors, these data suggest that chronic back pain patients are more easily influenced by operant conditioning factors than healthy controls.

There are some limitations in this area of research that should be considered. First, the experimental research has almost exclusively focused upon the conditioning of self-report. It is still unclear whether the above findings also generalize to other pain behaviors (Keefe and Dunsmore 1992). Second, the role of contingency awareness has not been systematically investigated. It is possible that participants are aware of the reinforcement of their pain ratings. It cannot be ruled out that results can be attributed to demand characteristics. Future studies should take into account the issue of contingency awareness in a more systematic and valid way (Lovibond and Shanks 2002). Third, the implicit assumption of operant conditioning that all pain behavior is learned by trial and error, occurring whenever the benefits outweigh the costs, is overly optimistic and also incorrect. For example, an intriguing repositioning of the operant conditioning of facial displays of pain is offered by Williams (2002). In her evolutionary account she reviews evidence that the facial display of pain is innate and hardwired. She convincingly argues that facial displays of pain are not shaped by social reinforcement, but that people learn to (partially) suppress and control the facial display of pain in particular situations. Such a form of learning, in which operant behavior does not emerge within a vacuum, but is firmly rooted within old phylogenetic motivational systems, is often overlooked in operant conditioning research (Crombez and Eccleston 2002).

2.2.2 The avoidance of aversive consequences

Much behavior is learned because it permits the person to avoid or postpone an aversive experience. Avoidance learning has long been recognized as a form of learning that may maintain or exacerbate clinical fear and anxiety (Davey, 1997a). Fordyce (1983) has recognized its potential in the development and maintenance of chronic pain problems. According to Fordyce, avoidance behavior is just another form of maladaptive pain behavior that develops when pain becomes chronic.

What exactly is avoided and reinforces the pain behavior may vary considerably between persons. An obvious example is that patients learn to avoid pain. Lethem *et al.* (1983) have provided the most elaborated version of this view in their fear-avoidance model of exaggerated pain perception. The central concept in this model is fear of pain. Lethem *et al.* (1983) postulated two extreme responses to pain, namely confrontation and avoidance. The former type of response typically leads to a reduction of fear with time, while the latter response usually leads to maintenance and exacerbation of fear, the end stage being a full-blown phobic state. The avoider is considered to be motivated to avoid any fresh exposure to pain. Therefore, when in time injury heals, patients often do not have corrective experiences. The avoidance behaviour prevents learning that certain movements do not harm or hurt anymore. A desynchrony between pain sensation, on the one hand, and pain experience and pain behavior, on the other hand, emerges. Furthermore, a low level of physical activity will have negative effects upon the physical condition of the patients. In extreme cases physical inactivity may result in a syndrome of physical deconditioning that may further contribute to the pain problem. Some patients do not avoid activities because of anticipated pain, but because they fear that these activities may lead to (re)injury (Kori *et al.* 1990; see also Chapter 9).

It may also be true that pain behaviors are maintained by the avoidance of aversive experiences that are not at all related to pain. A popular example is that pain behavior and, in particular, sick leave, may be reinforced and maintained by the avoidance of aversive and unsatisfying work conditions. Whenever these extra benefits outweigh the costs of pain behavior, one talks about secondary gain. Although clinical practice suggests that secondary gain does occur, its incidence is probably overestimated. It is often overlooked that the presence of pain also induces or creates distress and frustration at work. Patients, for whom pain interferes with their valued professional activities, may not resume work because they avoid these distressing and frustrating experiences.

A critical question is *how and why avoidance occurs and persists*. In the pain literature, it is often assumed that there is a close link between fear and avoidance. In that respect, some cognitive–behavioral models have been described as fear-avoidance models (Lethem *et al.* 1983; Waddell *et al.* 1993; Vlaeyen and Linton 2000; see also Chapter 1). It is taken for granted that fear is strongly associated with *avoidance*. Thus, initially, a patient may *escape* from pain by stopping his or her ongoing behavior. He or she may further learn to fear these behaviors or activities. It will be no surprise that the person who fearfully anticipates pain during physical activities, will avoid performing these activities. A strong and close link between fear and avoidance was also at the core of the two-factor theory of avoidance learning by Mowrer (1947). His model may appear outdated as Mowrer vigorously avoided the use of mentalistic/cognitive terms, but it clarifies an intriguing puzzle of avoidance behavior: Why does avoidance behavior not extinguish as it is followed by nothing? Or, in other words, what reinforces avoidance behavior?

The answer of Mowrer was straightforward. He proposed that avoidance was the result of two learning processes. The first process was related to classical conditioning, the second to operant conditioning. According to Mowrer (1947), organisms first experience the temporal relationship between an event (CS) and the aversive experience (UCS). In line with classical conditioning, organisms learn to respond with conditioned fear in these situations. Once classical conditioning has taken place, operant conditioning comes into play. The organism will learn to escape from the conditioned fear that is elicited by the CS. As a consequence, the UCS is also avoided. According to Mowrer, the reduction of conditioned fear by its escape is the fundamental drive of the maintenance of avoidance behavior. His model generated considerable research. However, the two-factor model has generally failed the test. Of particular importance, is the consistent failure of experimental studies to demonstrate that conditioned fear is responsible for avoidance behavior. There is indeed no strong relationship between fear and avoidance behavior. Most often avoidance takes place without the presence of fear.

Let us return to our clinical example. The guarding behaviors of patients may be successful in avoiding pain or injury, but there is often no conjunct experience of fear. Thus, avoidance persists even when fear is not experienced. Some critical experiments even point at the fear-inhibiting property of avoidance behavior. Starr and Mineka (1977) have demonstrated that the occurrence of avoidance behavior facilitated the extinction of conditioned fear. It is, therefore, no surprise that in studies with pain patients a desynchrony between avoidance behaviors and fear responses may occur (see Vlaeyen et al. 1995).

2.2.3 Conclusions

Fordyce (1976) was one of the first to apply the operant conditioning principles to pain behavior. A core assumption is that pain behavior emerges whenever the benefits outweigh the costs. Both experimental and clinical research has focused on the social reinforcement of pain behavior and on the instigation of avoidance behavior by pain-related fear. Although pain-related fear and avoidance behavior are two core constructs in many cognitive–behavioral models of chronic pain, there is no detailed and experimental research about the precise and dynamic processes underlying the interrelationship between pain-related fear and avoidance. Overall, the often assumed strong and close relationship between overt fear and anxiety, on the one hand, and avoidance, on the other hand, does not hold. The straightforward but simple idea that fear is responsible for persistent avoidance behavior is wrong, and needs further elaboration (see later).

3 New learning accounts of conditioned fear and avoidance

Classical and operant conditioning have been discussed within their historical context. Also some major research areas, in which the two learning accounts have been applied to the problem of pain, have been reviewed. Although it is well-documented in clinical studies with chronic pain patients that negative appraisals of pain are associated with avoidance (Crombez *et al.* 1999; Vlaeyen and Linton 2000), a fundamental understanding of the emergence and maintenance of avoidance behavior in relationship to pain-related fear is generally lacking. It is our conviction that the absence of a debate about this issue is a reflection of the ignorance about recent ideas within learning psychology. We will introduce new ideas and apply them to the problem of pain. The focus will be mainly on fear conditioning and avoidance (for other advances in the area of instrumental learning see Chapter 3). Wherever possible, available evidence will be discussed. However, as will be noted, there is almost no research of conditioning and avoidance in the area of pain. The main objective of the next section is more about stimulating thoughts than about reviewing data.

During the last decades, the role of cognitive factors in the process of learning has been increasingly recognized. Individuals learn to detect signals of impending pain and are able to verbally report upon these relationships. The dynamics of learning have been further stressed by affective–motivational accounts of learning. Classical conditioning is not a learning of "cold" cognitions, but involves an affective preparation for action. Indeed, the evolutionary significance of anticipatory fear is a preparation to defend or to escape. Which response will emerge, is still a poorly understood mechanism. It is, however, a consensus that the CR is never an exact replica of the UCR. It seems to be dependent upon a variety of factors. Finally, new insights about the nature of extinction have implications for the treatment of chronic pain.

3.1 Contingency and contingency-awareness

In a traditional model of classical conditioning, the temporal co-occurrence or contiguity between CS and UCS was long considered to be a necessary and sufficient condition for learning. It has, however, become clear that organisms do not learn about any possible co-occurrence of events. Most often learning is optimal whenever the CS proved to be a specific and sensitive signal for the UCS. Organisms are, therefore, not only sensitive to co-occurrences between the CS and the UCS, but also to the absence of co-occurrences. In other words, not the temporal coincidence, but the logical association between two events (i.e. contingency) is of importance.

The cognitive repositioning of the learning process has led to much debate about the role of awareness of the contingency between the CS and the UCS in learning (Brewer 1974). Dawson and Shell (1987) have repeatedly demonstrated that fear conditioning in humans occurs only when participants are able to verbalize the relationship between the CS and the UCS. There seem to be rare exceptions to this position (Öhman and Soares 1998) (for a review on the role of awareness in classical conditioning see Lovibond and Shanks 2002).

In line with the idea that fear conditioning is cognitively mediated, research has shown that fear conditioning is facilitated by verbal information about the contingency. Experiments have demonstrated that informing participants about the CS–UCS contingency generated fear conditioning prior to any pairings of CS and UCS (Dawson and Grings 1968; Wilson 1968). Accordingly, persons do not have to experience the pairings of CS and UCS. These findings have implications for clinical pain situations. Cultural beliefs about the relationship between events, or stories about origins of pain, may all fuel fearful apprehension of impending pain.

3.2 Characteristics of the UCS, UCS-inflation, and UCS revaluation

Although everyone experiences pain as an unpleasant and aversive experience, the extent of aversion and the specific nature of the threat vary substantially between individuals. An episode of moderate pain may be perceived as an aversive event with severe consequences by an athlete on the eve of an important competition, but an employee may experience the pain as a temporary nuisance and continue to work. Patients who think that "pain means damage to my body" will behave differently in anticipation of pain than patients who interpret pain as temporary discomfort. Price (1999) has tried to capture these multiple affective dimensions of pain affect. In his multistage model of pain processing, he distinguished between the immediate affective dimension of pain and the subsequent stage of pain affect. The immediate affective dimension of pain comprises the moment-by-moment unpleasantness of pain as well as other emotional feelings that pertain to the present or short-term future, such as distress, annoyance, or fear. In contrast, the secondary stage of pain-related affect is based on more elaborate reflection and relates to memories and imagination about the implications of having pain, such as the way pain interferes with different aspects of one's life, the difficulty enduring pain over time, and concern for the long-term consequences. It is reasonable to conclude that in most situations the characteristics that drive fear conditioning are not the sensory attributes of pain but its often idiosyncratic and multilayered affective characteristics (see also Chapter 9). In support of this idea is the finding that catastrophizing about pain, which is conceived as a cognitive style that involves the tendency to misinterpret and exaggerate the threat value of pain, amplifies fear of impending pain beyond pain intensity in both experimental and clinical situations (Crombez *et al.* 1998, 1999; Sullivan *et al.* 2001).

In a similar vein, Davey (1997*b*) has stressed that coping strategies may devalue the aversive nature of traumatic events. Examples are downward comparison (e.g. "Other people are worse off than me") (Wills 1981), positive reappraisal (e.g. "In every problem there is something good") (Davey 1993), cognitive disengagement (e.g. "The problems involved in this situation simply aren't important enough to get upset about"), optimism (e.g. "Everything will work itself out in the end") (Scheier and Carver 1992), faith in social support (e.g. "I have others who can help me through this"), denial (e.g. "I refuse to believe this is happening"), and life perspective (e.g. "I can put up with these problems as long as everything else in my life is okay").

We can thus conclude that the meaning of pain is not static, but dynamic, and often changes depending upon information from other sources. The animal conditioning literature suggests that fear responses change when the meaning of the UCS changes, even when this change in meaning occurs in the absence of the CS. A well-known illustration of this principle is *UCS-inflation* (Mackintosh 1983). After conditioning with a low intensity UCS, a few experiences with a high intensity UCS are introduced in the absence of the original CS. Most often anticipatory fear in response to the CS will change accordingly and will become more intense. It looks like the original UCS is reevaluated as more aversive and that this revaluation is taken into account on future presentations of the CS. Initially a certain movement (e.g. lifting) may elicit only weak pain. When a back pain patient experiences a sudden increase in pain without CS, subsequently the CS might evoke a stronger reaction. Thus, a new and more severe episode of back pain (UCS-inflation), even if this is not associated with lifting (CS), may lead to increased fear of lifting (CR).

A change in meaning of the UCS may also occur by *socially or verbally transmitted* information about the UCS (Baeyens *et al.* 1992; Davey 1997*b*). Hearing stories of patients who have become crippled and handicapped may inflate fear of pain. Caregivers, who inform patients about the potential damage, or "wear and tear," of the neck or back may inflate fearful anticipations of pain on future occasions. Changing the meaning of an UCS by verbal information appears to be an asymmetric process. It is relatively easy to produce large increases in fear as a result of verbal information, leading to inflation of the aversiveness of the UCS, but less easy to produce UCS devaluation effects as a result of verbal information about the UCS (Davey 1997*b*). Indeed, clinical practice shows that it is difficult to change the belief that "pain means injury" in patients with chronic pain. Alternatively, ambiguous advice to pick up daily activities, but to be careful to do movements in an appropriate way, easily inflates fear. Yet another way to inflate the meaning of the UCS is to worry or ruminate about the UCS and its possible consequences. Individuals suffering from phobia and anxiety disorders have a tendency to focus on and to rehearse all possible aversive outcomes of phobic encounters (Marks 1987). This ruminative and catastrophic tendency may inflate the aversive nature of the UCS, and may fuel fear responses to CSs (Norton and Asmundson 2003).

3.3 Characteristics of the CS, affective modulation, and occasion-setting

Which stimuli become signals for the UCS may vary to a large extent between persons. Of primordial importance is the often idiosyncratic learning context or history (but see also Garcia and Koelling 1966). In the case of pain, likely CSs are activities and movements that once elicited pain. But, interoceptive stimuli may also serve as CS. The occurrence of a pain episode is a conditioning trial that allows the individual to associate internal diffuse somatic sensations with the pain experienced. This is called interoceptive conditioning (Razran 1961). Diffuse somatic sensations give rise to anticipation anxiety (CR). They signal the possible occurrence of a new pain episode. So pain may be associated with interoceptive correlates of early stages of pain itself (see also Norton and Asmundson 2003).

As mentioned earlier, CRs often are not identical to UCRs. Which type of CR is elicited is often determined by the nature of the CS. Some CSs afford particular CRs (Pinel *et al.* 1980). Konorski (1967) has stressed the impact of the CS duration upon the selection of the CR. He argued that discrete and stimulus-specific defensive reflexes such as eye blink, withdrawal reflex, or muscle twitches occur only with CSs of short duration (e.g. half a second). Whenever the CS has a long duration, more generic defensive reactions (e.g. freezing) or a more diffuse preparation for defence may be observed as CRs. According to Konorski (1967), this more diffuse preparation for defence is the quintessence of conditioned fear. Its function is to prepare for action, and to sensitize lower-order, but more stimulus-specific, defensive responses. There is, therefore, a dynamic and specific interaction between different types of CRs (Konorski 1967; Wagner and Brandon 1989). Specific muscle twitches as CR will be intensified in situations of fearful anticipation of pain. The idea that conditioned fear may potentiate or sensitize other CRs (Wagner and Brandon 1989) has been the starting point for two new research areas in the domain of emotions and in the domain of animal learning.

In his affective–motivational theory of emotions, Lang (Lang *et al.* 1990; Lang 1995) conceives of emotions as action dispositions, which are primitively associated with either a behavioral set favoring approach (positive emotions) or a behavioral set disposing the organism to avoid or to escape (negative emotions). Furthermore, he emphasized that the relation between the action disposition and the actual response is not one to one. He contended that the actual response is not merely the consequence of the vigour of the action disposition, but is profoundly affected by contextual information. Thus, while a tendency to withdraw is the central feature of any aversive state, the actual response might be either approach to attack (fight) or escape (flight). Clear evidence for this position is found in etho-experimental animal research which indicated that, depending on the context and on the learning history, the rat's defensive response can include anxious vigilance, freezing, running, climbing, jumping, displacement, or attack on a fellow rat (see Blanchard and Blanchard 1987).

Following the idea of Konorski (1967), Lang and colleagues proposed specific hypotheses about the functional relevance of emotional states. According to Lang, an emotional state (1) sensitizes low-level reflexes with a matching affective tone, and (2) inhibits the reflexes with a mismatching affective tone. Thus, during negative emotions defensive reflexes will be intensified, whereas reflexes with a positive emotional value will be inhibited. These predictions have already received considerable support from several human studies (Vrana *et al.* 1988; Lang *et al.* 1990, 1992; Crombez *et al.* 1997) and animal studies (see Davis 1986) which primarily employed a startle inducing stimulus (an intense burst of white noise) prompting a protective-defensive reflex. It may, therefore, be expected that responses to pain or CRs will depend upon the background emotion. Elation and pleasant affective states may inhibit fearful apprehension in anticipation of pain, or even pain responses. Anxiety, stress, and fear may, on the other hand, potentiate conditioned fear and pain responses, and inhibit responses to pleasant stimuli. It is unknown whether a background experience of chronic pain has similar effects as a background experience of anxiety or fear. With acute pain as background experience, Crombez *et al.* (1997) found an intensification of a defensive startle reflex to a noise burst during high-intensity (painful) heat stimuli in comparison with the low-intensity (non-painful) heat stimuli.

Animal learning experiments have revealed that, in some circumstances, stimuli may not become a CS, but acquire a kind of high-order function. Holland (1992) calls these stimuli occasion-setters as they inform whether or not a CS predicts the UCS. In a typical experiment, a short-duration CS signals the UCS only when a background noise (occasion-setter) is present. Whenever the background noise is absent, the CS is not followed by the UCS. Almost any event (discrete stimuli of long duration, context, drug states, and emotional states) can become an occasion-setter. Intriguingly, occasion-setters do not elicit any CRs. They are, therefore, often overlooked in natural situations. However, they may account for some contradictory findings, in particular when CSs do not systematically elicit conditioned responding, and when extinction seems to be ineffective. Indeed, extinction of conditioned responding is only effective when it occurs in the presence of the original occasion-setter. The idea of occasion-setting has not yet been introduced in the area of pain. It may, however, further our understanding about the dynamics of conditioned fear and avoidance. In particular, the idea that pain may act as an occasion-setter has potential relevance. Indeed, patients often do not respond to CSs when pain-free, but are extremely sensitive to signals of further pain and vigorously avoid pain-worsening situations when in pain. It follows that therapy may be successful only in the presence of the occasion-setter—pain.

3.4 Extinction of conditioned fear, renewal, and generalization

Some mathematical accounts of classical conditioning consider extinction as the weakening or even disappearance of the associative strength between the CS and the UCS (Rescorla and Wagner 1972). However, there is a growing consensus that extinction does not result in simple unlearning or forgetting of the association between a CS and a UCS (Bouton and Swartzentruber 1991; Bouton 1994, 2000). Several experimental phenomena convincingly illustrate that extinction does not involve the destruction of the original learning, but instead may leave the acquired CS–UCS association intact: A formerly extinguished fear response may spontaneously reappear after a certain time (spontaneous recovery); there is often a swift reacquisition with an extinguished CS (rapid reacquisition); and one new UCS experience, even in the absence of the CS, may reanimate the CS–UCS association (reinstatement) (Baeyens *et al.* 1995).

Of particular theoretical and clinical relevance is the finding that extinction is often context-specific. This finding is best exemplified by the procedure of renewal. In this procedure, a CS is extinguished in a context B which is different from the acquisition context (context A). When after successful extinction in context B, the CS is reintroduced in context A, a strong recovery or renewal of conditioned responding toward the CS is observed (Bouton 2000). This phenomenon strongly indicates that extinction is often specific to its context. Rather than forgetting that the CS signals the UCS, the organism learns that "in this particular context, the CS–UCS relation does not hold" (cf., occasion-setting). Research in the area of phobia has substantiated the clinical relevance of this phenomenon (Mineka *et al.* 1999; Rodriguez *et al.* 1999). In the study of Mineka *et al.* (1999), 36 human participants who were phobic of spiders received one session of exposure therapy and were tested for return of fear 1 week later in either the same or a different context. The results indicated that participants tested in the new context showed a greater return of fear than participants tested in the same context. This context-specificity implies that the extinction of fear is difficult to generalize to other contexts. It will be no surprise that therapeutic effects in particular contexts, such as physiotherapy, will remain context-specific and will not generalize toward other situations.

Bouton (2000) has convincingly demonstrated that the notion of context should be broadly defined, including location, time, and internal state. According to Bouton and Swartzentruber (1991), the stimulus itself or some of its features may also have a similar function as a context. Recent research on chronic pain has supported the idea that extinction is stimulus-specific (Crombez *et al.* 2002; Goubert *et al.* 2002). Although back pain patients corrected their pain expectancies after just one exposure to a back-stressing movement, the corrections of pain expectancies tended not to generalize to another back-stressing movement. When asked to perform a second, new movement, overpredictions of pain reoccurred, implying a lack of generalization of extinction.

The fact that extinction is context- or stimulus-specific has clinical implications. For individuals suffering from excessive fears and phobias, exposure therapy has been shown to be the most effective treatment (Davey 1997*a*). Also in the case of pain-specific fear, exposure therapy is effective in the clinical rehabilitation of chronic pain patients with high pain-related fear (see Chapter 14). Further research should address how to generalize the effects of exposure. Classical conditioning suggests some promising avenues to increase the generalizability of extinction: (1) conducting exposure therapy in several different contexts (Gunther *et al.* 1998; Bouton 2000), (2) varying the stimulus during exposure (Rowe and Craske 1998*b*), and (3) distributing exposure sessions rather widely over time (Rowe and Craske 1998*a*; Bouton 2000; Tsao and Craske 2000). Applied to pain, exposure therapy should take place in different contexts, such as in a clinic, in the home situation, and so on. Second, a wide variety of movements should be selected for exposure therapy. This can be accomplished by making a fear hierarchy of movements that are successively practiced. Finally, exposure sessions could be distributed over time.

3.5 Avoidance, safety signals, and rule-governed behavior

How and why does avoidance occur and persist? The two-factor model of Mowrer (1947) has been largely unsuccessful in addressing this question. The idea that there is a strong relationship between fear and avoidance is wrong. Evidence points at the opposite: Avoidance behavior has a fear-inhibiting property (Starr and Mineka 1977). Recent views of avoidance have taken this property into account. They have argued that avoidance behavior or some of its features become "safety signals." Technically speaking, safety signals are the result of an inhibitory conditioning procedure. In such a procedure, stimuli correlate with the non-appearance of a UCS, and become signals of absence of the UCS (Mackintosh 1983). When the UCS is an aversive experience, the CS signals safety. In animal conditioning it has been repeatedly demonstrated that safety signals inhibit fear. The basic idea is that stimuli that are present during avoidance behavior become inhibitory stimuli. These stimuli signal that the aversive outcome will not occur, and inhibit fear. When these safety signals are absent, fear immediately resurfaces.

Sharp (2001) has pointed out that the "safety seeking behaviors" construct has been virtually ignored in the area of pain. He suggests that pain research could benefit from integrating this construct in to psychological models of pain. Sharp (2001) argued that fear is maintained via the effect that avoidance and other safety behaviors have on the cognitions and beliefs underlying (or associated with) the fear. That is, if a patient with chronic low back pain is afraid that lifting will result in (re)injury, then avoiding lifting will maintain the belief that lifting may lead to further damage. If patients continue to avoid lifting and other activities, there is no opportunity to disconfirm the belief.

There still remains a puzzle in many clinical instantiations of avoidance. Why do patients avoid aversive events that they have never experienced? The above explanation of avoidance behaviour assumes at least some experiences with the aversive event. Probably, this is the reason why early avoidance models in the area of pain focused upon the fear of pain and upon avoidance of pain (e.g. Lethem *et al.* 1983). However, patients with chronic pain often avoid movements in order to prevent injury, or in order to not become crippled or handicapped. In these cases, the dreaded future (e.g. become crippled) has never been experienced. Here, the distinction between behaviors that are contingency-shaped (learned through direct experience) and behaviors that are acquired via verbal mechanisms, so-called rule-governed behavior, is relevant (Skinner 1988). Humans generate rules regarding schedules of reinforcement, and these rules profoundly affect behavior (Hayes and Ju 1998). For example, someone who experiences pain may generate the rule "I must be careful that I don't make a wrong movement, otherwise I will injure myself." This rule may govern the behavior of pain patients, without having actually experienced injury due to a "wrong" movement. This rule may force patients to rest and to be careful. A potential problem of rule-governed learning is that humans become less sensitive to the actual contingency between behavior and out-come (Hayes and Ju 1998): Behavior may persevere despite its devastating effects. Many forms of clinical behaviors—including pain behaviors—show such persistence despite the experienced or potential negative consequences of these behaviors. Pain patients may follow the rule "if I search long enough, I will find a solution that relieves my pain." The persistent and unsuccessful search to find the solution for their pain may only fuel further frustration and distress (Aldrich *et al.* 2000).

4 **Conclusion**

In this chapter, we provided an overview of traditional conceptualizations of classical and operant conditioning as applied to pain. Concerning classical conditioning, most studies have focused upon the putative role of muscle tension as a CR in the process of chronification of pain, and upon the question of whether pain experiences can be directly conditioned. For both theses, empirical evidence proved to be limited. In the area of operant conditioning, traditional theories of avoidance behavior were reviewed as well as the impact of social consequences upon pain behavior. From this overview, it appears that the often-assumed strong and close relationship between pain-related fear and avoidance does not hold because most often avoidance takes place without the presence of fear. A fundamental understanding of the emergence and mainte-nance of avoidance behavior in relationship to pain-related fear is generally lacking, and, in our view, this is a reflection of the lack of knowledge about recent ideas within learning psychology.

Therefore, we outlined several new ideas on conditioning and applied these to pain and especially to pain-related fear and avoidance. As research findings in the domain of pain are limited, our aim was primarily to stimulate the reader in taking along the new thoughts into future research and clinical practice. During the last decades, the role of cognitive factors in the process of learning, and especially in fear conditioning, has been increasingly recognized. Fear conditioning is facilitated by verbal information about the contingency between CS and UCS. Furthermore, the aversive meaning of the UCS pain may differ across individuals (e.g. catastrophic thoughts about pain enhance the threat value of pain), its aversive meaning may be devaluated by the use of certain coping strategies (e.g. downward comparison), and the meaning of pain often changes depending upon information from other sources, such as socially or verbally transmitted information.

We also discussed that a preparation for defense or action is the quintessence of conditioned fear. Further, we introduced the idea that conditioned fear may potentiate or sensitize other CRs, which has been the starting point for two new research areas in the domain of emotions and in the domain of animal learning. In his affective–motivational theory of emotions, Lang *et al.* (1990) proposed that during negative emotions defensive reflexes are intensified, whereas reflexes with a positive emotional value are inhibited. It may, therefore, be expected that responses to pain will depend upon the background emotion. It is yet unknown whether a background experience of chronic pain has similar effects as a background experience of anxiety or fear. Suggestions that this may be the case are provided by the findings of Crombez *et al.* (1997), who used acute pain as background experience. In the domain of animal learning, the finding of the existence of occasion-setters has been found to account for some contradictory findings, and has led to the understanding that extinction of CRs is effective only when it occurs in the presence of the occasion-setter. Introducing this idea in the domain of pain may further our understanding about the dynamics of conditioned fear and avoidance. Furthermore, there is growing consensus that extinction does not result in simple unlearning or forgetting of the association between a CS and a UCS. Rather, the organism learns that "in this particular context, the CS–UCS relation does not hold." In accordance with therapy of excessive fears or phobias, exposure has been shown an effective treatment for chronic pain patients with high pain-related fear. Some suggestions were made how to generalize the effects of exposure.

Finally, a new view on avoidance behavior was introduced, in which it is assumed that avoidance behavior has a fear-inhibiting property. Avoidance behavior or stimuli that are present during avoidance behavior become "safety signals," which signal that the aversive outcome will not occur and inhibit fear. The only problem that remains unexplained by the "safety signals" construct is the observation that patients also avoid aversive events that they have never experienced. An explanation in terms of behaviors that are acquired via verbal mechanisms, so-called rule-governed behavior, may provide an answer in these instances of maintenance of avoidance behavior.

References

Aldrich, S., Eccleston, C., and Crombez, G. (2000). Worrying about chronic pain: Vigilance to threat and misdirected problem solving. *Behaviour Research and Therapy*, **38**, 457–70.

Baeyens, F., Eelen, P., Van den Bergh, O., and Crombez, G. (1992). The content of learning in human evaluative conditioning: Acquired valence is sensitive to US-revaluation. *Learning and Motivation*, **23**, 200–24.

Baeyens, F., Eelen, P., and Crombez, G. (1995). Pavlovian associations are forever: On classical conditioning and extinction. *Journal of Psychophysiology*, **9**, 127–41.

Blanchard, R.J. and Blanchard, D.C. (1987). An ethoexperimental approach to the study of fear. *The Psychological Record*, **37**, 305–16.

Block, A., Kremer, E., and Gaylor, M. (1980). Behavioral treatment of chronic pain: The spouse as a discriminative cue for pain behavior. *Pain*, **9**, 243–52.

Bolles, R.C. and Fanselow, M.S. (1980). A perceptual-defensive-recuperative model of fear and pain. *Behavioral and Brain Sciences*, **3**, 291–301.

Bouton, M.E. (1994). Conditioning, remembering, and forgetting. *Journal of Experimental Psychology: Animal Behavior Processes*, **20**, 219–31.

Bouton, M.E. (2000). A learning theory perspective on lapse, relapse, and the maintenance of behavior change. *Health Psychology*, **19**, 57–63.

Bouton, M.E. and Swartzentruber, D. (1991). Sources of relapse after extinction in pavlovian and instrumental learning. *Clinical Psychology Review*, **11**, 123–40.

Bouton, M.E., Mineka, S., and Barlow, D.H. (2001). A modern learning theory perspective on the etiology of panic disorder. *Psychological Review*, **108**, 4–32.

Brewer, W.F. (1974). There is no convincing evidence for operant or classical conditioning in adult humans. In W.B. Weiner and D.S. Palermo (eds.), *Cognition and the Symbolic Processes*. Hillsdale, NJ: Erlbaum.

Chapman, C.R. and Gagliardi, G.J. (1980). Clinical implications of Bolles, and Fanselow's pain/fear model. *Behavioral and Brain Sciences*, **3**, 305–6.

Crombez, G. and Eccleston, C. (2002). Comment on facial expression of pain: An evolutionary account. *Behavioral and Brain Sciences*, **25**, 457–8.

Crombez, G., Baeyens, F., and Eelen, P. (1994). Klassieke conditionering en geconditioneerde pijn [Classical conditioning and conditioned pain]. *Gedragstherapie*, **27**, 97–107.

Crombez, G., Vervaet, L., Baeyens, F., Lysens, R., and Eelen, P. (1996). Do pain expectancies cause pain in chronic low back pain patients? A clinical investigation. *Behaviour Research and Therapy*, **34**, 919–25.

Crombez, G., Baeyens, F., Vansteenwegen, D., and Eelen, P. (1997). Startle intensification during painful heat. *European Journal of Pain*, **1**, 87–94.

Crombez, G., Eccleston, C., Baeyens, F., and Eelen, P. (1998). When somatic information threatens, catastrophic thinking enhances attentional interference. *Pain*, **75**, 187–98.

Crombez, G., Vlaeyen, J.W.S., Heuts, P.H.T.G., and Lysens, R. (1999). Pain-related fear is more disabling than pain itself: Evidence on the role of pain-related fear in chronic back pain disability. *Pain*, **80**, 329–39.

Crombez, G., Eccleston, C., Vlaeyen, J.W.S., Vansteenwegen, D., Lysens, R., and Eelen, P. (2002). Exposure to physical movement in low back pain patients: Restricted effects of generalization. *Health Psychology*, **21**, 573–8.

Davey, G.C.L. (1993). A comparison of three cognitive appraisal strategies: The role of threat devaluation in problem-focused coping. *Personality and Individual Differences*, **14**, 535–46.

Davey, G.C.L. (1997a). *Phobias. A Handbook of Theory, Research and Treatment*. Chichester, New York, Weinheim, Brisbane, Singapore, Toronto: John Wiley & Sons Ltd.

Davey, G.C.L. (1997b). A conditioning model of phobias. In GCL Davey (ed.), *Phobias. A Handbook of Theory, Research and Treatment*, pp. 301–22. Chichester, New York, Weinheim, Brisbane, Singapore, Toronto: John Wiley & Sons Ltd.

Davis, M. (1986). Pharmacological and anatomical analysis of fear conditioning using the fear-potentiated startle paradigm. *Behavioral Neuroscience*, **100**, 814–24.

Dawson, M.E. and Grings, W.W. (1968). Comparison of classical conditioning and relational learning. *Journal of Experimental Psychology*, **76**, 227–31.

Dawson, M.E. and Shell, A.M. (1987). Human autonomic and skeletal classical conditioning: The role of conscious factors. In G.C.L. Davey (ed.), *Cognitive processes and Pavlovian Conditioning in Humans*, pp. 27–57. New York, NY: Wiley.

Eccleston, C., Williams, A.C.de C., and Rogers, W.S. (1997). Patients' and professionals' understandings of the causes of chronic pain: Blame, responsibility and identity protection. *Social Science and Medicine*, **45**, 699–709.

Epstein, S. (1973). Expectancy and magnitude of reaction to a noxious UCS. *Psychophysiology*, **10**, 100–7.

Flor, H. and Birbaumer, N. (1994). Acquisition of chronic pain. Psychophysiologic mechanisms. *APS Journal*, **3**, 119–27.

Flor, H. and Turk, D.C. (1989). Psychophysiology of chronic pain: Do chronic pain patients exhibit symptom-specific psychophysiological responses? *Psychological Bulletin*, **105**, 215–59.

Flor, H., Turk, D.C., and Birbaumer, N. (1985). Assessment of stress-related psychophysiological reactions in chronic back pain patients. *Journal of Consulting and Clinical Psychology*, **53**, 354–64.

Flor, H., Birbaumer, N., Schugens, M.M., and Lutzenberger, W. (1992). Symptom-specific psychophysiological responses in chronic pain patients. *Psychophysiology*, **29**, 452–60.

Flor, H., Breitenstein, C., Birbaumer, N., and Fürst, M. (1995). A psychophysiological analysis of spouse solicitousness towards pain behaviors, spouse interaction, and pain perception. *Behavior Therapy*, **26**, 255–72.

Flor, H., Knost, B., and Birbaumer, N. (2002). The role of operant conditioning in chronic pain: An experimental investigation. *Pain*, **95**, 111–18.

Fordyce, W.E. (1976). *Behavioral Methods for Chronic Pain and Illness*. St Louis: The C.V. Mosby Company.

Fordyce, W.E. (1983). Behavioral conditioning concepts in chronic pain. In J.J.E.A. Bonica (ed.), *Advances in Pain Research and Therapy*, Vol. **5**, pp. 781–8. New York, NY: Raven Press.

Fordyce, W.E. (1988). Pain and suffering. *American Psychologist*, **43**, 276–83.

Garcia, J. and Koelling, R.A. (1966). The relation of cue to consequence in avoidance learning. *Psychonomic Science*, **4**, 123–4.

Garvey, C.R. (1933). A study of conditioned respiratory changes. *Journal of Experimental Psychology*, **4**, 471–503.

Gentry, W.D. and Bernal, G.A.A. (1977). Chronic pain. In R. Williams and W.D. Gentry (eds.), *Behavioral Approaches to Medical Treatment*, pp. 173–82. Cambridge, MA: Ballinger.

Goubert, L., Francken, G., Crombez, G., Vansteenwegen, D., and Lysens, R. (2002). Exposure to physical movement in chronic back pain patients: No evidence for generalization across different movements. *Behaviour Research and Therapy*, **40**, 415–29.

Gunther, L.M., Denniston, J.C., and Miller, R.R. (1998). Conducting exposure treatment in multiple contexts can prevent relapse. *Behaviour Research and Therapy*, **36**, 75–91.

Hayes, S.C. and Ju, W. (1998). The applied implications of rule-governed behavior. In W.T. O'Donohue (ed.), *Learning and Behavior Therapy*, pp. 374–91. MA: Allyn & Bacon.

Holland, P.C. (1990). Event representation in Pavlovian conditioning: Image and action. *Cognition*, 37, 105–31.

Holland, P.C. (1992). Occasion setting in Pavlovian conditioning. *Psychology of Learning and Motivation—Advances in Research and Theory*, 28, 69–125.

Hollis, K.L. (1982). Pavlovian conditioning of signal-centered actionpatterns and autonomic behavior: A biological analysis of function. *Advances in the Study of Behavior*, 12, 1–64.

Jaynes, J. (1985). Sensory pain and conscious pain. *Behavioral and Brain Sciences*, 8, 61–3.

Keefe, F.J. and Dunsmore, J. (1992). The multifaceted nature of pain behavior. *APS Journal*, 1, 112–14.

Knost, B., Flor, H., Birbaumer, N., and Schugens, M.M. (1999). Learned maintenance of pain: Muscle tension reduces central nervous system processing of painful stimulation in chronic and subchronic pain patients. *Psychophysiology*, 36, 755–64.

Konorski, J. (1967). *The Integrative Activity of the Brain*. Chicago: The University of Chicago Press.

Kori, S.H., Miller, R.P., and Todd, D.D. (1990). Kinisiophobia: A new view of chronic pain behavior. *Pain Management*, Jan./Feb., 35–43.

Lang, P.J. (1995). The emotion probe: Studies of motivation and attention. *American Psychologist*, 50, 372–85.

Lang, P.J., Bradley, M.M., and Cuthbert, B.N. (1990). Emotion, attention, and the startle reflex. *Psychological Review*, 97, 377–95.

Lang, P.J., Bradley, M.M., and Cuthbert, B.N. (1992). A motivational analysis of emotion: Reflex–cortex connections. *Psychological Science*, 3, 44–9.

Lethem, J., Slade, P.D., Troup, J.D.G., and Bentley, G. (1983). Outline of a fear-avoidance model of exaggerated pain perceptions. *Behaviour Research and Therapy*, 21, 401–8.

Leuba, C. (1940). Images as conditioned sensations. *Journal of Experimental Psychology*, 26, 345–51.

Linton, S.J. and Götestam, K.G. (1985). Controlling pain reports through operant conditioning: A laboratory demonstration. *Perceptual and Motor Skills*, 60, 427–37.

Linton, S.J., Melin, L., and Götestam, K.G. (1985). Behavioral analysis of chronic pain and its management. In M. Hersen, A. Bellack, and H. Eisler (eds.), *Progress in Behaviour Modification*, Vol. 18. New York, NY: Academic Press.

Lousberg, R., Schmidt, A.J.M., and Groenman, N.H. (1992). The relationship between spouse solicitousness and pain behavior: Searching for more experimental evidence. *Pain*, 51, 75–9.

Lovibond, P.F. and Shanks, D.R. (2002). The role of awareness in Pavlovian conditioning: Empirical evidence and theoretical implications. *Journal of Experimental Psychology: Animal Behavior Processes*, 28, 3–26.

Mackintosh, N.J. (1983). *Conditioning and Associative Learning*. Oxford, England: Oxford University Press.

Marks, I.M. (1987). *Fears, Phobias and Rituals*. New York, NY: Academic Press.

Melzack, R. and Wall, P.D. (1965). Pain mechanism: A new theory. *Science*, 150, 971–7.

Mineka, S., Mystkowski, J.L., Hladek, D., and Rodriguez, B.I. (1999). The effects of changing contexts on return of fear following exposure therapy for spider fear. *Journal of Consulting and Clinical Psychology*, **67**, 599–604.

Mowrer, O.H. (1947). On the dual nature of learning—reinterpretation of "conditioning" and "problem-solving." *Harvard Educational Review*, **17**, 102–48.

Norton, P.J. and Asmundson, G.J.G. (2003). Amending the fear-avoidance model of chronic pain: What is the role of physiological arousal? *Behavior Therapy*, **34**, 17–30.

Öhman, A. and Soares, J.J.F. (1998). Emotional conditioning to masked stimuli: Expectancies for aversive outcomes following nonrecognized fear-relevant stimuli. *Journal of Experimental Psychology: General*, **127**, 69–82.

Pinel, J.P., Treit, D., Ladak, F., and MacLennan, A.J. (1980). Conditioned defensive burying in rats free to escape. *Animal Learning and Behavior*, **8**, 447–51.

Price, D.D. (1999). The dimensions of pain experience. In D.D. Price (ed.), *Psychological Mechanisms of Pain and Analgesia*, pp. 43–70. Seattle, WA: IASP Press.

Razran, G. (1961). The observable unconscious and the inferable conscious in current Soviet psychophysiology: Interoceptive conditioning, semantic conditioning, and the orienting reflex. *Psychological Review*, **68**, 81–147.

Rescorla, R.A. and Wagner, A.R. (1972). A theory of Pavlovian conditioning: Variations in the effectiveness of reinforcement and nonreinforcement. In A.H. Black and W.F. Prokasy (eds.), *Classical Conditioning II: Current Research and Theory*, pp. 64–99. New York, NY: Appleton-Century-Crofts.

Rodriguez, B.I., Craske, M.G., Mineka, S., and Hladek, D. (1999). Context-specificity of relapse: Effects of therapist and environmental context on return of fear. *Behaviour Research and Therapy*, **37**, 845–62.

Romano, J.M., Jensen, M.P., Turner, J.A., Good, A.B., and Hops, H. (2000). Chronic pain patient–partner interactions: Further support for a behavioral model of chronic pain. *Behavior Therapy*, **31**, 415–40.

Rowe, M.K. and Craske, M.G. (1998a). Effects of an expanding-spaced versus massed exposure schedule on fear reduction and return of fear. *Behaviour Research and Therapy*, **36**, 701–17.

Rowe, M.K. and Craske, M.G. (1998b). Effects of varied-stimulus exposure training on fear reduction and return of fear. *Behaviour Research and Therapy*, **36**, 719–34.

Scheier, M.F. and Carver, C.S. (1992). Effects of optimism on psychological and physical well-being: Theoretical overview and empirical update. *Cognitive Therapy and Research*, **16**, 201–28.

Sharp, T.J. (2001). The "safety seeking behaviours" construct and its application to chronic pain. *Behavioural and Cognitive Psychotherapy*, **29**, 241–4.

Skinner, B.F. (1988). An operant analysis of problem solving. In A.C. Catania and S. Harnard (eds.), *The Selection of Behaviour: The Operant Behaviorism of B.F. Skinner: Comments and Consequences*, pp. 218–77. New York, NY: Cambridge University Press.

Sokolov, Y.N. (1963). *Perception and the Conditioned Reflex*. Oxford: Pergamon Press.

Spence, S.H., Sharpe, L., Newton-John, T., and Champion, D. (2001). An investigation of symptom-specific muscle hyperreactivity in upper extremity cumulative trauma disorder. *The Clinical Journal of Pain*, **17**, 119–28.

Starr, M.D. and Mineka, S. (1977). Determinants of fear over the course of avoidance learning. *Learning and Motivation*, **8**, 332–50.

Sternbach, R.A. (1978). Clinical aspects of pain. In R.A. Sternbach (ed.), *The Psychology of Pain*, pp. 241–64. New York, NY: Raven Press.

Sullivan, M.J.L., Thorn, B.E., Haythornthwaite, J., Keefe, F.J., Martin, M., Bradley, L., and Lefebvre, J.C. (2001). Theoretical perspectives on the relation between catastrophizing and pain. *The Clinical Journal of Pain*, **17**, 52–64.

Tsao, J.C.I. and Craske, M.G. (2000). Timing of treatment and return of fear: Effects of massed, uniform, and expanding-spaced exposure schedules. *Behavior Therapy*, **31**, 479–97.

Turkkan, J.S. (1989). Classical conditioning: The new hegemony. *Behavioral and Brain Sciences*, **12**, 121–79.

Vlaeyen, J.W.S. and Linton, S.J. (2000). Fear-avoidance and its consequences in chronic musculoskeletal pain: A state of the art. *Pain*, **85**, 317–32.

Vlaeyen, J.W.S., Kole-Snijders, A.M.J., Boeren, R.G.B., and van Eek, H. (1995). Fear of movement/(re)injury in chronic low back pain and its relation to behavioural performance. *Pain*, **62**, 363–72.

Vrana, S.R., Spence, E.L., and Lang, P.J. (1988). The startle probe response: A new measure of emotion? *Journal of Abnormal Psychology*, **97**, 487.

Waddell, G., Newton, M., Henderson, I., Somerville, D., and Main, C.J. (1993). A Fear-Avoidance Beliefs Questionnaire (FABQ) and the role of fear-avoidance beliefs in chronic low back pain and disability. *Pain*, **52**, 157–68.

Wagner, A.R. and Brandon, S.E. (1989). Evolution of a structured connectionist model of Pavlovian conditioning (AESOP). In S.B. Klein and R.R. Mowrer (eds.), *Contemporary Learning Theories: Pavlovian Conditioning and the Status of Traditional Learning Theory*, pp. 149–90. Hillsdale, NJ: Lawrence Erlbaum Associates.

Williams, A.C. de C. (2002). Facial expression of pain: An evolutionary account. *Behavioral and Brain Sciences*.

Wills, T.A. (1981). Downward comparison principles in social psychology. *Psychological Bulletin*, **90**, 245–71.

Wilson, G.D. (1968). Reversal of differential GSR conditioning by instructions. *Journal of Experimental Psychology*, **76**, 491–3.

Chapter 3

A behavioral analysis of pain-related fear responses

Lance M. McCracken

1 Introduction

The importance of the pain sufferer's behavior in adjustment to chronic pain has been recognized for many years. Early developments of this notion included Fordyce's first published trial of operant methods (Fordyce *et al.* 1968) and his volume on behavioral methods for chronic pain (Fordyce 1976). These methods have been criticized over the years including recently (e.g. Sharp 2001). Criticisms often employ overly simplistic notions of "pain behavior" and fail to recognize that there have been considerable changes in the theoretical and empirical basis for current behavioral approaches in the past 30 years. Clarifying these developments may advance our understanding of chronic pain in general and pain-related fear and avoidance in particular.

Many believe that behavior therapy is an outdated version of therapy, replaced by popular cognitive–behavioral therapy. Cognitive–behavioral therapy, in turn, is thought to have subsumed much of the value of behavior therapy plus an added appreciation for thoughts, beliefs, and other cognitive processes. Unfortunately, cognitive–behavioral therapy has lost the link with basic behavioral and learning research that was the unique strength of behavior therapy in the past (Wolpe 1989). Cognitive–behavioral therapists turned rather to developments in social and experimental psychology (Bandura 1969; Lang 1977) and to other cognitive approaches developed within clinical contexts (Ellis 1974). What today's cognitive–behavioral practitioners and researchers may fail to realize is that basic behavioral and learning research, and research by clinical behavior analysts, has continued to develop in substantial ways, now addressing psychological issues that might surprise the larger group (O'Donohue 1998*a*). These developments appear to have particular relevance for chronic pain management and the role of fear and anxiety-related processes.

This chapter will review selected contemporary behavioral accounts that may have particular applicability to fear and anxiety responses associated with chronic pain. After this review a model analysis will be outlined, demonstrating how these accounts, and clinical methods derived from behavioral theories, might guide study, understanding, and management of pain-related fear responses.

2 History, philosophy, and integration

Behavioral approaches today are an outgrowth of the conditioning approaches of the past but have grown to include such topics as choice, self-control, behavioral economics, rule-governed behavior, stimulus equivalence, nonconscious learning, and even memory and categorization (O'Donohue 1998b). Behavior therapists in a range of specialty areas have called for a reintegration of contemporary treatment approaches with behavior theory and basic behavioral and learning research (Eifert and Plaud 1993; Wilson *et al.* 1997). The potential benefits from integration are clearly significant, but the historical reasons for the split are similarly stubborn (Hayes and Hayes 1992; Dougher 1995). Typically, the barrier to integration involves the causal status of cognition (Wilson *et al.* 1997). It is useful to briefly review the debate that has hampered integration.

Cognitively oriented therapists and researchers argue that thoughts are initiating causes of behavior and feelings while behavior analytically trained and radical behaviorists have argued that they are not. Clinical behavior analysts particularly have argued that cognitions are a form of human behavior and are the proper dependent variable of study or treatment, not simply the cause of other behavior. Certainly, cognitive processes can play an important role in the regulation and influence of other behavior, but an understanding of initiating causes must come from analyzing the context in which cognitive responses, and their relations with other behaviors, occur (Hayes and Wilson 1995; Wilson *et al.* 1997). This account posits that it is not enough to know what a person was thinking when they acted in a particular way or when they experienced a particular emotion. Finding the actual causes of the thought, action, and feeling requires identification of environmental and historical features that gave rise to them and to their interrelations. While contemporary behaviorally oriented therapists and clinical behavior analysts will freely admit a lack of attention to thoughts and verbal processes during the early history of behavior therapy, they can now highlight significant advancements in the past 10 years. And, despite well-known philosophical differences, it is argued that real opportunity for integration exists on issues related to empirical research and clinical outcome (Wilson *et al.* 1997).

In addition to arguments on philosophical and ontological grounds, increasing data shed doubt on the central role of cognition in other behavior change.

Burns and Spangler (2001) used structural equation modeling to examine possible causal links between dysfunctional attitudes and anxiety and depression in a large sample of outpatients receiving cognitive–behavioral therapy. They found that dysfunctional attitudes were correlated with levels of depression and anxiety; however, they did not find that change in dysfunctional attitudes led to changes in anxiety and depression during treatment. Numerous studies demonstrate that a range of treatment methods, including exposure therapy alone, can produce change in cognitive variables, and direct attempts to restructure thoughts are not necessary (Chambless and Gillis 1993; Newman *et al.* 1994; Abramowitz 1997). Similarly, a component analysis of cognitive–behavioral treatment for depression did not demonstrate a central role of strategies to change automatic thoughts or dysfunctional schemas but, rather, highlighted the importance of overt behavior change (Jacobsen *et al.* 1996). On the practical side, it is argued that cognitive variables are hypothetical constructs and difficult to measure and test (Lee 1992) and difficult or impossible to manipulate except by manipulating the patient/client's environment (including social or verbal environment). Thus, approaches to behavior change that emphasize the role of cognition simply do not yield the same degree of precise behavior influence and control (Forsyth *et al.* 1996).

3 Contemporary behavioral analysis of pain-related fear and avoidance

The history of current approaches to fear and avoidance began with Mowrer (1947) and Dollard and Miller (1950) and what is known as two-factor or two-process theory. In this account, classical conditioning leads to fear responses in the presence of a conditioned stimulus, and operant conditioning produces persistent avoidance, negatively reinforced by fear reduction. Two-factor theory was frequently criticized for its reliance on intervening variables (Hineline 1973), for the fact that fear and phobic behavior often appeared to arise in the absence of any relevant direct conditioning experience (Rachman 1977), and doubts about the reinforcing effects of escape and avoidance (DeSilva and Rachman 1984). However, Ayres (1998) has argued that criticisms of classical (Pavlovian) fear conditioning have been unsound. He presents a contemporary conditioning theory of fear that is not based on cognition or expectancy. This chapter will focus away from classical conditioning (see Chapter 2) and toward less frequently considered verbal, emotional, nonconscious, and social behavioral processes. Varied types of fear behavior will be considered, not just overt avoidance.

3.1 **Verbal processes**

It has long been recognized that fear and avoidance can be acquired by multiple mechanisms. Rachman (1977) referred to the three pathways as conditioning, modeling, and instruction. Wolpe (1981) referred to fear as "classical conditioned" and "cognitively learned." In either case, it was recognized that fear and avoidance could be acquired through verbal mechanisms. The distinction between behavior that is shaped by exposure to environmental contingencies versus acquired via verbal mechanisms, so-called rule-governed behavior, is not a new one (Skinner 1988) but it has received renewed attention. Recent work by behavior analysts recognizes special properties of verbal stimuli and how they can participate in the influence of other behavior and emotions (e.g. Hayes and Hayes 1992; Hayes and Wilson 1993, 1995; Dougher 1998).

It is clear that verbal processes can contribute to the fear and avoidance of chronic pain sufferers. They may respond with fear in pain-related situations due to threats associated with those situations by descriptions they heard, instructions they were given, or rules that are self-generated. Importantly, the fearful pain sufferer need not consciously remember, recite, or think about any of this verbal material in the context of their other fear and avoidance behavior for these other responses to occur (Hayes 1986). For instance, patients routinely follow the general rule "hurt equals harm." At some stage or other after an injury, patients are often given the instruction, "if it hurts, don't do it." They are often provided with descriptions of the workings of their back or other body parts, such as during health care visits, that equate movement with further tissue injury and from there, further suffering, disability, and even paralysis or death. The fact that these associations are acquired is readily shown by responses to measures of fear of pain (McCracken *et al.* 1992). Patients routinely report during assessments that their "spine is crumbling," that they may "damage a nerve," or may in some way or other make their pain worse, if they are not careful. Again, once initiated by verbal processes, fear responses may become more or less automatic in contexts that have acquired these functions to elicit and cue fear and avoidance responses, with no need for continued awareness of the "reason" for the response (Bouton *et al.* 2001).

Basic behavioral research into a phenomenon called "stimulus equivalence" begins to shed light on important aspects of cognition and learning (Sidman and Tailby 1982). Stimulus equivalence, and its various implications for human behavior problems, has been discussed in detail elsewhere (e.g. Hayes and Hayes 1992; Hayes and Wilson 1993; Dougher 1998). Briefly, stimulus equivalence offers an account of how verbal stimuli come to acquire influences (cueing, emotion evoking, motivating, and reinforcing) over other behavior by participation in equivalence relations with the events they represent. During learning and use of language we all learn matches between particular words or symbols and the real life events they represent. In turn we will learn additional "equivalence" between those initial members of an equivalence class and other words and events, through instruction or direct conditioning. Once an equivalence class is established in this way, any behavior influencing function trained for one member will transfer, without direct training, to all members of the class. Dougher and Hackbert (1994) present a useful application of stimulus equivalence to depression. In terms of fear and avoidance, this process helps explain, in behavioral terms, how consequences that have never been encountered (paralysis, crumbling spines, and (re)injury) can nonetheless exert a powerful influence. If pain is a felt event, and pain and injury have been associated in the past, such as through a description from a cautious health care provider, pain will occasion responses as if it is an injury event.

On the positive side, great convenience comes from the capacity to learn new behavior from hearing a description that associates that behavior with a set of consequences. Through this mechanism people need not contact pain and hardship to avoid them in some circumstances. We need not acquire lung cancer to avoid smoking, acquire skin cancer to learn sunscreen use, get injured in a car accident to learn seatbelt use, or have a heart attack to learn the virtues of exercise and a prudent diet. However, along with the conveniences of rules for the quick acquisition of steady behavior comes a considerable downside, a particular insensitivity to environmental contingencies. It has been demonstrated in laboratory studies that subjects given instructions show less behavior change than uninstructed subjects when their circumstances change and their behaviour becomes much less effective (Shimnoff *et al.* 1981; Hayes *et al.* 1986). It has been noted that many types of significant human behavior problems, such as addiction, anxiety disorders, borderline personality disorder, show this same rigidity, persistence of a particular pattern of behavior despite negative consequences (Hayes *et al.* 1996).

All therapy rationales are essentially rules that maintain patient behavioral effort until results of therapy become self-sustaining. The rule implied by the instruction, "if you continue to exercise, your ability to function will eventually improve" can help the fearful pain sufferer continue on a course of rehabilitation even if that course presents them with regular discomfort. A rule implying that "hurt equals harm" or "pain equals damage," on the other hand, is likely to lead to generalized avoidance. New therapy approaches may need to help patients discriminate rule-following that leads to healthy behavior from rule-following that leads to unhealthy behavior.

3.2 Emotional avoidance

Emotional avoidance has been recognized as a contributing issue or core problem issue in many common behavior problems including fear-related behavior problems (Foa *et al.* 1984; Linehan 1993; Hayes *et al.* 1996, 1999*a*). It has been argued that emotional avoidance is a pervasive reaction because of the nature of human language. It is a feature of language that thinking about or talking about, painful events can lead one to re-experience the aversive aspects of the event (Hayes and Wilson 1993; Hayes *et al.* 1996). Furthermore, people will try to control, suppress, or avoid their own negative emotional experiences, a strategy that appears momentarily successful but, in the long run often produces the opposite effect (e.g. Wegner *et al.* 1987). As a result people may attempt to prevent themselves from having completely appropriate emotional reactions, such as actively mourning a loss or experiencing anxiety in an uncertain situation. In turn, needed change and adjustments do not occur, and the situations that evoke these emotions retain their ability to do so when contacted in the future (Hayes *et al.* 1996). This process could help maintain fear and avoidance of pain or interfere with treatment.

There is another implication of how aspects of emotional responding can themselves take on aversive qualities. If persons who respond fearfully to pain also have acquired particular fear and intolerance of their own feelings of fear, the aversiveness and threat of the entire situation will be compounded. During the experience of pain they likely will not discriminate how much of their feelings of threat are evoked by the pain and how much by their various interoceptive experiences of fear itself. In either case, the compound aversiveness of the pain and anxiety experiences are likely to strengthen the inclination to avoid (Asmundson and Taylor 1996). Similar considerations are included in the "fear of fear" concept applied to panic disorder (Chambless *et al.* 1984) and to anxiety sensitivity which has been applied broadly to anxiety disorders (Reiss 1987) and to chronic pain (Asmundson and Norton 1995; Asmundson and Taylor 1996).

3.3 Social processes

Fordyce (1976) discussed both the role of social reinforcement and modeling in the acquisition of the broader class of pain behavior, including avoidance. It is recognized that modeling, sometimes referred to as vicarious conditioning, is one method of fear acquisition (Rachman 1977; Ost and Hugdahl 1981). However, careful consideration of current behavioral theory and findings may reveal additional social influences on pain-related fear and avoidance.

It was mentioned above that intolerance for the interoceptive features of emotional distress could compound the aversiveness of exposure to pain-related circumstances for the significantly pain-fearful patient. This could, in turn, enhance the reinforceability of avoidance. Intolerance of social scrutiny could have a similar effect. The patient with significant fear of pain who finds it aversive to be observed while having pain and appearing distressed is likely to have added distress in social situations and demonstrate more frequent avoidance. Asmundson *et al.* (1996) showed that 11 percent of a sample of disabled workers with chronic pain met standard criteria for social phobia. This is interesting because it is higher than would be expected in a community sample. Those with social phobia did not show greater disability than those without, however, they did report less social support. Their study did not investigate potential combined influences of fear of pain and social phobia. It remains possible that a significant proportion of pain sufferers with significant fear of pain engage in avoidance of activity due to combined influences of pain-related circumstances and aversive social influences. Certainly, histories of humiliation or embarrassment related to pain and histories that associate physical or emotional threat with pain can be brought together to produce fear and avoidance. One set of influences does not preclude the other.

Pain management programs often treat patients in group formats. This arrangement clearly provides an opportunity for highly fearful patients to observe successful exercise and other confrontation with pain-related circumstances by patients who demonstrate no harm. This may constitute vicarious exposure treatment. Similarly, patients' fearful behavior typically does not meet reinforcing forms of attention or help in treatment contexts. Thus, the effects of social reinforcement for fearful responses may be weakened.

Pain management is a social process, a process in which the treatment provider is sometimes the audience. An interesting study of undergraduate participants exposed to experimentally induced pain demonstrated the potential importance of social influences on responses to pain (Hayes and Wolf 1984). Experimental participants were given coping self-statements to read, memorize, and use during exposure (e.g. "I'll just relax and I'll be able to keep my hand in the water."). In the "public" group, participants also gave the statement to the experimenter to read while in the "private" group they did not. Results demonstrated significantly greater pain tolerance for the public group compared to a control group. The private group, on the other hand, did not differ from the control group. Although coping statements may be conceptualized in a number of ways, as self-instruction, attention diversion, or direct emotionally calming stimuli, none of these mechanisms can explain the effect of the private versus public manipulation. These authors concluded that tolerance was enhanced by "social standard setting" similar to the effect of public

commitment (Hayes and Wolf 1984). Clinicians appear to accept the therapeutic value of patient models and public commitments, or social standard
setting arrangements. Behavioral clinicians have in fact developed therapy
approaches that incorporate specific social mechanisms responsible for
the process of therapeutic change (Kohlenberg and Tsai 1991; Follette *et al.*
1996).

3.4 Nonconscious learning

Three methods through which fear and anxiety responses are acquired have
been mentioned, direct conditioning, modeling, and verbal mechanisms. There
is arguably another distinction to make. Some learning can be nonconscious
(Mineka and Ben Hamida 1998). A study of 106 patients with animal, social,
and claustrophobias showed that 15 percent could not recall any specific experiences that led to their fear (Ost and Hugdahl 1981). Among social phobias,
26 percent could not recall a specific onset event. Some have suggested that
significant rates of failure to recall onset circumstances imply another method
of fear acquisition (Ost and Hugdahl 1981). And, that fear responses may be
acquired based on learning that occurs automatically, unintentionally, and
without conscious awareness (Mineka and Ben Hamida 1998).

There are early examples and accumulating data on this issue of nonconscious learning. A covert thumb twitch response, detectable by physiological
monitoring, can be acquired when it produces termination of an aversive
noise without subjects being able to describe the relationship between the
response and the reinforcer (Hefferline *et al.* 1959). A person's speech can be
shaped to include more words of specified types when these word types
produce the response "mmm-hmm" from the experimenter. Later the subjects
have no awareness of the change in their behaviour, or the role of the experimenter's response (Greenspoon 1955). People can show fear responses to
conditioned stimuli even when these stimuli are not consciously perceived
(Ohman 1996). Patients with agoraphobia can demonstrate symptom improvement from subliminal exposure to agoraphobic scenes (Lee *et al.* 1983).

Nonconscious acquisition of fear may have implications for assessment and
management of pain-related fear and avoidance. First, certainly the absence of
a pain experience that could constitute a fear conditioning experience need
not lead the clinician to doubt a role of fear in the patient's problems. The
patient may not be aware of the experiences or reasons for their fear. Second,
ways that fear is acquired may have implications for treatment (Ost 1985). It
is possible that conscious, cognitive change methods such as education or
cognitive therapy may be less effective for changing behavior that is acquired
automatically and nonconsciously. Exposure-based or other experience-based

techniques, on the other hand, may effectively address nonconscious processes (Mineka and Ben Hamida 1998). A focus on nonconscious processes is useful because it forces us to remain aware of all of the interplay between behavior and the environment and helps prevent an unhealthy overemphasis solely on verbal mechanism or processes within conscious awareness. Those who are interested in cognitive-processing biases in chronic pain (see Pincus and Morley 2001 for a review) may find that results from the study of nonconscious learning are pertinent. There are many challenges in the study of non-consicous learning and clearly more work is needed.

3.5 Choice

Many will certainly have forgotten their learning classes during training when they memorized Herrnstein's (1970) version of the law of effect known as the *matching law*. Simply stated the matching law describes that the frequency of a particular response depends on the rate of reinforcement for that response as well as the rate of reinforcement for alternate responses. This law implies that in order to understand why a person behaves in a particular way in a situation, we must understand all sources of reinforcement, including extra-neous reinforcement for all other behaviors. Herrnstein's matching law is stated quantitatively; frequency of a defined response is equal to total response rate (total behavior output in the situation) multiplied by reinforcement rate of the defined response divided by the rate of reinforcement for the defined response plus the rate of all extraneous, concurrent reinforcement. Notice that response frequency is negatively related to the overall reinforcement rate and the shape of the function will happen to be hyperbolic (monotonic, increasing, and negatively accelerated). This equation implies that ease of behavior change will differ depending on the overall density of reinforcement in the environment. Relatively low rate reinforcement will provoke significant change of response frequency in an environment where overall reinforcement rate is lean (Plaud 1992).

Fernandez and McDowell (1995) tested the matching law in a sample of 12 patients with chronic pain. They measured frequency of pain behaviors, well behaviors, and rates of reinforcement for each from significant others. Their results demonstrated that, in both cases, pain behavior and well behav-ior, Hernstein's quantitative matching law was a good descriptive model of response rate. In both cases it was found that response rate was hyperbolically related to rate of reinforcement. The implication of their work is that the pain behavior of chronic pain sufferers can be reduced by reducing reinforcement for it or by increasing the rate of reinforcement freely delivered *or* contingent on well behavior (Fernandez and McDowell 1995). The distressed and avoidant responses entailing significant fear of pain clearly fall in the larger class of pain behavior and are controlled by the consequences they meet in the environment. Thus, these considerations of overall reinforcement rates, and rates of reinforcement for alternate behaviors, have implications for pain-related fear and avoidance.

4 Functional analysis of pain-related fear

Nearly 30 years ago Charles Ferster published a paper in the *American Psychologist* in which he conducted a thoughtful functional analysis of depression in terms of behavior and environment relations (Ferster 1973). Some years later Dougher and Hackbert (1994) conducted a similar, updated analysis, again relying on a behavior analytic approach. It does not appear that an account of fear has been done in this same way although it would be readily possible, as it would be possible to conduct a functional analysis specifically focusing on pain-related fear responses.

Current models of pain-related fear and disability clearly help us to under-stand the role of fear and avoidance in the larger scheme of emotional distress, exaggerated pain perception, and disability of chronic pain sufferers (Lethem *et al.* 1983; Asmundson *et al.* 1999; Vlaeyen and Linton 2000). They show how persistent fear and avoidance can lead to a cycle of decreasing functioning. They are of great use to organize research and are easily translated into treat-ment methods (Vlaeyen *et al.* 2001). However, there are limitations inherent in these models. They rely heavily on cognitive processes, such as expectancies and catastrophizing. These variables are completely acceptable from a behavioral view, as they can be readily understood in terms of known verbal-behavioral process, such as discussed earlier. The problem with these accounts is that the contextual influences on these cognitive processes, and their relations with other behaviors, while receiving mention (Vlaeyen and Linton 2000), have not been fully appreciated.

Table 3.1 details a functional analysis of pain-related fear responses. It utilizes the concept of a *response class*. This is a set of perhaps topographically dissimilar responses that nonetheless tend to operate on the environment in the same fashion or are controlled by the same environmental influences. The table illustrates 9 types of responses from the larger class of pain-related fear responses and 10 types of behavioral processes that may play a role in their acquisition and maintenance. Five of these behavioral processes are consid-ered direct and five are considered secondary or contributory. For the first five processes, pain and fear stimuli are the most pertinent contextual fea-tures while for the second five processes, social and other emotional stimuli

Table 3.1 A behavioral analysis of pain-related fear responses: Potentially important, primary (pain and fear of pain-related) and secondary (social, emotional, and other interoceptive) influences

Response types	Primary behavioral processes					Contributing behavioral influences				
	Elicitation or cueing by threatening pain situation	Establishment of reinforceability by aversive emotional or physical state	Negative reinforcement by reduction of exposure to pain	Negative reinforcement by reduction of pain-related fear	Verbal influences[a]	Elicitation or cueing by other aversive physical or emotional situation	Negative reinforcement by reduction of other interoceptive or emotional influences[b]	Negative reinforcement by reduction of exposure to an aversive social situation	Positive reinforcement by attention, sympathy, support	Weak or lacking alternate or competing response
Reduced physical activity	X	X	X	X	X	X	X		X	X
Reduced social activity	X	X			X	X		X		X
Complaints, help-seeking	X	X		X	X	X	X		X	X
Sedative use	X	X		X	X	X	X			X
Anxious facial expressions, gestures, postures	X				X	X		X	X	X
Anxious feelings	X				X	X				
Hypervigilance and pain focus	X	X			X	X				X
Fearful thoughts	X				X	X				X
Physiological arousal	X				X	X				

a These verbal influences can take the form of covert verbal cues, instructional or self-instructional influences, or verbally transferred behavioral influences on fear and avoidance of pain due to participation in equivalence classes.

b These emotional influences can be non-fear-related or non-pain-related emotional states such as reactions to restraint, loss, or mistreatment by others. Interoceptive influences can be any private feelings of distress or fatigue.

predominate. Each of the behavioral processes listed is based on principles established in laboratory and clinical research (see O'Donohue 1998*b*; Bouton *et al.* 2001 for reviews and discussions of these processes). The purpose of the table is to highlight the range of behaviors that may fall into this broader class and the range of interacting influences that may come to contribute to their frequency and persistence.

The response types listed are selected based on their topography and potential function. It is a presumption that these behaviors could form a functionally related response class. Inclusion of particular response types may appear to be more obvious than others. Some might rather classify help-seeking or medication consumption in another class, such as in the class of coping responses (e.g. Larsen *et al.* 1997). However, if these responses are emitted during exposure to a threat, if they are maintained by a history of negative reinforcement, or if they are provide relief from feelings of threat from pain, then they are functionally the same as avoidance of physical activity and, thus, need to be considered members of the class. In fact, we know that help-seeking and medication use form part of the item set for the avoidance subscale of the Pain Anxiety Symptoms Scale (PASS; McCracken *et al.* 1992) and achieve reasonable corrected total correlations, each above $r = 0.41$ (McCracken, unpublished data). A significant correlation between help-seeking and avoidance, as measured by the PASS, has been demonstrated in the past (McCracken *et al.* 1996). Hypervigilance can be considered a fear response with similar reasoning. When exposed to threat, a person naturally engages in this type of orienting, preparatory, and pre-problem-solving behavior. It is likely to co-occur with other fear responses and occur under the control of the same situational features. It is this behavior that selectively brings other behavior in contact with the environment for the function of minimizing harm, similar to the functions of overt avoidance, escape, or complaints.

Table 3.1 is incomplete in several respects. It does not fully clarify how the consequences of some fear responses can occasion other fear responses. For example, we have previously noted that pain-related physiological responses may produce increased complaints of physical symptoms and may increase hypervigilance or health care use (McCracken *et al.* 1998). Similarly, hypervigilance may contribute to avoidance since it may entail less attention to broad features of life situations, may lead the pain sufferer to be less in contact with natural contingencies, and may lead to other behaviors that are ineffective (McCracken 1997; Aldrich *et al.* 2000). For example, it is difficult to pay careful attention to pain and either perform a complex physical task or carry on a successful conversation at the same time. And, failure experiences will likely punish continued efforts and encourage further avoidance.

Each component response type in the larger class of pain-related fear responses can be seen as clearly disability engendering. These processes are difficult to include in Table 3.1 as well. Table 3.2 illustrates some of these influences. Some of these issues have been previously noted, such as the fear-avoidance-disuse-depression relationship (Lethem *et al.* 1983; Crombez *et al.* 1998; Asmundson *et al.* 1999; Vlaeyen and Linton 2000), effects of hyper-vigilance on functioning (McCracken 1997; Vlaeyen and Linton 2000;

Table 3.2 Disability engendering consequences of pain-related fear response types

Response type	Consequences
Reduced physical activity	1. Loss of physical capacity. 2. Physical discomfort with movement. 3. Reduced contact with stimulating activity. 4. Depression.
Reduced social activity	1. Reduced social support. 2. Reduced enjoyment of collateral activities. 3. Depression.
Complaints and help-seeking	1. Reduced responsibilities. 2. Reduced sense of achievement. 3. Disturbance of normal social relations. 4. Discouragement of social contacts from others:
Medication use	1. Reinforcement of "sick role." 2. Side Effects.
Anxious facial expressions, gestures, postures	1. "Unhelpful" attention or help. 2. Discouragement of social contacts from others.
Anxious feelings	1. Control attempts that may be unsuccessful. 2. Distraction from more useful efforts.
Hypervigilance	1. Distraction from useful situations in wider life context. 2. Failure experiences.
Fearful thoughts	1. Other anxious behavior of all types and consequences from those behaviors.
Physiological arousal	1. Increased physical discomfort. 2. Fatigue. 3. Perception of more physical symptoms. 4. Increased hypervigilance. 5. Increased health care use.

see Eccleston and Crombez 1999 for a review), and effects of physiological fear responses (McCracken *et al*. 1998; Vlaeyen and Linton 2000).

The problem with pain-related fear and avoidance responses is that they are not working for the pain sufferer in the long run. They are not getting patients consequences that entail good healthy functioning. It may seem contradictory, on the one hand, to claim that fear behaviors are selected and maintained by the consequences they meet yet, on the other hand, to describe the suffering and disability they produce. It may be important to clarify a behavioral view of consequences because this notion often creates confusion. In everyday thinking it is often considered that people do what they do because of what will happen next. For the behavioral researcher or clinician people do what they do in a particular context because of a history of consequences for similar behavior in that context in the past. The person may very well make a prediction about what result they will get, but both that prediction and other actions they take are determined by the interplay of history and situation. Unhealthy behavior often persists because circumstances change but the person's behavior never contacts those new circumstances. Isolating effects of avoidance and rule-following, as described earlier, are clear contributors to that result. Also, the types of insidious suffering and disability experiences that accumulate over time exert little helpful control in comparison to whatever immediate results responses appear to meet. The history that determines the probabilities of response in a particular context thus remains functionally intact, unrevised by experience.

5 Conclusion

Behavioral approaches have much to offer to the study of pain-related fear and avoidance. While there are numerous reasons for the failure of integration of contemporary behavioral theory and methods into this important area of research and clinical development, the opportunity exists to begin to redress this failure.

This chapter briefly reviewed some topics from contemporary behavior therapy and clinical behavior analysis. These include accounts of verbal processes, emotion, social processes, nonconscious learning, and choice. Behavioral processes in each of these areas are based on increasingly persuasive experimental evidence. Research into verbal processes such as rule governance and stimulus equivalence has already given rise to coherent treatment approaches for a range of behavior problems (Hayes *et al*. 1999*a*). Renewed attention from behavioral clinicians into social processes of therapy also has led to exciting treatment developments (Kohlenberg and Tsai 1991; Follette *et al*. 1996). It is worth considering what these developments might have to offer for our understanding and management of pain-related fear and avoidance in chronic pain sufferers.

A behavior analytic or radical behavioral approach to behavior problems is inherently functional, contextual, and pragmatic. As such, it places thinking and other cognitive processes primarily in the category of things to explain, not in the category of explanations. This chapter presented a preliminary typology of pain-related fear responses. This typology attempts to incorporate the notion of a response class, multiple situational influence, and behavior–behavior relations. Pain-related fear responses, like other important clusters of patient behavior, can be considered as a response class based on the way they are a product of the same history and controlling circumstances. Pain, associated external stimuli, and the various interoceptive stimuli of fear and anxiety elicit, occasion, motivate, and consequate, and thus evoke, shape, and maintain the members of the response class of fear responses. However, there are clearly coherent behavior accounts of verbal processes, other emotional processes, social influences, and effects of competing behavioral choices that can guide improved understanding of additional contributory processes as well. These basic verbal, emotional, and social influences on pain-related fear responses have remained almost untouched by research approaches to this point. These clearly deserve further study, study that may take the form of experimental investigations of verbal processes influencing pain responses (e.g. Hayes *et al.* 1999*b*) or investigations of novel treatment approaches, such as acceptance based treatments (Hayes *et al.* 1999*a*).

Finally, any coherent appreciation of a behavior problem must include a description of how it can create problems for the individual. A full situational analysis of the class of pain-related fear responses shows the many disability creating consequences in the physical, emotional, and social environment of the chronic pain sufferer. Further understanding of this web of interrelated effects seems likely to help us undo the mechanisms that set it in place.

References

Abramowitz, J.S. (1997). Effectiveness of psychological and pharmacological treatments for obsessive-compulsive disorder: A quantitative review. *Journal of Consulting and Clinical Psychology*, 65, 44–52.

Aldrich, S., Eccleston, C., and Crombez, G. (2000). Worrying about pain: Vigilance to threat and misdirected problem-solving. *Behaviour Research and Therapy*, 38, 457–70.

Asmundson, G.J.G., Jacobson, S.J., Allerdings, M.D., and Norton, G.R. (1996). Social phobia in disabled workers with chronic musculoskeletal pain. *Behaviour Research and Therapy*, 34, 939–43.

Asmundson, G.J.G. and Norton, G.R. (1995). Anxiety sensitivity in patients with physically unexplained chronic pain: A preliminary report. *Behaviour Research and Therapy*, **33**, 771–7.

Asmundson, G.J.G., Norton, P.J., and Norton, G.R. (1999). Beyond pain: The role of fear and avoidance in chronicity. *Clinical Psychology Review*, **19**, 97–119.

Asmundson, G.J.G. and Taylor, S. (1996). Role of anxiety sensitivity in pain-related fear and avoidance. *Journal of Behavioral Medicine*, **19**, 577–86.

Ayres, J.B.J. (1998). Fear conditioning and avoidance. In W. O'Donohue (ed.), *Learning and Behavior Therapy*, pp. 122–45. Boston, MA: Allyn and Bacon.

Bandura, A. (1969). *Principles of Behavior Modification*. New York, NY: Holt, Rinehart & Winston.

Bouton, M.E., Mineka, S., and Barlow, D.H. (2001). A modern learning theory perspective on the etiology of panic disorder. *Psychological Review*, **108**, 4–32.

Burns, D.D. and Spangler, D.L. (2001). Do changes in dysfunctional attitudes mediate changes in depression and anxiety in cognitive behavioral therapy? *Behavior Therapy*, **32**, 337–69.

Chambless, D.L., Caputo, G.C., Bright, P., and Gallagher, R. (1984). Assessment of fear in agoraphobia: The Body Sensations Questionnaire and the Agoraphobic Cognitions Questionnaire. *Journal of Consulting and Clinical Psychology*, **52**, 1090–7.

Chambliss, D.L. and Gillis, M.M. (1993). Cognitive therapy of anxiety disorders. *Journal of Consulting and Clinical Psychology*, **61**, 248–60.

Crombez, G., Vervaet, L., Lysens, R., Baeyens, F., and Eelen, P. (1998). Avoidance and confrontation of painful, back-straining movements in chronic back pain patients. *Behavior Modification*, **22**, 62–77.

DeSilva, P. and Rachman, S. (1984). Does escape behavior strengthen agoraphobis avoidance? A preliminary study. *Behaviour Research and Therapy*, **22**, 87–91.

Dollard, J. and Miller, N.E. (1950). *Personality and Psychotherapy: An Analysis in Terms of Learning, Thinking, and Culture*. New York, NY: McGraw Hill.

Dougher, M.J. (1995). A bigger picture: Cause and cognition in relation to differing scientific frameworks. *Journal of Behavior Therapy and Experimental Psychiatry*, **26**, 215–19.

Dougher, M.J. (1998). Stimulus equivalence and the untrained acquisition of stimulus functions. *Behavior Therapy*, **29**, 577–91.

Dougher, M.J. and Hackbert, L. (1994). A behavior-analytic account of depression and a case report using acceptance-based procedures. *The Behavior Analyst*, **17**, 321–34.

Eccleston, C. and Crombez, G. (1999). Pain demands attention: A cognitive-affective model of the interruptive function of pain. *Psychological Bulletin*, **125**, 356–66.

Eifert, G.H. and Plaud, J.J. (1993). From behavior theory to behavior therapy: The contributions of behavioral theories and research to the advancement of behavior therapy. *Journal of Behavior Therapy and Experimental Psychiatry*, **24**, 101–5.

Ellis, A. (1974). *Humanistic Psychotherapy: The Rational Emotive Approach*. New York, NY: Julian Press.

Fernandez, E. and McDowell, J.J. (1995). Response–reinforcement relationships in chronic pain syndrome: Applicability of Herrnstein's law. *Behaviour Research and Therapy*, **33**, 855–63.

Ferster, C.B. (1973, October). A functional analysis of depression. *American Psychologist,*
    28, 857–70.

Foa, E.B., Steketee, G., and Young, M.C. (1984). Agoraphobia: Phenomenological aspects,
    associated characteristics, and theoretical considerations. *Clinical Psychology Review,*
    4, 431–57.

Follette, W.C., Naugle, A.E., and Callaghan, G.M. (1996). A radical behavioral
    understanding of the therapeutic relationship in effecting change. *Behavior Therapy,*
    27, 623–41.

Fordyce, W.E. (1976). *Behavioral Methods for Chronic Pain and Illness.* St Louis, MO:
    The C.V. Mosby Company.

Fordyce, W.E., Fowler, R.S., Lehman, J.F., and DeLateur, B.J. (1968). Some implications
    of learning in problems of chronic pain. *Journal of Chronic Disease,* **21,** 179–90.

Forsyth, J.P., Lejuez, C.W., Hawkins, R.P., and Eifert, G.H. (1996). Cognitive vs. contextual
    causation: Different world views but perhaps not irreconcilable. *Journal of Behavior
    Therapy and Experimental Psychiatry,* **27,** 369–76.

Greenspoon, J. (1955). The reinforcing effect of two spoken sounds on the frequency
    of two responses. *American Journal of Psychology,* **68,** 409–16.

Hayes, S.C. (1986). The case of the silent dog—verbal reports and the analysis of rules:
    A review of Ericsson and Simon's protocol analysis: Verbal reports as data.
    Journal of the Experimental Analysis of Behavior, **45,** 351–63.

Hayes, S.C. and Hayes, L.J. (1992). Some clinical implications of contextualistic
    behaviorism: The example of cognition. *Behavior Therapy,* **23,** 225–49.

Hayes, S.C. and Wilson, K.G. (1993). Some applied implications of a contemporary
    behavior-analytic account of verbal events. *The Behavior Analyst,* **16,** 283–301.

Hayes, S.C. and Wilson, K.G. (1995). The role of cognition in complex human behavior:
    A contextualistic perspective. *Journal of Behavior Therapy and Experimental Psychiatry,*
    26, 241–8.

Hayes, S.C. and Wolf, M.R. (1984). Cues, consequences and therapeutic talk: Effects of
    social context and coping statements on pain. *Behaviour Research and Therapy,*
    22, 385–92.

Hayes, S.C., Brownstein, A.J., Haas, J.R., and Greenway, D. (1986). Instruction, multiple
    schedules, and extinction: Distinguishing rule-governed behavior from schedule
    controlled behavior. *Journal of the Experimental Analysis of Behavior,* **46,** 137–47.

Hayes, S.C., Wilson, K.G., Gifford, E.V., Follette, V.M., and Strosahl, K. (1996).
    Experiential avoidance and behavioral disorders: A functional dimensional approach
    to diagnosis and treatment. *Journal of Consulting and Clinical Psychology,* **64,** 1152–68.

Hayes, S.C., Strosahl, K.D., and Wilson, K.G. (1999a). *Acceptance and Commitment
    Therapy: An Experiential Approach to Behavior Change.* New York, NY:
    The Guilford Press.

Hayes, S.C., Bissett, R.T., Korn, Z., Zettle, R.D., Cooper, L.D., and Grundt, A.M. (1999b).
    The impact of acceptance versus control rationales on pain tolerance.
    The Psychological Record, **49,** 33–47.

Hefferline, R.F., Keenan, B., and Harford, R.A. (1959). Escape and avoidance conditioning
    in human subjects without their observation of the response. *Science,* **130,** 1338–9.

Herrnstein, R.J. (1970). On the law of effect. *Journal of the Experimental Analysis
    of Behavior,* **13,** 243–66.

Hineline, P.N. (1973). Varied approaches to aversion: A review of Aversive Conditioning and Learning, edited by F. Robert Brush. *Journal of the Experimental Analysis of Behavior*, **19**, 531–40.

Jacobson, N.S., Dobson, K.S., Traux, P.A., Addis, M.E., Koerner, K., Gollan, J.K., Gortner, E., and Prince, S.E. (1996). A component analysis of cognitive behavior treatment for depression. *Journal of Consulting and Clinical Psychology*, **64**, 295–304.

Kohlenberg, R.J. and Tsai, M. (1991). *Functional Analytic Psychotherapy: Creating Intense and Curative Therapeutic Relationship*. New York, NY: Plenum Press.

Lang, P.J. (1977). Imagery in therapy: An information processing approach. *Behavior Therapy*, **8**, 862–86.

Larsen, D.K., Taylor, S., and Asmundson, G.J.G. (1997). Exploratory factor analysis of the Pain Anxiety Symptoms Scale in patients with chronic pain complaints. *Pain*, **69**, 27–34.

Lee, C. (1992). On cognitive theories and causation in human behavior. *Journal of Behavior Therapy and Experimental Psychiatry*, **23**, 257–68.

Lee, I., Tyrer, P., and Horn, S. (1983). A comparison of subliminal, supraliminal a faded phobic cine-films in the treatment of agoraphobia. *British Journal of Psychology*, **143**, 356–61.

Lethem, J., Slade, P.D., Troup, J.D.G., and Bentley, G. (1983). Outline of fear-avoidance model of exaggerated pain perception-I. *Behaviour Research and Therapy*, **21**, 401–8.

Linehan, M.M. (1993). *Cognitive Behavioral Treatment for Borderline Personality Disorder*. New York, NY: Guilford Press.

McCracken, L.M. (1997). "Attention" to pain in persons with chronic pain: A behavioral approach. *Behavior Therapy*, **28**, 271–84.

McCracken, L.M., Faber, S.D., and Janeck, A.S. (1998). Pain-related anxiety predicts non-specific physical complaints in persons with chronic pain. *Behaviour Research and Therapy*, **36**, 621–30.

McCracken, L.M., Gross, R.T., Aikens, J., and Carnrike, C.L.M. (1996). The assessment of anxixety and fear in persons with chronic pain: A comparison of instruments. *Behaviour Research and Therapy*, **34**, 927–33.

McCracken, L.M., Zayfert, C., and Gross, R.T. (1992). The pain anxiety symptoms scale: Development and validity of a scale to measure fear of pain. *Pain*, **50**, 67–73.

Mineka, S. and Ben Hamida, S. (1998). Observational and nonconscious learning. In W. O'Donohue (ed.), *Learning and Behavior Therapy*, pp. 421–39. Boston: Allyn and Bacon.

Mowrer, O.H. (1947). On the dual nature of learning: A reinterpretation of "conditioning" and "problem-solving." *Harvard Educational Review*, **17**, 102–48.

Newman, M.G., Hoffman, S.G., Trabert, W., Roth, W.T., and Taylor, C.B. (1994). Does treatment of social phobia lead to cognitive changes? *Behavior Therapy*, **25**, 503–17.

O'Donohue, W. (1998a). Conditioning and third-generation behavior therapy. In W. O'Donohue (ed.), *Learning and Behavior Therapy*, pp. 1–14. Boston: Allyn and Bacon.

O'Donohue, W. (1998b). *Learning and Behavior Therapy*. Boston: Allyn and Bacon.

Ohman, A. (1996). Preferential preattentive processing of threat in anxiety: Preparedness and attentional bias. In R. Rapee (ed.), *Current Controversies in the Anxiety Disorders*, pp. 253–90. New York, NY: Guilford Press.

Ost, L.G. (1985). Ways of acquiring phobias and outcome of behavioral treatments. *Behaviour Research and Therapy*, **23**, 683–9.

Ost, L.G. and Hugdahl, K. (1981). Acquisition of phobias and anxiety reponse patterns in clinical patients. *Behaviour Research and Therapy*, **19**, 439–47.

Pincus, T. and Morley, S. (2001). Cognitive-processing bias in chronic pain: A review and integration. *Psychological Bulletin*, **127**, 599–617.

Plaud, J.J. (1992). The prediction and control of behavior revisited: A review of the matching law. *Journal of Behavior Therapy and Experimental Psychiatry*, **23**, 25–31.

Rachman, S. (1977). The conditioning theory of fear-acquisition: A critical reappraisal. *Behavior Research and Therapy*, **15**, 375–87.

Reiss, S. (1987). Theoretical perspectives on the fear of anxiety. *Clinical Psychology Review*, **7**, 585–96.

Sharp, T.J. (2001). Chronic pain: A reformulation of the cognitive-behavioral model. *Behaviour Research and Therapy*, **39**, 787–800.

Shimnoff, E., Catania, C., and Matthews, B.A. (1981). Uninstructed human responding: Sensitivity to low-rate performance to schedule contingencies. *Journal of the Experimental Analysis of Behavior*, **36**, 207–20.

Sidman, M. and Tailby, W. (1982). Conditional discrimination versus matching to sample: An expansion of a testing paradigm. *Journal of the Experimental Analysis of Behavior*, **37**, 5–22.

Skinner, B.F. (1988). An operant analysis of problem solving. In A.C. Catania and S. Harnard (eds.), *The Selection of Behavior: The Operant Behaviorism of B.F. Skinner: Comments and Consequences*. New York, NY: Cambridge University Press.

Vlaeyen, J.W.S., de Jong, J., Geilen, M., Heuts, P.H.T.G., and van Breukelen, G. (2001). Graded exposure *in vivo* in the treatment of pain-related fear: A replicated single-case experimental design in four patients with chronic low back pain. *Behavior Research and Therapy*, **39**, 151–66.

Vlaeyen, J.W.S. and Linton, S.J. (2000). Fear-avoidance and its consequences in chronic musculoskeletal pain: A state of the art. *Pain*, **85**, 317–32.

Wegner, D.M., Schneider, D.J., Carter, S.R., and White, T.L. (1987). Paradoxical effects of thought suppression. *Journal of Personality and Social Psychology*, **53**, 5–13.

Wilson, K.G., Hayes, S.C., and Gifford, E.V. (1997). Cognitions in behavior therapy: Agreements and differences. *Journal of Behavior Therapy and Experimental Psychiatry*, **28**, 53–63.

Wolpe, J. (1981). The dichotomy between classically conditioned and cognitively learned anxiety. *Journal of Behavior Therapy and Experimental Psychiatry*, **12**, 35–42.

Wolpe, J. (1989). The derailment of behavior therapy: A tale of conceptual misdirection. *Journal of Behavior Therapy and Experimental Psychiatry*, **20**, 3–15.

Chapter 4

The role of hypervigilance in the experience of pain

Stefaan Van Damme, Geert Crombez,
Christopher Eccleston, and Jeffrey Roelofs

1 Introduction

The role of fear of pain in the experience of pain is well-documented in
research with clinical and healthy samples. An increased level of pain-related
fear is associated with more intense pain (McCracken *et al.* 1996), more avoidance of activity (Crombez *et al.* 1998*c*; Waddell 1998), and greater functional
impairments (McCracken *et al.* 1993; Crombez *et al.* 1999*b*). Several authors
have also argued that fear of pain induces a hypervigilance for pain or other
somatic sensations (Eccleston and Crombez 1999; Aldrich *et al.* 2000; Vlaeyen
and Linton 2000). Hypervigilance for pain, or overalertness for pain, has been
understood in different ways. In this chapter we examine the concept
of hypervigilance to pain in normal and clinical pain samples. We focus in
particular upon recent functional and evolutionary accounts of attention to
threatening information, and upon the different attentional components
involved. We argue that (1) hypervigilance to pain can be usefully understood
within a context of "normal" attentional processes to pain, that (2) attention
to pain is a particular instantiation of attention to threat, and that (3) several
components of attention may be related to hypervigilance to pain. However,
before addressing these issues, we trace the historical roots of the concept of
hypervigilance.

2 Hypervigilance for pain: Defining and assessing the construct

2.1 Defining the concept of hypervigilance

Hypervigilance refers to "a heightened vigilance." The term *vigilance* was introduced in experimental psychology by Mackworth (1950). It was defined as the
predisposition to attend to certain classes of events, or the readiness to select

and respond to a certain kind of stimulus from the external or internal environment. According to Mackworth, vigilance is a learned phenomenon in which previous experience determines the current perception of certain stimuli. However, it was also thought possible to induce vigilance by instructing participants to attend to a particular event. Early experiments investigated the extent to which participants were able to sustain attention to weak external signals (such as visual or auditive stimuli) in a monotonous situation. Vigilance tasks have been applied as part of theory development in a wide range of clinical and nonclinical domains, such as attention deficit hyperactive disorder (Hall and Kataria 1992), work stress (Scerbo 2001), sleep deprivation (Corsi *et al.* 1996), and the use of drugs and medication (Lieberman *et al.* 1998).

One of the first authors to apply the construct of (hyper)vigilance to somatic sensations and pain was Richard Chapman (1978). He referred to hypervigilance as a perceptual habit of scanning of the body for somatic sensations. Hypervigilance was thought to be an emergent property of the threat value of pain. People who appraise bodily sensation as dangerous were thought to be more likely to develop a habit of scanning the body for threatening sensations. Hypervigilance, defined as a continuous scanning, is similar to the view expressed by Watson and Pennebaker (1989). In their seminal paper, these authors explored diverse explanations for the robust relationship between the disposition to experience negative affect and low mood (negative affectivity, NA) on the one hand and somatic complaints on the other. Indeed, an impressive number of studies have revealed that NA is strongly associated with symptom reporting and a heightened self-report of all types of physical sensations and symptoms, even in the absence of differences in medical markers of disease. Watson and Pennebaker argued that this relationship is best explained by a hypervigilance to somatic information in persons with high levels of NA: "First, [individuals with] high NAs may be more likely to notice and attend to normal body sensations and minor aches and pains. Second, because their scanning is fraught with anxiety and uncertainty, [individuals with] high NAs may interpret normal symptoms as painful or pathological (Watson and Pennebaker 1989: 247)."

Hypervigilance has also been used to account for medically unexplained symptoms and complaints. Barsky and Klerman (1983) suggest that an amplifying perceptual style explains symptom reporting in hypochondriasis. According to them, bodily complaints are maintained and amplified because persons are overalert for somatic sensations. A similar idea of perceptual amplification has been introduced in fibromyalgia (e.g. McDermid *et al.* 1996). Rollman and Lautenbacher (1993) argued that patients with fibromyalgia—a medically unexplained syndrome characterized by whole body pain as the primary feature—show a generalized pattern of hypervigilance, characterized by an increased attention to a variety of external and internal noxious sensations and, in particular, pain. A similar perceptual style is assumed to explain the bodily symptoms in persons with the irritable bowel syndrome (Chang *et al.* 2000).

Hypervigilance has become a key theoretical and clinical construct in explaining high symptom reporting, especially in situations of medically unexplained or ambiguous sensations. We should, however, be careful in equating high symptom reporting with hypervigilance. Hypervigilance is only one explanation for high symptom reporting. Other explanations using central nervous processes are possible. It is also presumptuous to conclude that a low pain threshold, a low pain tolerance, and high pain sensitivity are sensitive and specific indicators of hypervigilance. It is useful to remind ourselves of the definitions of these variables as described by the International Association for the Study of Pain Task Force on Taxonomy (1994):

1. Pain threshold is the minimal intensity at which a certain stimulus becomes painful for a person.
2. Pain tolerance is the maximal intensity at which a painful sensation is bearable for a person.
3. Pain sensitivity is an increased response to a stimulus which is normally painful.

These variables are measured with a number of different pain procedures, such as cold-pressor (e.g. Janssen *et al.* 2001), heat stimulation (e.g. Lautenbacher *et al.* 1999), and pressure (e.g. Pauli *et al.* 1999). They are frequently used as indicators for hypervigilance for pain, but often it has not been established that attentional processes are critically involved.

Hypervigilance as a construct may only be inferred based upon diverse sources of information and, most importantly, when it is demonstrated that attentional processes are involved. As such, the assessment of hypervigilance is similar to the assessment of emotions (Öhman 1987). Multiple processes are involved and these can be assessed by several methods, including self-reports, psychophysiological measures, and behavioral (experimental) measures. We briefly review these methods.

2.2 Assessing (hyper)vigilance

2.2.1 Self-report measures

There are two types of self-report instruments of hypervigilance to somatic sensations. Some questionnaires assess the consequences of hypervigilance (i.e. to what extent persons are aware of particular bodily sensations)

(Pennebaker Inventory of Limbic Languidness (PILL), Pennebaker 1982; Modified Somatic Perceptions Questionnaire (MSPQ), Main 1983). It is apparent that this type of instrument may suffer from alternative interpretations. Also, one should be aware of potential confounding between the item content of these questionnaires and the diagnostic criteria of syndromes. For instance, the diagnostic criteria for fibromyalgia and chronic fatigue include multiple somatic complaints.

The second type of questionnaires assesses more directly the experience of heightened vigilance to somatic sensations (Body Consciousness Questionnaire (BCQ) Miller et al. 1981; Body Vigilance Scale (BVS) Schmidt et al. 1997; Pain Vigilance and Awareness Questionnaire (PVAQ) McCracken 1997). The PILL (Pennebaker 1982) is a frequency inventory of 54 physical symptoms and complaints (e.g. racing heart, chest pain, and indigestion). It has most often been used in nonclinical samples. The MSPQ (Main 1983) is a 22-item measure of the frequency and breadth of diffuse somatic complaints. The MSPQ was developed specifically and validated for use with chronic low back pain patients. The BCQ (Miller et al. 1981) is a 15-item measure of awareness of one's body. It contains the subscales "private body consciousness" (awareness of internal sensations) and "public body consciousness" (awareness of observable aspects of the body). Particularly interesting is the private body consciousness subscale, which consists of 5 items such as "I am sensitive to internal bodily tensions." This questionnaire is validated for nonclinical populations. The BVS (Schmidt et al. 1997) is a 4-item questionnaire assessing attentional focus to internal bodily sensations during the past week. An example of an item is "I am the kind of person who pays close attention to internal sensations." This questionnaire is validated for nonclinical samples and anxiety disorder patients. The PVAQ (McCracken 1997) assesses vigilance for pain sensations. It contains 16 items (e.g. "I am quick to notice changes in pain intensity") of which respondents are asked to indicate how frequently it was true for them during the past 2 weeks. This questionnaire is validated in a sample of chronic low back pain patients.

2.2.2 Psychophysiological measures

Another method to assess hypervigilance for pain is by the use of psychophysiological measures, in particular, the measurement of event-related potentials (ERP). It is widely recognized that changes in P300 (P3) amplitude are associated with selective attention (Muller-Gass and Campbell 2002), vigilance (Portin et al. 2000), and the allocation of attentional resources (Kok 2001). The P300 component in response to painful stimuli has been studied as a direct measure of attention to pain (Dowman 2001). It was found that P300 amplitude increased when pain stimuli were presented (Zaslansky et al. 1996b;

Becker *et al.* 2000). Furthermore, it was found that such pain-evoked potentials reflect the emotional component (fear) rather than the sensory component (pain intensity) associated with attention to pain (Zaslansky *et al.* 1996*a*). However, this P300 procedure requires an experimental control of discrete and short-lasting pain stimuli. In situations of chronic pain this is not possible. Therefore, other paradigms, such as the oddball-paradigm, have been applied to indirectly assess attention to pain.

In an oddball-paradigm, individuals are required to detect a rare deviant stimulus (e.g. high pitch tone) amongst a series of stimuli (e.g. low pitch tones). It is known that the detection of the deviant target stimulus elicits a P300 response. The amplitude of this P300 response is, however, moderated by background variables such as pain. More specifically, the experience of pain diminishes the P300 response to the deviant stimulus. It is reasoned that the experience of pain demands attentional resources that cannot be allocated to the detection of the deviant stimulus. In a study by Lorenz and Bromm (1997), pain-free volunteers performed an auditory oddball task during experimental pain of long duration and control conditions. They found that the P300 amplitude in response to the deviant stimulus decreased during pain. This indicates that the attentional demand of pain diminishes the amount of attention allocated to a concurrent cognitive task. Lorenz *et al.* (1997) used a similar oddball task in chronic pain patients. They found that the P300 amplitude from the auditory oddball task was enlarged in patients during morphine-induced analgesia, possibly indicating that performance on the oddball task improved due to the removal of pain.

2.2.3 Behavioral measures

A third approach to assess hypervigilance for pain involves the use of behavioral indicators of attention. This method is most often used in experimental paradigms in which the consequences of selecting pain upon the attentional system are investigated. Before elaborating the results of this approach, it is helpful to first discuss the normal attentional selection of pain-related information.

3 Understanding hypervigilance for pain requires an understanding of normal attention for pain

In understanding the concept of hypervigilance, it is important to consider normal attention to pain. In essence, hypervigilance can be viewed as a deviation from normal attention. There is a range of "normal" attentional theories including neuropsychological (e.g. Posner and Petersen 1990), structural (e.g. Kahneman and Treisman 1984), and functional views (e.g. Allport 1989). We focus upon a functional perspective because it allows a swift implementation of affective and behavioral issues, and an easy formulation of implications for clinical practice. Within cognitive psychology, Allport (1989) has provided one of the most detailed functional accounts of attention, working primarily through the example of visual attention. Accepting the basic axiom that attention is about the selection of information at the expense of other information, he discussed attention within the context of the need of the organism to behave in a purposeful and coherent way. He argued that an efficient attentional system must fulfill two apparently conflicting requirements—the need for continuity against the need for interruptibility of attentional engagement (Allport 1989). First, it is important that current behavior and attentional engagement are maintained and protected from less important demands during the course of activity. At the same time, in an environment that is unpredictable and potentially dangerous, it is necessary that this engagement or ongoing behavior can be interrupted by new, more important demands such as threat (Norman and Shallice 1986). An effective balance between both attentional requirements is necessary for survival: Failure to shift attentional engagement to environmental threats is hazardous and possibly fatal, whereas constant shifting to each environmental event results in chaotic behavior (Allport 1989). From this functional perspective, Allport argues that attention is a dynamic mechanism of selection for action.

Eccleston and Crombez (1999) have developed a cognitive–affective model of the interruptive function of pain. In line with the core ideas of Allport (1989), Eccleston and Crombez (1999) argued that pain imposes an overriding priority for attentional engagement by activating a primitive defensive system that urges escape from somatic threat. Pain is designed to interrupt attention, even in environments with multiple demands. It is a signal of danger that enables an organism to respond promptly to the perceived source of threat (Wall 1994). Eccleston and Crombez (1999) proposed that the interruptive function of pain is not mediated by its sensory characteristics, but by its affective characteristics, especially its threat value.

In order to experimentally investigate the variables that affect the "normal" interruptive function of pain, a primary-task paradigm was developed (Crombez et al. 1994). The rationale is that the selection of pain in favor of other demands will result in a decreased attention to other task demands. In this paradigm participants are asked to perform an attentionally demanding task (e.g. a detection task or a discrimination task). During the task, a painful stimulus is administered and participants are instructed to ignore it. The degradation of task performance during pain, in terms of speed and accuracy, is considered a measure of attentional disruption by pain. Interruption of attention may be facilitated due to pain characteristics as well as to environmental characteristics.

3.1 Pain characteristics

Several variables that amplify the attentional disruption by pain in healthy volunteers have been identified using this paradigm.

1. *Novelty.* In pain-free students, it was found that a painful heat stimulus of which none of the participants had prior experience produced large task interference. This task interference was more pronounced at the beginning of the pain stimulus compared with the end of the stimulus (Crombez *et al.* 1994, 1996, 1997).

2. *Threat value.* In a sample of undergraduate students, performing an auditory discrimination task while being repeatedly exposed to low-intensity electrocutaneous stimuli, it was found that participants who were threatened with the possibility that highly intense painful stimuli would also be applied, showed a larger disruption of task performance immediately after the onset of a low-intensity electrocutaneous stimulus, compared with participants who were not threatened with high-intensity pain stimuli (Crombez *et al.* 1998*a*).

3. *Catastrophic thinking about pain.* In a study with pain-free students that were threatened with high-intensity pain stimuli, it was found that disruption of the primary task by low-intensity pain stimuli was more pronounced in students with a high level of catastrophic thinking about pain, compared with participants low in catastrophic thinking about pain (Crombez *et al.* 1998*b*).

The above-mentioned studies have all relied on healthy individuals. As pain is designed to interrupt, it is reasonable to assume that high-intensity pain will also interrupt task performance in pain patients. Indeed, despite the fact that, in many situations of chronic pain, pain can be considered as a "false alarm," it cannot be switched off, and remains interruptive. In line with this idea, Eccleston (1994, 1995) found that, in samples of chronic pain patients, those patients with high-intensity pain showed significant decrements in the performance of a high demanding task compared with those with low-intensity pain and pain-free controls. Furthermore, there is preliminary evidence that in chronic pain situations the interruptive function of pain is mediated by its threat value. In a study by Crombez *et al.* (1999*a*) it was found that patients who are fearful about their intense pain show decrements in task performance.

3.2 Environmental characteristics

Another crucial feature of the cognitive–affective model of pain, as proposed by Eccleston and Crombez (1999), is that interruption of ongoing behavior by pain is considered as the selection of information *at the expense of other demands in the environment.* Attentional interruption by pain is always the result of a dynamic interaction between the characteristics of the painful event and the characteristics of the other demands of the environment. It is, therefore, also affected by the characteristics of other demands in the environment. It follows that pain will interrupt more in environments with fewer competing demands. In the context of symptom reporting this idea was introduced by Pennebaker (1982) as the principle of cue competition: Individuals are most likely to notice physical sensations when there is a lack of external cues to compete with internal cues. This may be particularly true in monotonous and unstimulating environments. Several studies have supported this hypothesis. Joggers run faster and are less fatigued in an interesting cross-country run in comparison with a repetitive running of laps (Pennebaker and Lightner 1980). Furthermore, in environments that lack stimulation, participants cough more (Pennebaker 1980), experience more extreme emotions (Pennebaker 1982), and are more aware of feelings of fatigue (Pennebaker and Brittingham 1982). However, little is known about how and when this principle applies to the more aversive experience of pain. Results concerning the mechanisms underlying distraction from pain are inconclusive (McCaul *et al.* 1992; Johnson *et al.* 1998). For example, Hadjistavropoulos *et al.* (2000) found that distraction only works for patients who are not anxious about their health. Leventhal (1992) proposed the emotional significance of other demands as the most important aspect of the environment. Evidence in support of this hypothesis has been inconclusive (Stevens *et al.* 1989).

In conclusion, pain is designed to demand attention and to interrupt ongoing behavior. Whether pain will interrupt is the result of both pain-related characteristics (i.e. intensity, novelty, catastrophizing about pain) and characteristics of other demands in the environment. According to Eccleston and Crombez (1999), the threat value of pain is the key mediating pain-related variable. From this perspective, it is difficult to draw a sharp delineation between vigilance and hypervigilance. Hypervigilance to pain seems not to result from an abnormal characteristic of the individual, such as NA. Available evidence suggests that hypervigilance emerges as the working of normal mechanisms in abnormal situations. Such situations are (1) the chronic presence of high-intensity pain, (2) monotonous environments or environments that lack external stimulation, and most importantly, (3) the high threat value of pain.

4 Attention to pain is a particular instantiation of attention to threatening information

The idea that threat demands attention has been well-documented in the anxiety literature. The phenomenon of selecting threatening information at the expense of other information is well-known and discussed as attentional bias to threat. From an evolutionary point of view, fear and pain share several characteristics. Fear facilitates the detection of danger in the environment and helps to respond promptly to the threat. These features are similar to the ones described above for pain. It is, therefore, reasonable to assume that pain is a particular instantiation of threatening information. In this section we explore the role of hypervigilance to threat in the fear and anxiety literature. We do this for two reasons. First, some theories about fear and anxiety have started to disentangle the different components of hypervigilance to threat. Second, sophisticated experimental paradigms have been developed to investigate attentional bias to threat. Both issues are relevant and have implications for a further discussion of hypervigilance to pain.

In several cognitive models of fear and anxiety, attentional bias to threat plays a critical role in the aetiology and maintenance of anxiety disorders (Eysenck 1992; Öhman 1993; Williams *et al.* 1988). Eysenck (1992) has provided one of the most elaborate accounts of the role of attention to threat in anxiety and fear. In his hypervigilance theory, Eysenck did not restrict hypervigilance to threat to an attentional scanning mechanism but suggested that it may become manifest in a variety of ways. Most importantly, these manifestations depend upon the temporal imminence of threat. The following example may clarify the different components of hypervigilance. Imagine a person, afraid of spiders, who has to retrieve a bottle of wine from the cellar. The thought of descending the cellar stairs will be sufficient to make him fearful. This thought may also make him distracted by several irrelevant stimuli in the environment (general hypervigilance). From the moment he descends the stairs, with the possibility of being confronted with a spider, he begins to scan the environment for the presence of spiders (broad attentional field and scanning). This will result in the rapid detection of a spider. Attention will be drawn automatically to the spider (specific hypervigilance), and once it is detected, the person will have serious difficulties disengaging attention from the spider and directing attention to other stimuli, such as the labels on the wine bottles (narrowing of attention).

One particular feature of the hypervigilance theory of Eysenck (1992) does not match with the cognitive–affective model of the interruptive function of pain (Eccleston and Crombez 1999). According to Eysenck, only persons with the stable disposition to experience anxiety (i.e. trait anxiety or NA) are vulnerable to hypervigilance for threat. In particular, in situations when state anxiety is high, hypervigilance emerges. Alternatively, persons scoring low on the disposition to experience anxiety would become avoidant and divert attention away from threat. The moderation of the effects of state anxiety by trait anxiety is, however, at odds with an evolutionary account of the functions of fear and anxiety. If threat is high and is reliably associated with danger, there is no survival advantage in ignoring threat, especially if the costs of vigilance are low. Even individuals low in trait anxiety should attend to stimuli with a high threat value. This comment has been more fully developed by Mogg and Bradley (1998). They suggest a nonlinear relationship between the level of threat and the attentional bias to threat. As long as the threat value is below a certain threshold, individuals will switch away from threat and continue to pursue their goals. When the threat value exceeds a threshold, an attentional bias to threat occurs. The moderation of the effects of state anxiety by trait anxiety can be explained by differences in threat appraisal. For persons with high trait anxiety, events and stimuli are appraised as more threatening. Although this hypothesis is highly plausible, it awaits empirical corroboration.

In conclusion, there are many similarities between the function of pain and the function of fear and anxiety upon the attentional system. Attention to pain can usefully be considered as one particular instantiation of attention to threat. Vigilance to threat is a dynamic process and consists of diverse components depending upon the imminence of threat, such as distractibility, selective attention, scanning, and difficulty disengaging. Scanning is only one possible attentional component of vigilance. In the fear and anxiety literature, more specific hypervigilance or attentional bias to threat is a common object of study. The same phenomenon with the same experimental paradigms has been investigated in patients with chronic pain. The results of this approach are reviewed in the next section.

5 Empirical evidence for attentional bias in chronic pain: Results from the modified Stroop task and the dot probe paradigm

Patients with almost all forms of emotional complaint (e.g. general anxiety disorder, phobia, obsessive–compulsive disorder, posttraumatic stress disorder, and depression) display an attentional bias to information that is specifically related to their emotional concerns (see Eysenck 1992; Williams *et al.* 1996 for a review). The modified Stroop paradigm and the dot probe paradigm are the most common experimental paradigms used in the investigation of attentional bias (Logan and Goetsch 1993). These paradigms have also been frequently applied in the area of pain (see Pincus and Morley 2001; Roelofs *et al.* 2002). We briefly summarize the results of the studies using the modified Stroop paradigm and the dot probe paradigm.

In a modified Stroop paradigm, categories of emotionally salient words and neutral words are presented in different colors. Response times to name the color of each word are measured. In an emotional variant of the paradigm, neutrally valent words are compared with emotionally valent words and the color-naming latency can be compared. Typically, color-naming is slowed when words are threatening and are relevant to the patients' concern. It is inferred that the emotional content of words interferes with color-naming these words. Instructing chronic pain patients to name the color of the print of pain-related words and neutral words should result in an interference effect that is larger for pain patients compared to healthy controls. Several studies have used the modified Stroop paradigm to investigate whether pain patients have an attentional bias to sensory or affective pain words (Pearce and Morley 1989; Boissevan 1994; Duckworth *et al.* 1997; Pincus *et al.* 1998; Crombez *et al.* 2000; Snider *et al.* 2000). Results of these studies only partially support the existence of an attentional bias to pain-related information in chronic pain patients. All studies using the modified Stroop paradigm are summarized in Table 4.1. Roelofs *et al.* (2002) conducted a meta-analysis on data from five Stroop studies of 101 chronic pain patients (i.e. Pearce and Morley 1989; Boissevain 1994; Pincus *et al.* 1998; Snider *et al.* 2000). Taken together, the meta-analysis indicated that chronic pain patients showed increased interference on both sensory and affective pain-related words compared to healthy controls.

Table 4.1 Studies using the modified Stroop task

Reference	Country	Research sample	N_r/N_c[a]	Attentional bias
Pearce and Morley (1989)	UK	Chronic pain patients	16/16	Sensory + affective pain words
Boissevan (1994)	Canada	Various types of pain patients	15/15	Sensory pain words
Duckworth et al. (1997)	USA	Chronic pain patients	10/10	No
Pincus et al. (1998), study A	UK	Chronic pain patients	20/20	No
Pincus et al. (1998), study B	UK	Chronic pain patients	17/17	No
Crombez et al. (2000)	Belgium	Chronic low back pain patients	25/0	Sensory pain words
Snider et al. (2000)	Canada	Chronic back/neck pain patients	33/33	Sensory + affective pain words

[a] N_r, number of participants in research sample; N_c, number of participants in control sample.

The second paradigm used to investigate information processing biases is the dot probe paradigm. Generally, in the dot probe paradigm, two words (an emotional word and a neutral word) appear on a screen simultaneously. Next, one of these two words is replaced by a small dot. Participants are instructed to react to this dot by indicating the location in which it appeared. In an emotional variant of the dot probe experiment, response times to the dot can be compared with attentional engagement with a preceding emotional or neutral word. A speeding up of detection time when the dot replaces the emotional word and a delay in detection time when it replaces the neutral word are indicative of selective attentional bias. In the case of chronic pain, detection time is expected to be faster when the dot replaces a pain word compared to a neutral word and this acceleration of detection time is expected to be larger in pain patients compared to healthy controls. Only one study has used the dot probe paradigm in chronic pain patients. Asmundson *et al.* (1997) found no evidence for an attentional bias to sensory and affective pain words. However, in two published studies (Keogh *et al.* 2001*a,b*) with nonclinical samples, an attentional bias was found in pain-free persons high in fear of pain or physical anxiety sensitivity. All studies using the dot probe paradigm are summarized in Table 4.2.

Empirical evidence for attentional bias in studies using a modified Stroop paradigm or a dot probe paradigm is weak. Some evidence suggests that pain-related fear and anxiety sensitivity are associated with attentional bias. Attentional bias, as measured with a modified Stroop task or a dot probe task, appears to represent a subtle phenomenon, which is difficult to replicate. Several issues need to be further addressed. First, modified Stroop tasks and dot probe tasks use words as pain stimuli. The use of words as valid and appropriate stimuli may be limited, as they are semantic representations of pain. In addition, the words used in these tasks should preferably match to the

Table 4.2 Studies using the dot probe paradigm

Reference	Country	Research sample	N_r/N_c[a]	Attentional bias
Asmundson *et al.* (1997)	Canada	Chronic pain patients	19/22	No
Keogh *et al.* (2001a)	UK	High fear of pain normals	18/17	Pain words
Keogh *et al.* (2001b)	UK	High physical anxiety normals	24/27	Physical threat words

[a] N_r, number of participants in research sample; N_c, number of participants in control sample.

current concerns of pain patients. Second, attentional biases have often been observed in emotional disorders. However, it has been shown that attentional bias can disappear when the phobic object or situation is in close temporal or physical proximity to patients (Matthews and Sebastian 1993). The presence of pain in patients who completed a modified Stroop task or a dot probe may have suppressed the attentional bias, and this may account for the inconsistent results. Third, pain researchers have neglected the heterogeneity amongst patients with chronic pain. In particular, in patients with high pain-related fear one should expect an attentional bias. As yet, almost no researchers have attempted to take into account the individual differences in the experience of chronic pain (Crombez *et al.* 2000).

In sum, both the modified Stroop paradigm and the dot probe paradigm have been frequently used to investigate attentional bias or specific hypervigilance to pain-related information. In sharp contrast to the findings in anxiety and fear, findings from both paradigms are subtle and difficult to replicate. Several methodological problems may explain these findings. One important challenge for future research is to capture the somatic threat within experimental paradigms. A disadvantage of both the modified Stroop paradigm and the dot probe paradigm is that threat is presented within the visual and not the somatosensory modality.

6 Hypervigilance to pain and pain signals: A diversity of attentional components

Evidence converges on the idea that hypervigilance to pain is not the result of an abnormal characteristic of the individual. Of most importance seems to be the threat-value of pain. Because the threat-value of pain is both biologically hardwired and culturally acquired, a sharp delineation between normal attention and hypervigilance to pain is not easy to make. Therefore, we propose not to focus upon the defining features of hypervigilance and normal attention, but to focus upon the contexts in which the diverse components of hypervigilance emerge, and upon the dynamic and functional interrelationships between these components.

To achieve this refocusing, we need new experimental paradigms that take into account the following three issues.

1. Hypervigilance to pain emerges in contexts with multiple demands. This requires experimental tasks in which pain is presented amongst other types of information, and in which attention towards or away from pain can be experimentally manipulated by task instructions. In this way, the involvement of attention in hypervigilance can be critically demonstrated.

2. Hypervigilance to pain consists of diverse attentional components: General hypervigilance or distractibility (tendency to attend to irrelevant and non-noxious somatic sensations), bodily scanning, specific hypervigilance or selective attention to threatening somatosensory sensations, broad attentional scanning in order to facilitate pain detection, and, finally, the narrowing of the attentional field in order to focus on pain.

3. Hypervigilance to pain requires information within the somatosensory modality.

Most often, paradigms (e.g. the dot probe paradigm) used to investigate visual or spatial attention have been adopted from anxiety and fear research. There is, however, a wealth of other paradigms beyond vision and spatial attention that can be adopted (Spence *et al.* 2001, 2002). An example of this approach is the body scanning paradigm (Peters *et al.* 2000). Patients suffering from fibromyalgia and pain-free volunteers were required to perform several tasks. One task was the detection of visual stimuli. A second task was the detection of somatosensory stimuli. In the first two phases, both tasks were performed separately. It was hypothesized that there would be no difference in the detection of the somatosensory stimuli between the patient and the control group. Indeed, it was reasoned that all participants were paying close attention to the somatosensory stimuli and to the visual stimuli. In a subsequent phase, both tasks were performed simultaneously. This phase was a critical test of the hypothesis that fibromyalgia patients are hypervigilant for somatosensory information. It was reasoned that the tendency to scan for somatic information would result in a faster detection of somatosensory information. However, there was no evidence for scanning and specific hypervigilance to somatosensory information in fibromyalgia patients. Of importance seemed to be the threat value of the somatosensory information. Independent of group, participants with pain-related fear were quicker to detect somatosensory information. This is in line with a recent questionnaire study which revealed that hypervigilance to pain is not a unique characteristic of fibromyalgia but, rather, is dependent upon the threat value of pain (Crombez *et al.* in press).

A similar approach was followed in a cueing paradigm (Van Damme *et al.* 2002). It is well-documented that the detection of targets is facilitated (retarded) when participants are (in)correctly cued for a target. Following this reasoning, Van Damme *et al.* (2002) cued the presence of an auditory target or a pain target (electrocutaneous stimulus) with a corresponding cue—the word *tone* or the word *pain*—in pain-free volunteers. It was reasoned that a valid cue would facilitate the detection of the target, and that an invalid cue (the word *tone* for a pain target) would slow down target detection. Of more importance was the hypothesis that participants would have fewer problems to respond to the pain target after the invalid tone cue. It was reasoned that the pain target would automatically draw attention, resulting in less problems to shift attention away from the invalid tone cue toward the pain target. Results were in line with this idea of a specific hypervigilance to pain.

It is reasonable to assume that hypervigilance to pain also extends to hypervigilance to signals of pain (Eccleston and Crombez 1999). Although early identification of pain will allow for efficient escape, successful avoidance of pain requires vigilance for reliable cues of impending pain. Attentional processes to signals of pain were also investigated in the cueing study of Van Damme *et al.* (2002). It was found that pain cues narrowed the attentional field, making it more difficult to attentionally disengage from these cues. This effect was more pronounced in person with high catastrophic thinking.

In sum, only recently have researchers begun to investigate hypervigilance as conceptualized in this chapter. However, a number of promising research paradigms have been introduced, capturing the different components of hypervigilance. Results of these recent studies suggest the following propositions: First, bodily scanning seems to be a characteristic of normal attention to somatic threat rather than a component of hypervigilance to pain. Second, there is evidence that hypervigilance for pain is associated with a narrowing of the attentional field and the difficulty to disengage attention from pain and shift toward other demands in the environment.

7 Conclusion

There is merit in the idea that attention to pain is a normal, evolutionary valuable process. However, when people become overalert for pain and for signals of impending pain, this may result in a persistent and dysfunctional disruption of attention and behavior. This overalertness, characterized as hypervigilance, will occur particularly in an environment poor in potential targets of sustained attentional engagement, and when somatic stimuli are perceived as being of high intensity. It was also found in recent research that hypervigilance is mediated by the threat value of pain, which may be affected by individual difference variables such as catastrophic thinking about pain and fear of pain. It appears that scanning of the body to threatening painful stimuli is not a component of hypervigilance for pain but, rather, a characteristic of normal, evolutionarily determined and valuable attention for pain. However, preliminary evidence suggests that hypervigilance is characterized by the fast shifting of attention to threatening painful stimuli, difficulties shifting attention away from pain once it is detected (attentional fixedness), and difficulty engaging with other important demands in the environment.

These findings have a number of important implications. First, hypervigilance for pain may be responsible for increased pain experience. It is possible that hypervigilance mediates the often observed relation between pain-related fear and experienced pain. Alternatively, it has also been argued that increased pain experience may lead to increased pain-related fear, resulting in hypervigilance for pain. Second, hypervigilance may be one mechanism by which fear of pain leads to avoidance. For patients with a high level of fear of pain, possible signals of impending pain, such as mild somatic sensations, may be very threatening. Because they expect that these signals will always result in high pain and disability, they will become fearful and overalert for these pain signals. As a result of this, they will avoid any movement they expect to result in pain. Third, hypervigilance will result in the more frequent report of symptoms. Fourth, as research shows that a high threat value of pain results in difficulty disengaging from pain and pain signals, cognitive interference will occur. For example, in a recent study by Kuhajda *et al.* (2002), it was found that headache adversely affected encoding and memory of words. Fifth, there is an important clinical implication: As hypervigilance seems to be mediated by the threat value of pain, distraction is probably not an effective treatment technique in patients with a high level of catastrophic thinking about pain. This was confirmed in the study by Hadjistavropoulos *et al.* (2000), who found that distraction was not effective in chronic pain patients with a high level of health anxiety. The clinical implications of an attentional model of pain-related fear processing deserve closer examination.

References

Aldrich, S., Eccleston, C., and Crombez, G. (2000). Worrying about chronic pain: Vigilance to threat and misdirected problem solving. *Behaviour Research and Therapy*, **38**, 457–70.

Allport, A. (1989). Visual attention. In: M.I. Posner (ed.), *Foundation of Cognitive Science*, pp. 631–82. Hillsdale, NJ: Erlbaum.

Asmundson, G.J.G., Kuperos, J., and Norton, G.R. (1997). Do patients with chronic pain selectively attend to pain-related information? Preliminary evidence for the mediating role of fear. *Pain*, **72**, 27–32.

Barsky, A.J. and Klerman, G.L. (1983). Overview: Hypochondriasis, bodily complaints, and somatic styles. *American Journal of Psychiatry*, **140**, 273–83.

Becker, D.E., Haley, D.W., Urena, V.M., and Yingling, C.D. (2000). Pain measurement with evoked potentials: Combination of subjective ratings, randomized intensities, and long interstimulus intervals produces a P300-like confound. *Pain*, **84**, 37–47.

Boissevain, M.D. (1994). *Information Processing in Chronic Pain: The Role of Depression.* Unpublished Thesis. University of Western Ontario, Canada.

Chang, L., Mayer, E.A., Johnson, T., Fitzgerald, L.Z., and Naliboff, B. (2000). Differences in somatic perception in female patients with irritable bowel syndrome with and without fibromyalgia. *Pain*, **84**, 297–307.

Chapman, C.R. (1978). Pain: The perception of noxious events. In R.A. Sternbach (ed.), *The Psychology of Pain*, pp. 169–202. New York: Raven Press.

Corsi, C.M., Arce, C.R., Lorenzo, I., and Guevara, M.A. (1996). Time course of reaction time and EEG while performing a vigilance task during total sleep deprivation. *Journal of Sleep Research and Sleep Medicine*, **19**, 563–9.

Crombez, G., Baeyens, F., and Eelen, P. (1994). Sensory and temporal information about impending pain: The influence of predictability on pain. *Behaviour Research and Therapy*, **32**, 611–22.

Crombez, G., Eccleston, C., Baeyens, F., and Eelen, P. (1996). The disruptive nature of pain: An experimental investigation. *Behaviour Research and Therapy*, **34**, 911–18.

Crombez, G., Eccleston, C., Baeyens, F., and Eelen, P. (1997). Habituation and the interference of pain with task performance. *Pain*, **70**, 149–54.

Crombez, G., Eccleston, C., Baeyens, F., and Eelen, P. (1998*a*). Attentional disruption is enhanced by the threat of pain. *Behaviour Research and Therapy*, **36**, 195–204.

Crombez, G., Eccleston, C., Baeyens, F., and Eelen, P. (1998*b*). When somatic information threatens, catastrophic thinking enhances attentional interference. *Pain*, **75**, 187–98.

Crombez, G., Vervaet, L., Lysens, R., Baeyens, F., and Eelen, P. (1998*c*). Avoidance and confrontation of painful, back-straining movements in chronic back pain patients. *Behaviour Modification*, **22**, 62–77.

Crombez, G., Eccleston, C., Baeyens, F., Van Houdenhove, B., and Van den Broeck, A. (1999*a*). Attention to chronic pain is dependent upon pain-related fear. *Journal of Psychosomatic Research*, **47**, 403–10.

Crombez, G., Vlaeyen, J.W.S., Heuts, P.H.T.G., and Lysens, R. (1999*b*). Pain-related fear is more disabling than pain itself: Evidence on the role of pain-related fear in chronic back pain disability. *Pain*, **80**, 329–39.

Crombez, G., Hermans, D., and Adriaensen, H. (2000). The emotional stroop task and chronic pain: What is threatening for chronic pain sufferers? *European Journal of Pain*, **4**, 37–44.

Crombez, G., Eccleston, C., Van den Broeck, A., Goubert, L., and Van Houdenhove, B. (in press). Hypervigilance to pain in fibromyalgia: The mediating role of pain intensity and catastrophic thinking about pain. *Clinical Journal of Pain*.

Dowman, R. (2001). Attentional set effects on spinal and supraspinal responses to pain. *Psychophysiology*, **38**, 451–64.

Duckworth, M.P., Iezzi, A., Adams, H.E., and Hale, D. (1997). Information processing in chronic pain disorder: A preliminary analysis. *Journal of Psychopathology and Behavioural Assessment*, **19**, 239–55.

Eccleston, C. (1994). Chronic pain and attention: A cognitive approach. *British Journal of Clinical Psychology*, **33**, 535–47.

Eccleston, C. (1995). The attentional control of pain: Methodological and theoretical concerns. *Pain*, **63**, 3–10.

Eccleston, C. and Crombez, G. (1999). Pain demands attention: A cognitive–affective model on the interruptive function of pain. *Psychological Bulletin*, **125**, 356–66.

Eysenck, M.W. (1992). *Anxiety: The Cognitive Perspective*, p. 195. Hillsdale, NJ: Lawrence Erlbaum Associates.

Hadjistavropoulos, H.D., Hadjistavropoulos, T., and Quine, A. (2000). Health anxiety moderates the effects of distraction versus attention to pain. *Behaviour Research and Therapy*, **38**, 425–38.

Hall, C.W., and Kataria, S. (1992). Effects of two treatment techniques on delay and vigilance tasks with attention deficit hyperactive disorder (ADHD) children. *Journal of psychology*, **126**, 17–25.

International Association for the Study of Pain Task Force on Taxonomy (1994). *Classification of Chronic Pain Syndromes and Definitions of Pain Terms*, 2nd edn. Seattle, WA: IASP Press.

Janssen, S.A., Spinhoven, P., and Brosschot, J.F. (2001). Experimentally induced anger, cardiovascular reactivity, and pain sensitivity. *Journal of Psychosomatic Research*, **51**, 479–85.

Johnson, M.H., Breakwell, G., Douglas, W., and Humphries, S. (1998). The effects of imagery and sensory detection distractors on different measures of pain: How does distraction works? *British Journal of Clinical Psychology*, **37**, 141–54.

Kahneman, D. and Treisman, A.M. (1984). Changing views of attention and automaticity. In R. Parasuraman and D.R. Davies (eds.), *Varieties of Attention*. New York, NY: Academic Press.

Keogh, E., Ellery, D., Hunt, C., and Hannent, I. (2001a). Selective attentional bias for pain-related stimuli amongst pain fearful individuals. *Pain*, **91**, 91–100.

Keogh, E., Dillon, C., Georgiou, G., and Hunt, C. (2001b). Selective attentional biases for physical-threat in physical anxiety sensitivity. *Journal of Anxiety Disorders*, **15**, 299–315.

Kok, A. (2001). On the utility of P3 amplitude as a measure of processing capacity. *Psychophysiology*, **38**, 557–77.

Kuhajda, M.C., Thorn, B.E., Klinger, M.R., and Rubin, N.J. (2002). The effect of headache pain on attention (encoding) and memory (recognition). *Pain*, **97**, 213–21.

Lautenbacher, S., Spernal, J., Schreiber, W., and Krieg, J.C. (1999). Relationship between clinical pain complaints and pain sensitivity in patients with depression and panic disorder. *Psychosomatic Medicine*, **61**, 822–7.

Leventhal, H. (1992). I know distraction works even though it doesn't. *Health Psychology*, **11**, 208–9.

Lieberman, H.R., Coffey, B., and Kobrick, J. (1998). A vigilance task sensitive to the effects of stimulants, hypnotics, and environmental stress: The Scanning Visual Vigilance Test. *Behaviour Research Methods, Instruments, and Computers*, **30**, 416–22.

Logan, A.C., and Goetsch, V.L. (1993). Attention to external threat cues in anxiety states. *Clinical Psychology Review*, **13**, 541–59.

Lorenz, J. and Bromm, B. (1997). Event-related potential correlates of interference between cognitive performance and tonic experimental pain. *Psychophysiology*, **34**, 436–45.

Lorenz, J., Beck, H., and Bromm, B. (1997). Cognitive performance, mood and experimental pain before and during morphine-induced analgesia in patients with chronic non-malignant pain. *Pain*, **73**, 369–75.

Mackworth, N.H. (1950). *Researches in the Measurement of Human Performance*. Medical Research Council Special Report Series, p. 268.

Main, C.J. (1983). The Modified Somatic Perception Questionnaire (MSPQ). *Journal of Psychosomatic Research*, **2**, 503–14.

Mathews, A. and Sebastian, S. (1993). Suppression of emotional Stroop effects by fear arousal. *Cognition and Emotion*, **7**, 517–30.

McCaul, K.D., Monson, N., and Maki, R.H. (1992). Does distraction reduce pain-produced distress among college students? *Health Psychology*, **11**, 210–17.

McCracken, L.M. (1997). "Attention" to pain in persons with chronic pain: A behavioral approach. *Behaviour Research and Therapy*, **28**, 271–84.

McCracken, L.M., Gross, R.T., Sorg, P.J., and Edmands, T.A. (1993). Prediction of pain in patients with chronic low back pain: Effects of inaccurate prediction and pain-related anxiety. *Behaviour Research and Therapy*, **31**, 647–52.

McCracken, L.M., Gross, R.T., Aikens, J., and Carnrike, C.L.M. Jr. (1996). The assessment of anxiety and fear in persons with chronic pain. *Behaviour Research and Therapy*, **34**, 927–33.

McDermid, A.J., Rollman, G.B., and McCain, G.A. (1996). Generalized hypervigilance in fibromyalgia: Evidence of perceptual amplification. *Pain*, **66**, 133–44.

Miller, L.C., Murphy, R., and Buss, A.H. (1981). Consciousness of body: Private and public. *Journal of Personality and Social Psychology*, **41**, 397–406.

Mogg, K., and Bradley, B.P. (1998). A cognitive-motivational analysis of anxiety. *Behaviour Research and Therapy*, **36**, 809–48.

Muller-Gass, A. and Campbell, K. (2002). Event-related potential measures of the inhibition of information processing: I. Selective attention in the waking state. *International Journal of Psychophysiology*, **46**, 177–95.

Norman, D.A. and Shallice, T. (1986). Attention to action: Willed and automatic control of behaviour. In R.J. Davidson, G.E. Schwarz, and D. Shapiro (eds.), *Consciousness and Self-regulation: Advances in Research and Theory*, Vol. 4, pp. 1–18. London: Plenum Press.

Öhman, A. (1987). The psychophysiology of emotion: An evolutionary-cognitive perspective. In P.K. Ackles, J.R. Jennings, and M.G.H. Coles (eds.), *Advances in Psychophysiology*, Vol. 2, pp. 79–127. Greenwich, CT: JAI Press.

Öhman, A. (1993). Fear and anxiety as emotional phenomena: Clinical phenomenology, evolutionary perspectives, and information processing mechanisms. In M. Lewis and J.M. Haviland (eds.), *Handbook of Emotions*. New York, NY: Guilford.

Pauli, P., Wiedemann, G., and Nickola, M. (1999). Pain sensitivity, cerebral laterality, and negative affect. *Pain*, **80**, 359–64.

Pearce, J. and Morley, S. (1989). An experimental investigation of the construct validity of the McGill Pain Questionnaire. *Pain*, **39**, 115–21.

Pennebaker, J.W. (1980). Perceptual and environmental determinants of coughing. *Basic and Applied Social Psychology*, **1**, 83–91.

Pennebaker, J.W. (1982). *The Psychology of Physical Symptoms*. New York, NY: Springer-Verlag.

Pennebaker, J.W. and Brittingham, G.L. (1982). Environmental and sensory cues affecting the perception of physical symptoms. In: A. Baum and J. Singer (eds.), *Advances in Environmental Psychology*, Vol. 4. Hillsdale, NJ: Erlbaum.

Pennebaker, J.W. and Lightner, J.M. (1980). Competition of internal and external information in an exercise setting. *Journal of Personality and Social Psychology*, **39**, 165–74.

Peters, M.L., Vlaeyen, J.W.S., and van Drunen (2000). Do fibromyalgia patients display hypervigilance for innocuous somatosensory stimuli? Application of a body scanning reaction time paradigm. *Pain*, **86**, 283–92.

Pincus, T. and Morley, S. (2001). Cognitive processing bias in chronic pain: A review and integration. *Psychological Bulletin*, **127**, 599–617.

Pincus, T., Fraser, L., and Pearce, S. (1998). Do chronic pain patients 'stroop' on pain stimuli? *British Journal of Psychology*, **37**, 49–58.

Portin, R., Kovala, T., Polo-Kantola, P., Revonsuo, A., Muller, K., and Matikainen, E. (2000). Does P3 reflect attentional or memory performances, or cognition more generally? *Scandinavian Journal of Psychology*, **41**, 31–40.

Posner, M.I. and Petersen, S.E. (1990). The attention system of the human brain. *Annual Review of Neuroscience*, **13**, 25–42.

Roelofs, J., Peters, M.L., and Vlaeyen, J.W.S. (2002). The modified Stroop paradigm as a measure of selective attention towards pain-related stimuli in chronic pain patients: A meta analysis. *European Journal of Pain*, **6**, 273–81.

Rollman, G.B. and Lautenbacher, S. (1993). Hypervigilance effects in fibromyalgia: Pain experience and pain perception. In H. Voeroy and H. Merskey (eds.), *Progress in Fibromyalgia and Myofascial Pain*, pp. 149–59. New York, NY: Elsevier Science Publishers BV.

Scerbo, M.W. (2001). Stress, workload, and boredom in vigilance: A problem and an answer. In P.A. Hancock and P.A. Desmond (eds.), *Stress, Workload, and Fatigue. Human Factors in Transportation*, pp. 267–78. Mahwah, NJ: Lawrence Erlbaum.

Schmidt, N.B., Lerew, D.R., and Trakowski, J.H. (1997). Body vigilance in panic disorder: Evaluating attention to bodily perturbations. *Journal of Consulting and Clinical Psychology*, **65**, 214–20.

Snider, B.S., Asmundson, G.J.G., and Wiese, K.C. (2000). Automatic and strategic processing of threat cues in patients with chronic pain: A modified stroop evaluation. *Clinical Journal of Pain*, **16**, 144–54.

Spence, C., Nicholls, M.E.R., and Driver, J. (2001). The cost of expecting events in the wrong sensory modality. *Perception and Psychophysics*, **63**, 330–6.

Spence, C., Bentley, D.E., Phillips, N., McGlone, F.P., and Jones, A.K.P. (2002). Selective attention to pain: A psychophysical investigation. *Experimental Brain Research*, **145**, 395–402.

Stevens, M.J., Heise, R.A., and Pfost, K.S. (1989). Consumption of attention versus affect elicited by cognitions in modifying acute pain. *Psychology Reports*, **64**, 284–6.

Van Damme, S., Crombez, G., and Eccleston, C. (2002). Retarded disengagement from pain cues: The effects of pain catastrophizing and pain expectancy. *Pain*, **100**, 111–18.

Vlaeyen, J.W.S. and Linton, S.J. (2000). Fear-avoidance and its consequences in chronic musculuskeletal pain: A state of the art. *Pain*, **85**, 317–32.

Waddell, G. (1998). *The Back Pain Revolution*. Edinburgh, London, New York, Philadelphia, Sydney, Toronto: Churchill Livingstone.

Wall, P.D. (1994). Introduction to the edition after this one. In P.D. Wall and R. Melzack (eds.), *The Textbook of Pain*, 3rd edn., pp. 1–7. Edinburgh: Churchill Livingstone.

Watson, D. and Pennebaker, J.W. (1989). Health complaints, stress, and distress: Exploring the central role of negative affectivity. *Psychological Review*, **96**, 234–54.

Williams, J.M.G., Mathews, A., and MacLeod, C. (1996). The emotional Stroop task and psychopathology. *Psychological Bulletin*, **120**, 3–24.

Williams, J.M.G., Watts, F.N., MacLeod, C., and Mathews, A. (1988). *Cognitive Psychology and Emotional Disorders*. Chichester: Wiley.

Zaslansky, R., Sprecher, E., Katz, Y., Rozenberg, B., Hemli, J.A., and Yarnitsky, D. (1996a). Pain-evoked potentials: What do they really measure? *Evoked Potentials—Electroencephalography and Clinical Neurophysiology*, **100**, 384–91.

Zaslansky, R., Sprecher, E., Tenke, C.E., Hemli, J.A., and Yarnitsky, D. (1996b). The P300 in pain evoked potentials. *Pain*, **66**, 39–49.

Chapter 5

Negative affectivity, catastrophizing, and anxiety sensitivity

Edmund Keogh and
Gordon J.G. Asmundson

1 Introduction

The role that emotions play in the perception and experience of pain is considered to be an important, though admittedly not well understood process (Riley and Robinson 1999; Price 1999, 2000; Rainville 2002). Research indicates that separate brain regions may control the sensory and emotional components of pain. For example, imaging studies suggest that the anterior association cortex plays an important role in affective pain (Rainville *et al.* 1997). Evidence is also emerging that indicates how cognitive and emotional factors influence descending control mechanisms of pain sensations (Millan 1999, 2002).

As is apparent from the chapters in this volume, fear of pain is acknowledged as being an important vulnerability factor in pain chronicity (see also Vlaeyen and Linton 2000). Alongside fear of pain, however, there have also been other anxiety- and fear-related constructs receiving attention. These include negative affectivity, catastrophizing, and anxiety sensitivity (see Chapter 9 for detailed reviews of measures associated with the latter two of these constructs). The primary objective of this chapter is to provide readers with a review of these other relevant emotional constructs, in both clinical and nonclinical pain groups, and consider how they relate to fear of pain. We shall also consider the potential relationship between these constructs, as well as address the moderating effect of gender. As will become clear, there are not only important differences between men and women in their experience of pain, but also in their emotional responses.

2 Conceptual framework

To begin we shall attempt to provide a conceptual overview of the potential relationship between negative affectivity, catastrophizing, anxiety sensitivity, and the fear of pain. However, this is not an easy task since these constructs are not generally considered together and there is potentially some overlap between them. We will, therefore, draw on recent work into the structure of personality (e.g. Watson and Clark 1992; Lilienfeld *et al.* 1993), which suggests these constructs should be considered as part of an interrelated hierarchy. The general higher-order construct of negative emotionality sits at the top of this hierarchy, whereas other more specific constructs such as anxiety sensitivity serve as specific lower-order factors (also see Taylor 1995). Figure 5.1 presents an adapted version of the hierarchical model outlined by Lilienfeld *et al.* (1993), with the addition of the pain-relevant constructs important to this chapter. Thus, anxiety sensitivity and injury sensitivity are conceptualized as second-order factors. We suggest also that pain catastrophizing and the fear of pain may act as first order factors that lie under the second order injury sensitivity

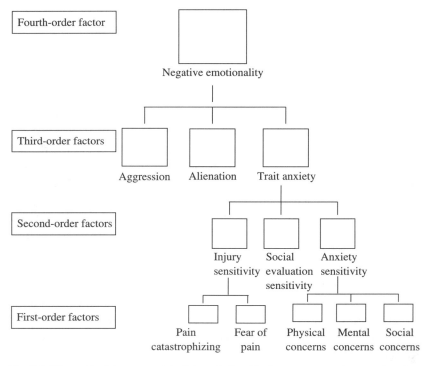

Fig. 5.1 Hierarchical factor model of the relationship between negative emotionality, and lower-order constructs. (Adapted with permission from *Advances in Behaviour research & Therpay,* **15**, S.O. Lilienfeld, R.G. Jacob, and S.M. Turner, "Anxiety sensitivity: An examination of theroetical and methodological issues," p. 172, Copyright (1993), with permission from Pergamon Press, Ltd.)

factor and may be expected to relate to more general fear of bodily (physical) sensations through the link between the second-order factors injury sensitivity and anxiety sensitivity. This view is, of course, entirely speculative at present. Nevertheless, we feel that this may be a good starting point to help readers conceptualize the potential interrelationship between these pain-relevant constructs. We will return to this model at the end of this chapter.

3 Negative affectivity

3.1 Definition

Negative affectivity is typically viewed as a general, stable, heritable trait-like tendency to experience a broad range of negative feelings such as worry, anxiety, self-criticisms, and a negative self-view (Clark and Watson 1991; Watson *et al.* 1988*a,b*; Mineka *et al.* 1998). It is related to a range of emotional disorders, the most commonly cited being the affective and anxiety disorders, and is used to explain the high correlation between measures of depression and anxiety (e.g. Watson *et al.* 1988*a*; Zinbarg and Barlow 1996; Spence 1997). Negative affectivity is often measured using the Positive and Negative Affect Schedule (PANAS; Watson *et al.* 1988*b*). However, it has been argued that measures such as the Spielberger State-Trait Anxiety Inventory (STAI; Spielberger *et al.* 1983) and the Beck Depression Inventory (BDI; Beck and Steer 1993) may also be considered as general measures of the construct (Foa and Foa 1982; Gotlib and Cane 1989; Watson and Kendall 1989). For the purposes of the current discussion, we shall include studies that use such general measures of anxiety and depression in our review.

3.2 Clinical pain studies

As is apparent to anyone involved in the management of pain, patients often report concurrent negative thoughts and feelings. Comprehensive reviews of the role of such negative emotions in pain patients have already been published and generally conclude that chronic pain is often associated with heightened levels of anxiety, depression, and anger (e.g. Banks and Kerns 1996; Robinson and Riley 1999; Keefe *et al.* 2001; Munafo and Stevenson 2001; Janssen 2002; Pincus *et al.* 2002). Numerous studies suggest that such negative moods are associated with a wide range of pain-related symptoms, including increased pain experiences (e.g., Taenzer *et al.* 1986; Geisser *et al.* 2000), disturbed physical functioning (e.g. Holzberg *et al.* 1996), stress-induced analgesia (e.g. de Bruin *et al.* 2001), disability (e.g. Dekker *et al.* 1993), post-surgical pain, and physical complaints both on ward and at home (e.g. de Groot *et al.* 1997; Kain *et al.* 2000), longer time to discharge and greater patient-controlled analgesia behaviors (Perry *et al.* 1994; Thomas *et al.* 1995).

A second observation is the link between gender differences in pain perception and gender differences in negative affectivity (Keogh 2001). The typical finding is that women report more negative pain-related experiences, different pain coping strategies, and different responses to analgesics when compared to men (e.g. Unruh 1996; Berkley and Holdcroft 1999; Ciccone and Holdcroft 1999; Fillingim and Ness 2000). It also seems as if there are important differences between men and women in emotional responses to stress (e.g. Leibenluft 1999). Given the link between stress, immunological functioning, and susceptibility to pain and illness (Kiecolt-Glaser *et al.* 2002*a,b*), it is very possible that gender differences in emotions play an important role in the relationship between negativity and pain experiences. However, there have been few attempts to directly assess gender differences in pain and emotion within the same study. For example, Edwards *et al.* (2000) examined gender differences in pain-related anxiety (measured using the Pain Anxiety Symptoms Scale (PASS); McCracken *et al.* 1992) and adjustment to chronic pain in patients referred to a multidisciplinary treatment center. They found that men high in pain-related anxiety reported greater pain severity, interference, and lower daily activity than males low in anxiety. No such effects were found amongst women. This finding is somewhat surprising given that females typically report more pain and more negative affectivity than men (Leibenluft 1999; Fillingim 2000).

With respect to the link between the fear of pain and negative affectivity, only a few studies have been conducted. However, of those that do exist it seems as if fear of pain measures may be strong predictors of chronicity. McCracken *et al.* (1992) found that the PASS explained additional variance in both pain-related interference and disability, once trait anxiety and depression had been controlled for. Burns *et al.* (2000) examined pain reports of 98 males with musckuloskeletal pain using the multidimensional pain inventory (MPI; Kerns *et al.* 1985), and found pain severity to be slightly more highly correlated with the PASS ($r = 0.31$) than the BDI ($r = 0.25$) and STAI-T ($r = 0.19$). Regression analysis revealed that fear of pain scores did *not* account for greater variance than general negative affectivity measures. However, these investigators also sought to predict behavioral measures of physical capacity (lifting and carrying), using regression analysis, entering BDI, STAI-T, and pain severity scores at step 1, and PASS scores at step 2. PASS scores were found to predict both variables even when controlling for trait anxiety, depression, and pain severity. Most recently, in a study involving 227 musculoskeletal injury patients seeking treatment at a physiotherapy clinic, Asmundson and Hadjistavropoulos (2001) found that the fearful appraisals subscale of the PASS, but not the STAI-T or Anxiety Sensitivity Index

(ASI; Reiss *et al.* 1986), explained unique variance in the prediction of avoidance behavior and functional limitations.

3.3 Experimental pain studies

One potential problem associated with investigating the role of negative affectivity in chronic pain patients is that it is often not possible to measure such emotions prior to the onset of the painful condition. It is, therefore, unclear whether the association between pain-related negativity and pain is present before the onset of pain. Has the painful condition increased negative affectivity? Or, was a tendency toward negative affectivity present prior to the onset of pain and, if so, does it act as a (possibility latent) vulnerability factor to negative pain behaviors? The use of experimental pain induction studies (Edens and Gil 1995) on healthy volunteers is one means of determining whether those high in negative affectivity are more sensitive to pain. Indeed, by experimentally controlling the type and amount of pain experienced, investigators can tease apart relationships between emotional factors and measures of pain sensitivity (e.g. pain threshold, pain tolerance).

Although only a few well-controlled studies of emotion and pain exist, the evidence suggests that manipulations of mood may influence experimentally manipulated pain experiences (for review and discussion see, Rhudy and Meagher 2001*b*). The general pattern of results is that negative moods increase pain sensitivity whereas positive moods have the opposite effect (e.g. Dougher *et al.* 1987; Cornwall and Donderi 1988; Zelman *et al.* 1991). For example, when Zelman *et al.* (1991) examined the effects of negative and positive mood inductions on cold pressor pain experiences, depressed mood reduced pain tolerance levels, whereas positive induction resulted in an increase.

Several recent studies have also shown that emotional priming has an influence on pain sensitivity. Meagher *et al.* (2001), for example, investigated the effect of pleasant and unpleasant pictures on pain when viewed just before a cold pressor pain task. A decrease in pain tolerance was found when viewing fear-related slides, whereas no change was observed when viewing relatively positive images. de Wied and Verbaten (2001) reported similar effects in that, when primed with pain-related images, participants exhibited reduced cold pressor pain tolerance levels. While the aforementioned findings are impressive, there are also studies that produce somewhat contradictory effects (e.g. al Absi and Rokke 1991; Rudy and Meagher 2000; Janssen *et al.* 2001), in that they report increases rather than decreases in pain sensitivity as a result of negative mood. Rhudy and Meagher (2000) have suggested that one possible reason for these differences may lie in the type of negative mood that is being examined. For example, they report a study in which they compared the effects of fear and anxiety on radiant heat pain thresholds. Fear, induced using expo-sure to brief shocks, was found to be associated with *decreased* pain responses. However, anxiety, induced by the threat of shock, was found to result in an *increase* in pain responsiveness. (The distinction between fear and anxiety is detailed in Chapter 1.)

Finally, there is evidence to suggest gender differences in the relationship between negative affectivity and pain (Jones and Zachariae 2002). Two recent studies have been reported, both of which may shed additional light on the mixed effects reported above. Rhudy and Meagher (2001*b*) investigated the effect of induced stress (loud noise) on hypoalgesic responses in men and women. Noise was, as expected, found to increase physiological and psycho-logical arousal levels. Noise also resulted in fear-related hypoalgesia in women, but not in men. Keogh and Witt (2001), using caffeine to induce changes in physiological and psychological arousal, have reported similar gender-dependent hypoalgesic effects. They found that caffeine increased arousal as well as pain threshold and tolerance levels. Interestingly, they also found gen-der differences. Women were not only found to report more caffeine-related decreases in composure (i.e. increased anxiety) than men, but also exhibited evidence for greater caffeine-related cardiovascular-hypoalgesia. This suggests that changes in arousal, and so possibly anxiety as well, may have differential effects for how men and women react to painful stimuli. Unfortunately, the few studies that directly compare fear of pain and general measures of nega-tive affectivity in healthy groups, mean that the relative role of fear and anxiety in experimentally induced pain is not yet clear.

3.4 Interim summary

Investigations into negative affectivity and pain collectively suggest that the two are closely related. It also seems that gender differences in negative affect-ivity and pain may be interrelated. Furthermore, evidence exists to suggest that the fear of pain may be an important determinant in the maintenance and possible development of negative pain experiences and pain-related behaviors in both acute and chronic pain patients. However, since few studies directly compare fear of pain and negative affectivity measures, it is unclear at present what the role of pain-related fear is in the pain experiences of other-wise healthy individuals. It is likely, however, that healthy individuals with a high fear of pain possess an important (and possibly) latent vulnerability fac-tor that predisposes them toward negative pain behaviors (Asmundson *et al.* 1999; Vlaeyen and Linton 2000). It is also possible that such susceptibility is more pronounced in women than men.

4 Catastrophizing

4.1 Definition

Interest into the concept of catastrophizing in the context of pain and pain-related coping strategies has also increased over the past few years (see Keefe *et al.* 2001; Sullivan *et al.* 2001). Catastrophizing is generally viewed as a negative cognitive process of exaggerated negative rumination and worry. It has both a cognitive and an affective component, and is thought to be an important negative coping strategy that is also related to how well patients recover from pain (see Boothby *et al.* 1999). Catastrophizing is often measured using the Pain Catastrophizing Scale (PCS; Sullivan *et al.* 1995) or the catastrophizing scale of the Coping Strategies Questionnaire (CSQ; Rosenstiel and Keefe 1983). The PCS comprises three subscales relating to rumination, magnification, and helplessness, whereas the CSQ comprises one global scale.

4.2 Clinical pain studies

Catastrophizing has been investigated in a wide range of different clinical settings. The basic finding is that catastrophizing is related to increased negative pain experiences (e.g. McCracken *et al.* 1992; Sullivan *et al.* 1995, 1998). For example, Sullivan *et al.* (1995; study three) found that when a clinical pain group experienced painful medical procedures (electrodiagnostic), catastrophizers were more likely to report greater pain and anxiety than non-catastrophizers. Similar relationships between catastrophizing and pain experiences have been reported in back pain (e.g. Turner *et al.* 2002), headaches (e.g. Ukestad and Wittrock 1996), dental treatment (e.g. Sullivan and Neish 1998, 1999), osteoarthritis (e.g. Keefe *et al.* 2000), and burn-related pains (e.g. Haythronthwaite *et al.* 2001). It also seems that catastrophizing is related to increased disability (e.g. Burton *et al.* 1995; Sullivan *et al.* 1998; Severeijns *et al.* 2001). For example, Severeijns *et al.* (2001) found that catastrophizing predicts pain intensity, disability, and distress, even when controlling for physical impairment. Finally, Geisser *et al.* (1994) found that catastrophizing mediates the relationship between depression and the emotional dimensions of pain, as measured by the affective component of the McGill Pain Questionnaire (Melzack 1975).

As with negative affectivity measures, there seem to be important gender differences in the tendency to catastrophize. Females seem to report a greater tendency to catastrophize than males. For example, Severeijns *et al.* (2001) found that in addition to catastrophizing, gender also predicted pain intensity in a group of mixed chronic pain patients. Osman *et al.* (2000) found that, amongst a pain outpatient group, women scored higher than men on the rumination scale of the PCS. Interestingly, Keefe *et al.* (2000) report a study on a group of osteoarthritis patients in which they not only found that women reported higher levels of pain and disability than men, but that the tendency to catastrophize mediated this relationship. This suggests that catastrophizing may not only act as an important psychological vulnerability factor in negative pain experiences, but may also help explain gender differences in pain perception.

With respect to the relationship between catastrophizing and fear of pain in chronic groups, only a few studies have been conducted to date (e.g. Vlaeyen *et al.* 1995). In the initial development of the PASS with pain patients attending a multidisciplinary pain management center, McCracken *et al.* (1992) reported strong correlations between the somatic, cognitive, and fearful appraisal subscales (all *r*'s around 0.67) and catastrophizing as measured on the CSQ. A smaller correlation was found with the PASS escape/avoidance subscale ($r = 0.42$). When McCracken and Gross (1993) investigated whether fear of pain was related to negative coping strategies amongst a chronic group predominantly made up of back pain patients, they found that the cognitive subscale was associated with less overall coping and that, of all the coping strategies, catastrophizing was related most strongly to PASS scores. Likewise, Vlaeyen *et al.* (1995) have reported that fear of movement and injury are related to catastrophizing and depression in chronic musculoskeletal pain patients, and Crombez *et al.* (1999) have reported that fear of pain and pain catastrophizing are more important in predicting disability than negative affectivity. Finally, Severeijns *et al.* (2001) found that catastrophizing predicted pain intensity, disability, and distress even when controlling for impairment.

In one of the few prospective investigations, Linton *et al.* (2000) examined the role of catastrophizing and fear-avoidance amongst a group of 415 adults (who were initially pain free) from the Middle-Sweden Back Pain Project. At 12-month follow-up, 19 percent reported developing pain around the spinal area. When Linton *et al.* (2000) investigated whether fear-avoidance and catastrophizing acted as risk factors in the spinal pain symptoms, fear-avoidance was found to have a two-fold increase in the risk of developing spinal pain if participants' fear-avoidance scores fell above the medium. For catastrophizing, however, a relatively weak risk was found. This pattern of results suggests that fear-avoidance rather than catastrophizing acts as a risk factor for spinal pain.

4.3 Nonclinical pain studies

There have also been attempts to investigate catastrophizing in the context of nonclinical settings. For example, in their original validation study of the PCS,

Sullivan *et al.* (1995; study two) compared non-clinical participants who were classified as either high or low in pain catastrophizing. Catastrophizers reported significantly more cold pressor pain than non-catastrophizers. They also reported more emotional distress. Similar results were reported by Sullivan *et al.* (1997) who looked at the effects of thought suppression on cold pressor pain reports. They found that both catastrophizing and thought suppression influenced reports of cold pressor pain.

Regarding gender differences in catastrophizing, similar patterns are found in non-clinical studies as reported for clinical groups (e.g. Sullivan *et al.* 1995; Osman *et al.* 1997, 2000, study one). In a student sample, Osman *et al.* (1997; study one and two) investigated gender differences in the PCS, and found that women reported more rumination, helplessness, and total catastrophizing scores than men. In a follow-up study in an adult community sample, these investigators found, as above, that women scored higher than men on the rumination and helplessness subscales as well as on the total PCS scale (Osman *et al.* 2000). Following administration of the cold pressor task to a group of healthy adults, Sullivan *et al.* (2000) found that catastrophizing mediated the differences between men and women in reported intensity and duration to cold pressor pain. While this adds weight to the argument that catastrophizing may help explain gender differences in pain perception, a study by Ellis and D'Eon (2002; study two) reports mixed findings. They examined the role of catastrophizing and gender on finger pressure pain sensitivity amongst undergraduates with and without regular monthly headaches. Results suggested that, while male and female catastrophizers did not differ in pain tolerance, the male non-catastrophizers tolerated pain for longer than females. Interestingly, for reported pain intensity at tolerance, men reported less pain than women and catastrophizers reported more pain than non-catastrophizers. Unfortunately, it is not reported whether there was a catastrophizing by gender interaction for pain severity at tolerance.

There also seems to be an association between catastrophizing and fear of pain in nonclinical groups. Sullivan *et al.* (1995; study 4) examined the relationship between PCS, trait anxiety, depression, and the fear of pain (measured using the Fear of Pain Questionnaire (FPQ); see McNeil and Rainwater 1998). As can be seen from Table 5.1, although catastrophizing was significantly correlated with depression ($r = 0.26$), trait anxiety ($r = 0.32$), and negative affect ($r = 0.32$), by far the largest correlation was found with the fear of pain ($r = 0.80$). Pain ratings were also taken during a cold pressor task. Only fear of pain and catastrophizing were significantly related to cold pressor pain ratings (FPQ = 0.37; PCS = 0.46), with regression analysis revealing that catastrophizing was the only significant predictor ($FPQ_{sr} = 0.01$; $PCS_{sr} = 0.29$).

Table 5.1 Correlations among individual differences measures

Scale	PCS	FPQ	NA	PA	STAI-T	BDI	Pain
PCS	—						
FPQ	0.80**	—					
NA	0.32*	0.33*	—				
PA	0.02	0.08	−0.08	—			
STAI-T	0.32	0.34**	0.73**	−0.42**	—		
BDI	0.26	0.27*	0.57**	−0.30*	0.72**	—	
Pain	0.46*	0.37**	0.11	−0.06	0.15	0.09	—

Note: $N = 60$; PCS = Pain Catastrophizing Scale; FPQ = Fear of Pain Questionnaire; NA = Negative Affectivity; PA = Positive Affectivity; STAI-T = State-Trait Anxiety Inventory; BDI = Beck Depression Inventory; Pain = Composite pain score computed by adding all three pain ratings. * $p < .05$. ** $p < .01$

Source: Reprinted from *Psychological Assessment, 7*, M.J.L. Sullivan, S.R. Bishop, and J. Pivik, "The pain catastrophizing scale: development and validation", p. 530, Copyright (1995), with permission from American Psychological Association.

While this suggests catastrophizing may be related to the fear of pain, Ellis and D'Eon (2002; study two) failed to find any significant FPQ differences between catastrophizers and non-catastrophizers. Group differences were, however, found with respect to state negative emotionality. This is surprising given that both studies made use of the FPQ.[1] Two studies have found evidence to suggest that catastrophizing may predispose individuals toward experiencing pain-related fear when threatened with intense pain (Eccleston, *et al.* 1998; Crombez *et al.* 2002). These same studies failed, however, to find that the effects of catastrophizing on attention to pain are mediated by negative affectivity. Together this suggests that it is currently unclear whether catastrophizing predisposes individuals toward pain fearfulness or vice versa.

4.4 Interim summary

In sum, catastrophizing is clearly associated with the fear of pain. Furthermore, it seems that catastrophizing may be an important mediator of gender differences in the perception and experience of both clinical and nonclinical pain states. However, it is unclear whether catastrophizing is a cause or a consequence of fear of pain. Unfortunately, given that few studies compare fear of pain and catastrophizing as predictors of pain experience in non-clinical groups, definite conclusions regarding their association cannot be made at this point in time. Future research that addresses the causal relationship between these variables is required.

[1] Sullivan *et al.* (1995) used the original FPQ, whereas Ellis and D'Eon (2002) used the revised FPQ-III.

5 **Anxiety sensitivity**

5.1 **Definition**

The final construct that we shall discuss in this chapter is anxiety sensitivity. Anxiety sensitivity is personality trait conceptualized as the fear of anxiety-related sensations (Reiss *et al.* 1986; Taylor 1999*a,b*). Those high in anxiety sensitivity are believed to be more likely to interpret sensations such as a rapidly beating heart, sweating, and memory loss as a sign of harm, whereas those low in anxiety sensitivity are more likely to interpret such sensations as being unpleasant, but not threatening. Anxiety sensitivity is most commonly measured using the ASI, from which three lower-order dimensions (relating to physical, social, and mental concerns) and one higher-order global fear dimension are determined (Zinbarg *et al.* 1997). While several expanded versions (i.e. having more items) of the ASI have been published (e.g. Taylor and Cox 1998), these are still in the early stages of development and they are yet to be used in studies of pain and pain populations.

Anxiety sensitivity is closely related to the emotional disorders, especially panic disorder, posttraumatic stress disorder (PTSD), and depression (e.g. Taylor *et al.* 1992). Furthermore, prospective studies suggest that anxiety sensitivity may actually predispose some individuals toward such disorders, even in the absence of a history of known psychopathology (e.g. Schmidt *et al.* 1997). Research is now emerging to suggest that anxiety sensitivity is not only related to the perception and experience of pain, but also related to the development of the fear of pain.

5.2 **Clinical pain studies**

Anxiety sensitivity is considered important in the experience of both acute and chronic pain (for reviews see Asmundson 1999; Asmundson *et al.* 1999*a*, 2001*b*). It has been related to a wide range of different pain-related conditions, including headaches, gastrointestinal disorder, lower-back pain, musculoskeletal pain, asthma, menstrual pain, and postpartum distress (e.g. Carr *et al.* 1994; Asmundson and Norton 1995; Sigmon *et al.* 1996; Asmundson *et al.* 1998*a,b*, 1999*b*; Plehn *et al.* 1998; Norton *et al.* 1999; Keogh *et al.* 2002; Greenberg and Burns 2003). The general pattern emerging from these studies is that patients high in anxiety sensitivity seem much more likely to report higher levels of pain and negative coping compared to patients low in anxiety sensitivity. For example, Asmundson and Norton (1995) found that lower back pain patients high in anxiety sensitivity were more likely to experience greater negative pain experiences (see also, Plehn *et al.* 1998). It has also been suggested that anxiety sensitivity should be associated with increased use of substances that have anxiety dampening effects, and so may also play a role in the development of analgesic use (McNally 1996). Confirming this hypothesis, Asmundson and Norton (1995) reported that patients with high anxiety sensitivity were far more likely to take analgesic medications than those with medium or low levels (71 versus 34 versus 25 percent, respectively). Asmundson and Taylor (1996) also found that the fear of pain, which was predicted from anxiety sensitivity, was associated with greater analgesic use in back pain patients. However, for patients with recurring headaches, Asmundson *et al.* (1999*b*, 2001*a*) failed to find convincing evidence that anxiety sensitivity is associated with increased analgesic use.

Research has also investigated the role of anxiety sensitivity in exacerbating psychopathological responses in both acute and chronic pain states (e.g. Asmundson *et al.* 1998*a,b*, 2000; Keogh *et al.* 2002; Greenberg and Burns 2003). For example, Asmundson *et al.* (1998*b*) report a study in which they investigated PTSD in pain patients with work-related injuries (e.g. strains, falls, crushes, lacerations). Whereas depression was related to the frequency of PTSD symptoms, anxiety sensitivity (as well as social fears and somatic attentional focus) was related to PTSD severity. More recently, Keogh *et al.* (2002) conducted a prospective study in which they found that antenatal levels of anxiety sensitivity measured at 36 weeks gestation predicted PTSD-type symptoms 2 weeks postpartum. This suggests that anxiety sensitivity may act as a predisposition factor in the development of psychopathological responses to painful events. Gender differences in the association between clinical pain states and anxiety sensitivity have yet to be conducted.

As well as being related to psychopathology, anxiety sensitivity is also related to the fear of pain (e.g. Asmundson and Taylor 1996; Asmundson *et al.* 1999*b*, 2000; Zvolensky *et al.* 2001). This is perhaps unsurprising given that both anxiety sensitivity and the fear of pain are related to the fear of bodily sensations, with the former being more general in nature. What is interesting, however, is that evidence suggests anxiety sensitivity may actually lead to the development of pain-related fear. Using structural equation modeling, Asmundson and Taylor (1996) found that the fear of pain was best predicted from anxiety sensitivity and pain severity. Fear of pain was then found to go on to predict negative coping behaviors such as avoidance and analgesic use (see Fig. 5.2). It is important to note that pain severity *did not predict negative coping behaviors, except indirectly through fear of pain*. Asmundson *et al.* (1999*b*) found that anxiety sensitivity, pain-related cognitive dysfunction, and sensory pain experiences predicted the fear of pain in a group of patients with recurring headaches. Finally, a study by Greenberg and Burns (2003) examined chronic musculoskeletal pain patients' cold pressor experiences, and found that anxiety sensitivity was a stronger predictor of pain responses than

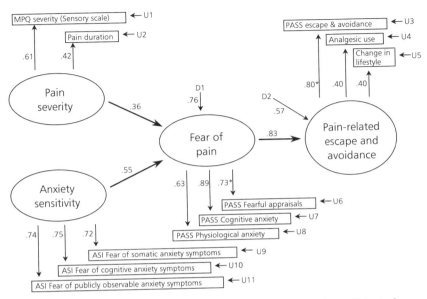

Fig. 5.2 Path diagram for final model showing standardized path coefficients for significant paths (all *P*'s < 0.001). Coefficients marked with an asterisk were fixed to identify the model. D = disturbance terms. U = uniqueness terms. (Reprinted from *Journal of Behavioral Medicine,* **19**, G.J.G. Asmundson and S. Taylor, "Role of Anxiety Sensitivity in Pain-Related Fear and Avoidance," p. 582, Copyright (1996), with permission from Plenum Publishing Corporation.)

pain anxiety (measured using the PASS). Although speculative, these latter results suggest that anxiety sensitivity *might* mediate the relationship between fear of pain and pain experience.

Together, these studies in clinical samples suggest that anxiety sensitivity may indeed act as a vulnerability factor in the development of pain-related fear, in much the same way as it acts as a susceptibility factor in the development of panic disorder and PTSD. It also seems as if anxiety sensitivity may be an important factor in the development of pain-related fear. Compelling evidence from non-clinical samples of children and adolescents, discussed below, supports this developmental vulnerability hypothesis.

5.3 Nonclinical pain studies

Convincing evidence for an association between anxiety sensitivity and pain are found in studies on healthy volunteers that use experimental pain induction procedures. Schmidt and Cook (1999) investigated the role of anxiety sensitivity on the pain responses of panic disorder patients when engaging in a cold pressor pain challenge. They found evidence to suggest that anxiety sensitivity mediated the relationship between diagnostic status (i.e. panic disorder or controls) and pain responses. Keogh and colleagues (Keogh and Birkby 1999; Keogh and Mansoor 2001; Keogh and Chaloner 2002; Keogh and Cochrane 2002) have also used the cold pressor task to investigate pain responses in non-clinical groups that vary in anxiety sensitivity. Keogh and Mansoor (2001) found that participants high in anxiety sensitivity reported more negative responses to self-reported sensory and affective pain (see Fig. 5.3). A similar pattern of results was reported by Keogh and Cochrane (2002), who found that anxiety sensitivity was negatively associated with pain thresholds. Finally, Keogh and Chaloner (2002) investigated the moderating role that anxiety sensitivity had on caffeine-induced hypoalgesia in healthy women. Caffeine (250 mg) was administered to women pre-selected as either high, medium, or low in anxiety sensitivity. Caffeine was used because, as well as having panicogenic properties, it is an analgesic adjuvant. Those low in anxiety sensitivity exhibited caffeine-induced improvement in negative mood (less depressed) and caffeine-related hypoalgesia, suggesting that the analgesic effects of caffeine may depend on anxiety sensitivity status.

With respect to gender differences in the relationship between anxiety sensitivity and pain, only one known study has been conducted to date. Keogh and Birkby (1999) investigated the role of anxiety sensitivity and gender on the perception of cold pressor pain, and found that although anxiety sensitivity

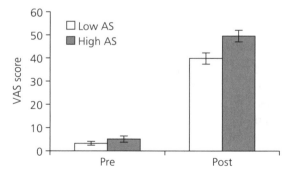

Fig. 5.3 The effect of coping instruction on visual analog pain scores before and after the cold pressor task. (Reprinted from *European Journal of Pain*, **5**, E. Keogh and L. Mansoor, "Investigating the effects of anxiety sensitivity and coping strategy on the perception of cold pressor pain in healthy women," p. 1363, Copyright (2001), with permission from European Federation of chapters of the International Association for the study of Pain.)

was associated with an increased vulnerability to painful events, it was moderated by gender. Specifically, women high in anxiety sensitivity were found to report higher sensory pain experiences to cold pressor pain than women low in anxiety sensitivity. No such effects were found for the more behavioral measures of pain tolerance and pain threshold. The fact that anxiety sensitivity was not related to pain experiences amongst men suggests that gender might be an important factor in the anxiety sensitivity–pain relationship. Additional research is required to clarify this issue.

There have also been a few studies that have investigated the link between anxiety sensitivity and the fear of pain in non-clinical groups. For example, McNeil and Rainwater (1998; study one) report that those high in fear of pain have higher anxiety sensitivity scores than those with a low fear of pain. Muris *et al.* (2001*a*) found that anxiety sensitivity was a better predictor of the fear of pain than trait anxiety amongst a group of children (see Table 5.2). Likewise, Muris *et al.* (2001*b*) found anxiety sensitivity to predict fear of pain amongst a group of adolescents. These investigators also found anxiety sensitivity to remain as a significant predictor of fear of pain when controlling for panic symptoms, trait anxiety, and panic disorder. Most recently, Keogh and Cochrane (2002) found, amongst healthy volunteers, a significant correlation between anxiety sensitivity and affective pain reports to cold pressor pain, even when controlling for fear of pain scores (partial $r = 0.20$). While a growing number of studies indicate that anxiety sensitivity is important in the fear of pain, there are still very few prospective studies that compare anxiety sensitivity and fear of pain, and so the direction of causation still remains unclear.

5.4 Interim summary

Taken together, investigations into the role of anxiety sensitivity and pain suggest, in both clinical and non-clinical pain groups, that the two are inter-related. Those high in anxiety sensitivity seem to be more likely to report greater negative pain experiences. Most important, it seems that anxiety sensitivity may be an important factor in the development of pain-related fear. That is, it may be a vulnerability factor that predisposes one to develop fear of pain and, in the context of certain situations, the development of chronic pain behavior. It is too early, however, to say whether this pain-related vulnerability is greater in women than men and whether it is heritable, learned, or both. It is also too early to say whether anxiety sensitivity is a stronger predictor of pain experiences than negative affectivity or catastrophizing. Again, the causal relationship between these interrelated constructs has yet to be adequately investigated.

Table 5.2 Correlations (corrected for gender and age) between anxiety sensitivity, trait anxiety, pain symptoms, somatization symptoms, and panic disorder symptoms, on the one hand, and fear of pain, on the other hand

	PASS scores				
	Total score	Somatic anxiety	Cognitive anxiety	Fear	Escape/ avoidance
CASI-R					
Total score	0.65	0.61	0.65	0.54	0.32
Fear of cardiovascular symptoms	0.59	0.55	0.51	0.53	0.36
Fear of publicly observable symptoms	0.39	0.39	0.43	0.31	0.15*
Fear of cognitive dyscontrol	0.54	0.49	0.58	0.42	0.26
Fear of respiratory symptoms	0.60	0.57	0.60	0.51	0.29
CSI					
Pain symptoms	0.40	0.44	0.40	0.31	0.14*
Other somatisation symptoms	0.50	0.50	0.49	0.42	0.21*
STATIC					
Trait anxiety	0.46	0.42	0.50	0.36	0.21*
RCADS					
Panic disorder symptoms	0.47	0.49	0.49	0.41	0.16*

Note: CASI-R, childhood anxiety index revised; PASS; CSI, children's somatization inventory; STAIC, state-trait anxiety inventory for children; RCADS, revised children's anxiety and depression scale; * $p < 0.05$, all other correlations were significant at $p < 0.05/45$, that is, Bonferroni correction.

Source: Reprinted from *Behaviour Research and Therapy*, **39**, P. Muris, J. Vlaeyen, and C. Meesters, "The relationship between anxiety sensitivity and fear of pain in healthy adolescents," p. 1363, Copyright (2001), with permission from Elsevier Science.

6 Conclusion

Evidence is now emerging to suggest that negative affect, catastrophizing, and anxiety sensitivity are all related to the fear of pain and fear-avoidance behaviors. Some of the evidence presented here suggests that anxiety sensitivity plays an important role in the development of pain-related fear and associated avoidance behavior. Other studies suggest that negative affectivity and catastrophizing also play a role in this regard. To date, few studies have incorporated measures of all of these constructs within a design that would allow evaluation of their relative and unique contributions to fear of pain and related negative coping behaviors. Further research is required to address this issue.

Research is also needed to determine the conceptual relationship between negative affectivity, catastrophizing, anxiety sensitivity, and related constructs such as injury sensitivity, and the association of each of these to fear of pain. This research might be rooted using a hierarchical model such as our modified depiction of the one proposed by Lilienfeld *et al.* (1993; see Fig. 5.1). For example, little research has considered injury sensitivity in this context. It would be of value to compare associations and predictive utility of the two second-order factors—anxiety sensitivity and injury sensitivity—relative to fear of pain and avoidance behavior and determine whether the fear of pain and catastrophizing about pain are indeed lower-order constructs specifically associated with injury sensitivity. Furthermore, some consideration as to the potential overlap of items in the measures used to examine these constructs would also seem necessary.

It also remains unclear how these constructs are causally related to the experience of pain. Unfortunately, no longitudinal studies have been conducted to examine the relative and unique roles of these constructs in the onset and maintenance of pain. Moreover, no treatment-outcome studies have investigated whether therapy-related changes in these constructs mediate changes in pain experiences. It is, therefore, currently difficult to speculate whether any one of these constructs should be recommended as a specific target for any intervention over the others. Additional research is needed to determine whether focusing on these constructs will produce clinically relevant changes, and if so, which ones are most beneficial.

What is also apparent from this review is that important differences may exist between men and women in the emotion–pain relationship. Further investigation is clearly required, directly investigating the potential interactive role gender and emotion have in moderating, and maybe mediating, fear-responses to pain. It is very possible that a different relationship exists between the various constructs reported for men and women. If so, then this may mean that we need to construct gender-specific psychotherapeutic treatments much in the same way as is currently being considered for pharmacological pain management interventions.

Evidence suggests that the constructs covered in this chapter are not only related in patients with acute and chronic pain conditions but also within otherwise healthy individuals. This suggests a shared vulnerability (also see Asmundson *et al.* 2002). If it is possible to understand the mechanisms that may predispose individuals toward fear-avoidance, we may be in a better position to develop interventions that combat such fears and anxieties at source, and even to 'inoculate' individuals against pathological states prior to the development of painful conditions.

Acknowledgments

Preparation of this article was supported, in part, by an operating grant and investigator award to the second author from the Canadian Institutes of Health Research (CIHR) and the Saskatchewan-CIHR Regional Partnerships Program.

References

al Absi, M. and Rokke, P.D. (1991). Can anxiety help us tolerate pain? *Pain*, **46**, 43–51.

Asmundson, G.J.G. (1999). Anxiety sensitivity and chronic pain: Empirical findings, clinical implications, and future directions. In S. Taylor (ed.), *Anxiety Sensitivity: Theory, Research and Treatment of the Fear of Anxiety*, London: Lawrence Erlbuam Associates.

Asmundson, G.J.G. and Hadjistavropoulos, H.D. (2001). Is anxiety sensitivity a better predictor of pain-specific fear, avoidance, and functional limitations than negative affectivity? *Pain Research and Management*, **6**(Suppl A), 19A.

Asmundson, G.J.G. and Norton, G.R. (1995). Anxiety sensitivity in patients with physically unexplained chronic back pain: A preliminary report. *Behaviour Research and Therapy*, **33**, 771–7.

Asmundson, G.J.G. and Taylor, S. (1996). Role of anxiety sensitivity in pain-related fear and avoidance. *Journal of Behavioural Medicine*, **19**, 577–86.

Asmundson, G.J.G., Frombach, I.K., and Hadjistavropoulos, H.D. (1998a) Anxiety sensitivity: Assessing factor structure and relationship to multidimensional aspects of pain in injured workers. *Journal of Occupational Rehabilitation*, **8**, 223–34.

Asmundson, G.J.G., Norton, G.R., Allerdings, M.D., Norton, P.J., and Larsen, D.K. (1998b). Posttraumatic stress disorder and work-related injury. *Journal of Psychosomatic Research*, **44**, 107–20.

Asmundson, G.J.G., Norton, P.J., and Norton, G.R. (1999a). Beyond pain: The role of fear and avoidance in chronically. *Clinical Psychology Review*, **19**, 97–119.

Asmundson, G.J.G., Norton, P.J., and Veloso, F. (1999b). Anxiety sensitivity and fear of pain in patients with recurring headaches. *Behaviour Research & Therapy*, **37**, 703–13.

Asmundson, G.J.G., Bonin, M.F., Frombach, I.K., and Norton, G.R. (2000). Evidence of a disposition toward fearfulness and vulnerability to posttraumatic stress in dysfunctional pain patients. *Behaviour Research and Therapy*, **38**, 801–12.

Asmundson, G.J.G., Wright, K.D., and Hadjistavropoulos, H.D. (2001b). Anxiety sensitivity and disabling chronic health conditions: State of the art and future directions. *Scandinavian Journal of Behaviour Therapy*, **29**, 100–17.

Asmundson, G.J.G., Wright, K.D., Norton, P.J., and Veloso, F. (2001*a*). Anxiety sensitivity and other emotionality traits in predicting headache medication use in patients with recurring headaches: Implications for abuse and dependency. *Addictive Behaviours*, **26**, 827–40.

Asmundson, G.J.G., Coons, M.J., Taylor, S., and Katz, J. (2002). Invited article (peer-reviewed). PTSD and the experience of pain: Research and clinical implications of shared vulnerability and mutual maintenance models. *Canadian Journal of Psychiatry*, **47**, 930–7.

Banks, S.M. and Kerns, R.D. (1996). Explaining high rates of depression in chronic pain: A diathesis–stress framework. *Psychological Bulletin*, **119**, 95–110.

Beck, A.T. and Steer, R.A. (1993). *Manual for the Revised Beck Depression Inventory*. San Antonio, TX: Psychological Corporation.

Berkley, K.J. and Holdcroft, A. (1999). Sex and gender differences in pain. In P. Wall and R. Melzack (eds), *Textbook of Pain*, 4th edn. London: Churchill Livingstone.

Boothby, J.L., Thorn, B.E., Stroud, M.W., and Jensen, M.P. (1999). Coping with pain. In R.J. Gatchel and D.C. Turk (eds.), *Psychosocial Factors in Pain*. Edinburgh: Guilford Press.

Burns, J.W., Mullen, J.T., Higdon, L.J., Mei Wei, J., and Lansky, D. (2000). Validity of the Pain Anxiety Symptoms Scale (PASS): Prediction of physical capacity variables. *Pain*, **84**, 247–52.

Burton, A.K., Tillotson, K.M., Main, C.J., and Hollis, S. (1995). Psychosocial predictors of outcome in acute and subchronic low back trouble. *Spine*, **20**, 722–8.

Carr, R.E., Lehrer, P.M., Rausch, R.L., and Hochron, S.M. (1994). Anxiety sensitivity and panic attacks in an asthmatic population. *Behaviour Research and Therapy*, **32**, 411–18.

Ciccone, G.K. and Holdcroft, A. (1999). Drugs and sex differences: A review of drugs relating to anaesthesia. *British Journal of Anaesthesia*, **82**, 255–65.

Clark, L.A. and Watson, D. (1991). Tripartite model of anxiety and depression: Psychometric evidence and taxonomic implications. *Journal of Abnormal Psychology*, **100**, 316–36.

Cornwall, A. and Donderi, D.C. (1988). The effect of experimentally induced anxiety on the experience of pressure pain. *Pain*, **35**, 105–13.

Crombez, G., Vlaeyen, J.W.S., Heuts, P.H., and Lysens, R. (1999). Pain-related fear is more disabling than pain itself: evidence on the role of pain-related fear in chronic back pain disability. *Pain*, **80**, 329–39.

Crombez, G., Eccleston, C., Van den Broeck, A., Van Houdenhove, B., and Goubert, L. (2002). The effects of catastrophic thinking about pain upon attentional interference by pain: No mediation of negative affectivity in healthy volunteers and in low back pain patients. *Pain, Research & Management*, 7, 31–9.

de Bruin, J.T., Schaefer, M.K., Krohne, H.W., and Dreyer, A. (2001). Preoperative anxiety, coping, and intraoperative adjustment: Are there mediating effects of stress-induced analgesia? *Psychology & Health*, **16**, 253–71.

de Groot, K.I., Boeke, S., van den Berge, J., Duivenvoorden, H.J., Bonke, B., and Passchier, J. (1997). The influence of psychological variables on postoperative anxiety and physical complaints in patients undergoing lumbar surgery. *Pain*, **69**, 19–25.

de Wied, M. and Verbaten, M.N. (2001). Affective pictures processing, attention, and pain tolerance, *Pain*, **90**, 163–72.

Dekker, J., Tola, P., Aufdemkampe, G., and Winckers, M. (1993). Negative affect, pain and disability in osteoarthritis patients: The mediating role of muscle weakness. *Behaviour Research and Therapy*, **31**, 203–6.

Dougher, M.J., Goldstein, D., and Leight, K.A. (1987). Induced anxiety and pain. *Journal of Anxiety Disorders*, **1**, 259–64.

Eccleston, C., Baeyens, F., and Eelen, P. (1998). When somatic information threatens, pain catastrophizing enhances attentional interference. *Pain*, **75**, 197–8.

Edens, J.L. and Gil, K.M. (1995). Experimental induction of pain: Utility in the study of clinical pain. *Behavior Therapy*, **26**, 197–216.

Edwards, R., Augustson, E.M., and Fillingim, R. (2000). Sex-specific effects of pain-related anxiety on adjustment to chronic pain. *Clinical Journal of Pain*, **16**, 46–53.

Ellis, J.A. and D'Eon, J.L. (2002). Pain, emotion, and the situational specificity of catastrophizing. *Cognition & Emotion*, **16**, 519–32.

Fillingim, R.B. (ed). (2000). Sex, gender and pain. *Progress in Pain Research and Management*, Vol. 17. Seattle, WA: IASP.

Fillingim, R.B. and Ness, T.J. (2000). Sex-related hormonal influences on pain and analgesic responses. *Neuroscience & Biobehavioural Reviews*, **24**, 485–501.

Foa, E.B. and Foa, U.G. (1982). Differentiating depression and anxiety: Is it possible? Is it useful? *Psychopharmacological Bulletin*, **18**, 62–8.

Geisser, M.E., Robinson, M.E., Keefe, F.J., and Weiner, M.L. (1994). Catastrophizing, depression and the sensory, affective and evaluative aspects of chronic pain. *Pain*, **59**, 79–83.

Geisser, M.E., Roth, R.S., Theisen, M.E., Robinson, M.E., and Riley, J.L. (2000). Negative affect, self-report of depressive symptoms, and clinical depression: relation to the experience of chronic pain. *Clinical Journal of Pain*, **16**, 110–20.

Gotlib, I.H. and Cane, D.B. (1989). Self-report assessment of depression and anxiety. In P.C. Kendall and D. Watson (eds.), *Anxiety and Depression: Distinctive and Overlapping Features*. London: Academic Press.

Greenberg, J. and Burns, J.W. (2003). Pain anxiety among chronic pain patients: Specific phobia or manifestation of anxiety sensitivity? *Behaviour Research and Therapy*, **41**, 223–40.

Haythronthwaite, J.A., Lawrence, J.W., and Fauerbach, J.A. (2001). Brief cognitive interventions for burn pain. *Annals of Behaviour Medicine*, **23**, 42–9.

Holzberg, A.D., Robinson, M.E., Geisser, M.E., and Gremillion, H.A. (1996). The effects of depression and chronic pain on psychosocial and physical functioning. *Clinical Journal of Pain*, **12**, 118–25.

Janssen, S.A. (2002). Negative affect and sensitization to pain. *Scandinavian Journal of Psychology*, **43**, 131–7.

Janssen, S.A., Spinhoven, P., and Brosschot, J.F. (2001). Experimentally induced anger, cardiovascular reactivity, and pain sensitivity. *Journal of Psychosomatic Research*, **51**, 479–85.

Jones, A. and Zachariae, R. (2002). Gender, anxiety, and experimental pain sensitivity: An overview. *Journal of the American Medical Women's Association*, **57**, 91–4.

Kain, Z.N., Sevarino, F., Alexander, G.M., Pincus, S., and Mayes, L.C. (2000). Preoperative anxiety and postoperative pain in women undergoing hysterectomy—A repeated-measures design. *Journal of Psychosomatic Research*, **49**, 417–22.

Keefe, F.J., Lefebvre, J.C., Egert, J.R., Affleck, G., Sullivan, M.J., and Caldwell, D.S. (2000). The relationship of gender to pain, pain behavior, and disability in osteoarthritis patients: The role of catastrophizing. *Pain*, **87**, 325–34.

Keefe, F.J., Lumley, M., Anderson, T., Lynch, T., Studts, J.L., and Carson, K.L. (2001). Pain and emotion: New research directions. *Journal of Clinical Psychology*, **57**, 587–607.

Keogh, E. (2001). Psychology, gender and pain. *Newsletter of the International Association for the Study of Pain Special Interest Group on Sex, Gender and Pain*, **3**, 3–5.

Keogh, E. and Birkby, J. (1999). The effect of anxiety sensitivity and gender on the experience of pain. *Cognition & Emotion*, **13**, 813–29.

Keogh, E. and Chaloner, N. (2002). The moderating effect of anxiety sensitivity on caffeine-induced hypoalgesia in healthy women. *Psychopharmacology*, **164**, 429–31.

Keogh, E. and Cochrane, M. (2002). Anxiety sensitivity, cognitive biases and the experience of pain. *The Journal of Pain*, **3**, 320–9.

Keogh, E. and Mansoor, L. (2001). Investigating the effects of anxiety sensitivity and coping strategy on the perception of cold pressor pain in healthy women. *European Journal of Pain*, **5**, 11–25.

Keogh, E. and Witt, G. (2001). Hypoalgesic effect of caffeine in normotensive men and women. *Psychophysiology*, **38**(6), 866–95.

Keogh, E., Ayers, S., and Francis, H. (2002). Does anxiety sensitivity predict post-traumatic stress symptoms following childbirth? A preliminary report. *Cognitive Behaviour Therapy*, **31**, 155–65.

Kerns, R.D., Turk, D.C., and Rudy, T.E. (1985). The West Haven-Yale Multidimensional Pain Inventory (WHYMPI). *Pain*, **23**, 345–56.

Kiecolt-Glaser, J.K., McGuire, L., Robles, T.F., and Glaser, R. (2002*a*). Emotions, morbidity, and mortality: New perspectives from psychoneuroimmunology. *Annual Review of Psychology*, **53**, 83–107.

Kiecolt-Glaser, J.K., McGuire, L., Robles, T.F., and Glaser, R. (2002*b*). Psychoneuroimmunology: Psychological influences on immune function and health. *Journal of Consulting & Clinical Psychology*, **70**, 537–47.

Leibenluft, E. (ed.) (1999). *Gender Differences in Mood and Anxiety Disorders: From Bench to Bedside*. Washington, DC: American Psychiatric Press.

Lilienfeld, S.O., Turner, S.M., and Jacob, R.G. (1993). Anxiety sensitivity: An examination of theoretical and methodological issues. *Advances in Behaviour Research and Therapy*, **15**, 147–83.

Linton, S.J., Buer, N., Vlaeyen, J., and Hellsing, A. (2000). Are fear-avoidance beliefs related to the inception of an episode of back pain? A prospective study. *Psychology & Health*, **14**, 1051–9.

McCracken, L.M. and Gross, R.T. (1993). Does anxiety affect coping with chronic pain? *Clinical Journal of Pain*, **9**, 253–9.

McCracken, L.M., Zayfert, C., and Gross, R.T. (1992). The Pain Anxiety Symptoms Scale: Development and validation of a scale to measure fear of pain. *Pain*, **50**, 67–73.

McNally, R.J. (1996). Anxiety sensitivity is distinguishable from trait anxiety. In R.M. Rapee (ed.), *Current Controversies in the Anxiety Disorders*. London: Guildford Press.

McNeil, D.W. and Rainwater, A.J. (1998). Development of the Fear of Pain Questionnaire—III. *Journal of Behaviour Medicine*, **21**, 389–410.

Meagher, M.W., Arnau, R.C., and Rhudy, J.L. (2001). Pain and emotion: Effects of affective picture modulation. *Psychosomatic Medicine*, **63**, 79–90.

Melzack, R. (1975). The McGill Pain Questionnaire: Major properties and scoring methods. *Pain*, **1**, 277–9.

Millan, M.J. (1999). The induction of pain: An integrative review. *Progress in Neurobiology*, **57**, 1–164.

Millan, M.J. (2002). Descending control of pain. *Progress in Neurobiology*, **66**, 355–474.

Mineka, S., Watson, D., and Clark, L.A. (1998). Comorbidity of anxiety and unipolar mood disorders. *Annual Review of Psychology*, **49**, 377–412.

Munafo, M.R. and Stevenson, J. (2001). Anxiety and surgical recovery. Reinterpreting the literature. *Journal of Psychosomatic Research*, **51**, 589–96.

Muris, P., Vlaeyen, J.W.S., Meesters, C., and Vertongen, S. (2001*a*). Anxiety sensitivity and fear of pain in children. *Perceptual Motor Skills*, **92**, 456–8.

Muris, P., Vlaeyen, J., and Meesters, C. (2001*b*). The relationship between anxiety sensitivity and fear of pain in healthy adolescents, *Behaviour Research and Therapy*, **39**, 1357–68.

Norton, G.R., Norton, P.J., Asmundson, G.J.G., Thompson, L.A., and Larsen, D.K. (1999). Neurotic butterflies in my stomach: The role of anxiety, anxiety sensitivity and depression in functional gastrointestinal disorders. *Behaviour Research Therapy*, **47**, 233–40.

Osman, A., Barrios, F.X., Gutierrez, P.M., Kopper, B.A., Merrifield, T., and Grittmann, L. (2000). The Pain Catastrophizing Scale: Further psychometric evaluation with adult samples. *Journal of Behavioural Medicine*, **23**, 351–65.

Osman, A., Barrios, F. X., Kopper, B. A., Hauptmann, W., Jones, J., and O'Neill, E. (1997). Factor structure, reliability, and validity of the Pain Catastrophizing Scale. *Journal of Behavioral Medicine*, **20**, 589–605.

Perry, F., Parker, R.K., White, P.F., and Clifford, P.A. (1994). Role of psychological factors in postoperative pain control and recovery with patient-controlled analgesia. *Clinical Journal of Pain*, **10**, 57–63.

Plehn, K., Peterson, R.A., and Williams, D.A. (1998). Anxiety sensitivity: Its relationship to functional status in patients with chronic pain. *Journal of Occupational Rehabilitation*, **8**, 213–22.

Pincus, T., Burton, A.K., Vogel, S., and Field, A.P. (2002). A systematic review of psychological factors as predictors of chronicity/disability in prospective cohorts of low back pain. *Spine*, **27**, E109–E120.

Price, D.D. (1999). *Psychological Mechanisms of Pain and Analgesia*. Edited by IASP Press. Seattle, WA: IASP Press.

Price, D.D. (2000). Psychological and neural mechanisms of the affective dimension of pain. *Science*, **288**, 1769–72.

Rainville, P. (2002). Brain mechanisms of pain affect and pain modulation. *Current Opinions in Neurobiology*, **12**, 195–204.

Rainville, P., Duncan, G.H., Price, D.D., Carrier, B., and Bushnell, M.C. (1997). Pain affect encoded in human anterior cingulate but not somatosensory cortex. *Science*, **277**, 968–71.

Reiss, S., Peterson, R.A., Gursky, D.M., and McNally, R.J. (1986). Anxiety sensitivity, anxiety frequency and the prediction of fearfulness. *Behaviour Research and Therapy*, **24**, 1–8.

Rhudy, J.L. and Meagher, M.W. (2000). Fear and anxiety: Divergent effects on human pain thresholds *Pain*, **84**, 65–75.

Rhudy, J.L. and Meagher, M.W. (2001*a*). Noise stress and human pain thresholds: Divergent effects in men and women. *The Journal of Pain*, **2**, 57–64.

Rhudy, J.L. and Meagher, M.W. (2001*b*). The role of emotion in pain modulation. *Current Opinion in Psychiatry*, **14**, 241–5.

Riley, M.E. and Robinson, J.L. (1999). The role of emotion in pain. In R.J. Gatchel and D.C. Turk (eds.), *Psychosocial Factors in Pain: Critical Perspectives*. London: Guildford.

Robinson, M.E., Riley, J.L., and Myers, C.D. (2000). Psychosocial contributions to sex-related differences in pain responses. In R.B. Fillingim (ed.), *Sex, Gender, and Pain. Progress in Pain Research and Management*, Vol. 17. Seattle, WA: IASP Press.

Rosenstiel, A.K. and Keefe, F.J. (1983). The use of coping strategies in chronic low back pain patients: Relationship to patient characteristics and current adjustment. *Pain*, **17**, 33–44.

Schmidt, N.B. and Cook, B.H. (1999). Effects of anxiety sensitivity on anxiety and pain during a cold pressor challenge in patients with panic disorder. *Behaviour Research and Therapy*, **37**, 313–23.

Schmidt, N.B., Lerew, D.R., and Jackson, R.J. (1997). The role of anxiety sensitivity in the pathogenesis of panic: Prospective evaluation of spontaneous panic attacks during acute stress. *Journal of Abnormal Psychology*, **106**, 355–64.

Severeijns, R., Vlaeyen, J.W.S., van den Hout, M.A., and Weber, W.E. (2001). Pain catastrophizing predicts pain intensity, disability, and psychological distress independent of the level of physical impairment. *Clinical Journal of Pain*, **17**, 165–72.

Sigmon, S.T., Fink, C.M., Rohan, K.J., and Hotovy, L.A. (1996). Anxiety sensitivity and menstrual cycle reactivity: Psychophysiological and self-report differences. *Journal of Anxiety Disorders*, **10**, 393–410.

Spence, S.H. (1997). Structure of anxiety symptoms among children: A confirmatory factor-analytic study. *Journal of Abnormal Psychology*, **106**, 280–97.

Spielberger, C.D., Gorsuch, R.L., Lushene, R., Vagg, P.R., and Jacobs, G.A. (1983). *Manual for the State-trait Anxiety Inventory (Form Y)*. Palo Alto, CA: Consulting Psychologists Press.

Sullivan, M.J. and Neish, N. (1998). Catastrophizing, anxiety and pain during dental hygiene treatment. *Community Dentistry & Oral Epidemiology*, **26**, 344–9.

Sullivan, M.J. and Neish, N. (1999). The effects of disclosure on pain during dental hygiene treatment: the moderating role of catastrophizing. *Pain*, **79**, 155–63.

Sullivan, M.J.L., Bishop, S.R., and Pivik, J. (1995). The Pain Catastrophizing Scale: Development and validation. *Psychological Assessment*, **7**, 524–32.

Sullivan, M.J.L., Rouse, D., Bishop, S., and Johnston, S. (1997). Thought suppression, catastrophizing, and pain. *Cognitive Therapy & Research*, **21**, 555–68.

Sullivan, M.J., Stanish, W., Waite, H., Sullivan, M., and Tripp, D.A. (1998). Catastrophizing, pain, and disability in patients with soft-tissue injuries. *Pain*, **77**, 253–60.

Sullivan, M.J.L., Tripp, D.A., and Santor, D. (2000). Gender differences in pain and pain behaviour: The role of catastrophizing. *Cognitive Therapy & Research*, **24**, 121–34.

Sullivan, M.J., Thorn, B., Haythornthwaite, J.A., Keefe, F., Martin, M., Bradley, L.A., and Lefebvre J.C. (2001). Theoretical perspectives on the relation between catastrophizing and pain. *Clinical Journal of Pain*, **17**, 52–64.

Taenzer, P., Melzack, R., and Jeans, M.E. (1986). Influence of psychological factors on postoperative pain, mood and analgesic requirements. *Pain*, **24**, 331–42.

Taylor, S. (1995). Anxiety sensitivity: Theoretical perspectives and recent findings. *Behaviour Research and Therapy*, **33**, 243–58.

Taylor, S. (1999*a*). Anxiety sensitivity: Theoretical perspectives and recent findings. *Behaviour Research and Therapy*, **33**, 243–58.

Taylor, S. (1999*b*). *Anxiety Sensitivity: Theory, Research and Treatment of the Fear of Anxiety*. London: Lawrence Erlbuam Associates.

Taylor, S. and Cox, B.J. (1998). An expanded Anxiety Sensitivity Index: Evidence for a hierarchic structure in a clinical sample. *Journal of Anxiety Disorders*, **12**, 463–84.

Taylor, S., Koch, W.J., and McNally, R.J. (1992). How does anxiety sensitivity vary across the anxiety disorders? *Journal of Anxiety Disorders*, **6**, 249–59.

Thomas, V., Heath, M., Rose, D., and Flory, P. (1995). Psychological characteristics and the effectiveness of patient-controlled analgesia. *British Journal of Anaesthesia*, **74**, 271–6.

Turner, J.A., Jensen, M.P., Warms, C.A., and Cardenas, D.D. (2002). Catastrophizing is associated with pain intensity, psychological distress, and pain-related disability among individuals with chronic pain after spinal cord injury. *Pain*, **98**, 127–34.

Ukestad, L.K. and Wittrock, D.A. (1996). Pain perception and coping in female tension headache sufferers and headache-free controls. *Health Psychology*, **15**, 65–8.

Unruh, A.M. (1996). Gender variations in clinical pain experience. *Pain*, **65**, 123–67.

Vlaeyen, J.W.S. and Linton, S.J. (2000). Fear-avoidance and its consequences in chronic musculoskeletal pain: A state of the art. *Pain*, **85**, 317–32.

Vlaeyen, J.W.S., Kole-Snijders, A.M., Boeren, R.G., and van Eek, H. (1995). Fear of movement/(re)injury in chronic low back pain and its relation to behavioral performance. *Pain*, **62**, 363–72.

Watson, D. and Clark, L.A. (1992). Affects separable and inseparable: On the hierarchical arrangement of the negative affects. *Journal of Personality & Social Psychology*, **62**, 489–505.

Watson, D. and Kendall, P.C. (1989). Understanding anxiety and depression: Their relation to negative and positive affective states. In P.C. Kendall and D. Watson (eds.), *Anxiety and Depression: Distinctive and Overlapping Features*. London: Academic Press.

Watson, D., Clark, L.A., and Carey, G. (1988*a*). Positive and negative affectivity and their relation to anxiety and depressive disorders. *Journal of Abnormal Psychology*, **97**, 346–53.

Watson, D., Clark, L.A., and Tellegen, A. (1988*b*). Development and validation of the brief measures of positive and negative affect: The PANAS scales. *Journal of Personality and Social Psychology*, **54**, 1063–70.

Zelman, D.C., Howland, E.W., Nichols, S.N., and Cleeland, C.S. (1991). The effects of induced mood on laboratory pain. *Pain*, **46**, 105–11.

Zinbarg, R.E. and Barlow, D.H. (1996). Structure of anxiety and the anxiety disorders: A hierarchical model. *Journal of Abnormal Psychology*, **105**, 181–93.

Zinbarg, R.E., Barlow, D.H., and Brown, T.A. (1997). Hierarchical structure and general factor saturation of the anxiety sensitivity index: Evidence and implications. *Psychological Assessment*, **9**, 277–84.

Zvolensky, M.J., Goodie, J.L., McNeil, D.W., Sperry, J.A., and Sorrell, J.T. (2001). Anxiety sensitivity in the prediction of pain-related fear and anxiety in a heterogeneous chronic pain population. *Behaviour Research and Therapy*, **39**, 683–96.

Chapter 6

Attitudes toward physical activity: The role of implicit versus explicit associations

Els L.M. Gheldof, Peter J. de Jong,
Jan Vinck, and Ruud M.A. Houben

1 Introduction

There is growing evidence that attitudes and beliefs play an important role in the etiology, chronification, and treatment outcomes of chronic low back pain. In this context, negative attitudes and beliefs toward daily and work-related physical activity have been studied extensively, validating cognitive–behavioral models explaining how exaggerated fear of pain/movement/injury may lead to avoidance of activities, disability, and depression (Vlaeyen and Linton 2000; see also Chapter 1).

Despite advances in our understanding of the role of fear/avoidance beliefs, a number of issues remain unsolved. Why, for instance, do some back pain patients tend to persist in avoiding (certain) activities, while knowing that immobility is harmful? In the same line, it is unclear why some clinicians, in contrast to what they know to be the right advice, and in contrast to what they explicitly proclaim, implicitly and subtly induce (or reinforce) activity-avoiding attitudes in their communication with low back pain patients. It is generally known that immobility (in the long run) is not helpful in back pain, and especially among physicians, it should be expected that they advise *against* immobility, although we know the opposite is often true (e.g. Goubert *et al.* 2003; also see Chapter 12).

In this chapter, we will explore the possibility that such "illogical" behavior (of both patients and clinicians) may be explained by the coexistence of incongruent explicit and implicit attitudinal components. Attitudes which are consciously expressed and endorsed are defined as *explicit attitudes* (Bohner and Wänke 2002), whereas attitudes of which the individual is not necessarily aware of (nor of their influence on his or her behavior) are referred to as *implicit attitudes* (de Houwer 2002). Measures believed to indirectly grasp on these rather automatic attitudes are called *indirect measures*. We will highlight some of these new paradigms, focusing on the complexities of attitudes and on differences between implicit and explicit measurement techniques, and will discuss consequences and future directions of this novel research area for the study of pain-related fear.

2 **Background**

Generally, attitudes are defined as "evaluative beliefs," usually thought of as comprising a cognitive, an affective, and a behavioral component (Ajzen 1988). It is widely accepted that attitudes are learned, have an evaluative character, include a readiness to respond toward the attitude object, have a motivating or driving force (toward behavior), and a relatively enduring nature (Oskamp 1977). Whenever an attitude is activated, it will trigger a process of selective perception and will serve as a filter that biases the individual's immediate perception of the situation, its information processing, and the definition of the event in the immediate situation (Fazio 1986). The attitude-construct is most often situated in the tradition of social psychology (Bohner and Wänke 2002). Largely comparable concepts, like "schemata," or "beliefs" stem from different, more clinical traditions (Teachman *et al.* 2001).

Recent advances in theorizing about attitudes show that they are complex. These complexities may help resolve the questions phrased before in the introduction. Indeed, it has become clear that attitudes, at times, might be arranged in a hierarchical order, in that more specific attitudes might be inferred from more general attitudes (Bohner and Wänke 2002). Further, people sometimes experience some degree of ambivalence toward a certain attitude object, so that attitudinal dimensions may be evaluatively inconsistent, in that one dimension may be rather positive and the other one rather negative. Accordingly, depending on situational cues or motivational state (being responsible for attitudinal selectivity in processing and recall), one may zoom in on a different aspect of the attitudinal object. Although it is clear that other attitudes, such as self-reliance (Tait and Chibnall 1998) or self-efficacy (Asghari and Nicholas 2001) play a role in low back pain, we will focus on fear-related attitudes and beliefs.

Before further exploring current understanding of the role of these attitudes and beliefs, we briefly look at what is known about the origin of these attitudes. As for attitudes in general, fear/avoidance beliefs may result from direct (painful) experiences (Goubert *et al.* 2003), from role models, education, or cultural factors (Waddell 1998), and from conflicting medical recommendations. More specifically, it appears that immobility and recuperative quiescence are primitive and "natural" responses to harm and pain (Keay *et al.* 2000; Morgan and Carrive 2001), by which the tendency to avoid movement as a response to pain or injury may be viewed as rather "instinctive." This may, then, easily become part of cultural attitudes that are reinforced by immediate pain relief and by social models. In the rest of this chapter, we try to provide an overview of recent evidence on some gains and gaps in our understanding and measurement of pain-related fear.

3 Deliberative reasoning versus spontaneity of day-to-day decisions

According to the theory of reasoned action (Ajzen and Fishbein 1980), the rational act of weighing salient costs and benefits of behavioral alternatives along with relevant normative guidelines, are believed to guide our behavior through the formation of behavioral intentions. Central to this and similar models is rationality as a determinant of behavior (Bodur *et al.* 2000). However, behavior is often guided by habitual and spontaneous evaluations of the environment (De Houwer 2003*b*), emotions (e.g. anticipated regret), personal norms, and influence of past behavior (Sabini 1995; Ajzen 2001) rather than by deliberative reasoning (Jacoby and Kelley 1990; Brug *et al.* 2000). In an effort to understand how attitudes can guide behavior beyond rationality, Fazio (1986) proposes implicit attitudes as object-evaluation associations (i.e. an association between a given attitude object and a given evaluation) which can be activated by the attitude object in a fully automatic fashion, facilitating smooth, relatively effortless functioning (Fazio 1990).

When people are motivated to make a "correct" decision (e.g. when they are concerned about being evaluated on the basis of their attitude or attitude-related behavior), and meanwhile have the opportunity (e.g. sufficient time) to weigh the available knowledge and the possible consequences of expressing an attitude, they are more likely to behave on the basis of their explicit attitude (i.e. conscious and deliberative reasoning) (see Fazio 1990). Conversely, in situations where people lack motivation or opportunity to monitor their attitude or behavior, knowledge and normative prescriptions are less likely to be activated, and they will spontaneously rely on their implicit "default" attitude, which enables them to evaluate choice alternatives, make a decision, and perform a behavior in a rather quick fashion (Sanbonmatsu and Fazio 1990). Under time constraints (e.g. physicians) and/or acute pain or emotions, implicit attitudes may be expected to rule behavior. In the context of health problems, this implies that under certain conditions the implicit dimension of attitudes may predominantly guide behavior. These implicit attitudes may be dysfunctional and may therefore (1) obstruct healthy behaviors, (2) prevent one from seeking treatment when symptoms occur, or (3) reduce therapy adherence once a disease is diagnosed (Sarafino 1998).

3.1 Indirect measures or self-reports: Some disadvantages

It might be clear by now that the type of measure we use to index individuals' attitudes is a crucial factor in the ability to predict behavior from attitudes (Sherman *et al.* 2003). Thus far, most studies on pain-related fear have relied on self-report measures. These include the Tampa Scale of Kinesiophobia (TSK; Kori *et al.* 1990), Pain Catastrophizing Scale (PCS; Sullivan *et al.* 1995), Pain Anxiety Symptoms Scale (PASS; McCracken *et al.* 1992), and Fear-Avoidance Beliefs Questionnaire (FABQ; Waddell *et al.* 1993). These instruments are described in detail in Chapter 9. They have proven to be very fruitful— empirically as well as clinically—in furthering our understanding of pain behavior and disability. However, it has been documented that answers on self-reports may be distorted by demand characteristics (de Jong 2002; Greenwald *et al.* 2002), attributional bias (Nisbett and Wilson 1977), contextual cues or normative guidelines (Fazio 1986), or by the assumed triggering of unintentional "reactivity" (Fazio *et al.* 1995). Moreover, evidence suggests that people may have little ability to report accurately about their cognitive processes (or about the influence of environmental stimuli on their responses). Instead, when people are asked to report how a specific stimulus influenced a specific response, they most often rely on *a priori* theories about the presumed causal relation between that particular type of stimulus on that type of response (Nisbett and Wilson 1977). Especially in the context of pain behavior and pain treatment, it might be the case that patients have generated an *a priori* theory about the causes and consequences of their pain, which most probably will reveal itself in the results of self-reports. Finally, the value of self-report attitude measures is limited in that they tell only part of the story due to the fact that the pertinent cognitions are simply not amenable to introspection, while, per definition, they give no information about implicit attitudes. Clearly, the assessment of pain-related attitudes and beliefs may benefit from indirect non-reactive measures, tapping attitude layers that may be inaccessible to conscious deliberation (Crosby *et al.* 1980; Banaji and Greenwald 1994; Fazio *et al.* 1995; Greenwald and Banaji 1995).

3.2 Indirect measures provide differential or additional predictive power

Indirect attitude measures are thought to bypass some of the well-known drawbacks of self-report measures. However, unlike some researchers proposing indirect measures as the ultimate method to disclose "one's true attitude" (Fazio *et al.* 1986), free from measurement bias or contextual and motivational factors, we assume direct and indirect measures both to be valid estimates of a person's evaluation (attitude) or cognition (belief), but reflecting different components of the attitude response (de Jong *et al.* 2001; Wiers *et al.* 2002). Germane to this, it has been argued that self-report measures are better predictors of strategic behavior (when social pressure is high, or when people have time and motivation to weigh pro's and con's), whereas indirect measures are better predictors of spontaneous or automatic behaviors (e.g. affective or physiological responses) over which individuals have little control (de Jong *et al.* 2001). Sustaining the idea that implicit and explicit measures may have differential predictive power, implicit self-esteem was found to be a better predictor of nonverbal anxiety (during a self-relevant interview), whereas explicit self-esteem had superior predictive power with respect to self-handicapping about the interview and individuals' own ratings of their anxiety (Spalding and Hardin 1999). Similarily, Asendorpf *et al.* (2002) recently demonstrated how an implicit measure of shyness (i.e. IAT, see below) was the superior predictor of subtle shy behaviors, whereas an explicit measure of shyness better predicted controllable shy behaviors. Relatedly, a recent study on fear-relevant associations in spider (non)fearful individuals demonstrated that self-reports were better predictors of avoidance behavior, as measured by a Behavioral Approach Test and implicit attitude estimates specifically predicted the automatic fear reaction (Huijding *et al.* submitted-*b*).

Following this, measures of implicit and explicit attitudes might also have differential predictive power in the context of back pain. That is, acts of avoidance or confrontation performed by back pain patients may be differently predicted on the basis of their implicit and explicit attitudes. Since recent studies indicated that the assessment of implicit associations may be responsive to contextual cues and motivational state (Gemar *et al.* 2001; Wittenbrink *et al.* 2001; Sherman *et al.* 2003), it seems important to take these factors into consideration when studying the predictive validity of implicit attitudes in the context of back pain.

4 Ambivalent and dual attitudes toward pain, movement, and activity

Unlike the idea that people hold only "one" attitude—be it implicit or explicit—toward an attitude object, it might be more realistic to assume that people often hold more complex attitudes. This applies also for people's attitudes toward pain, movement, and activity. First, people can hold different (ambivalent) implicit attitudes toward different aspects of the attitudinal object

(Sherman *et al.* 2003). This implies that back pain patients may come to adopt a complex pattern of differential implicit associations toward pain, treatment, physical activity, and movement, depending on context or motivational cues. Second, individuals may not only be characterized by ambivalent implicit attitudes but also by so-called dual attitudes (Wilson *et al.* 2000). That is, people may be characterized by discongruent implicit and explicit associations. For example, there is evidence that people may have a non-fearful attitude toward spiders at the explicit level along with a negative affective association regarding spider cues at the implicit level (de Jong *et al.* 2003). These different attitudes may come to surface as a function of contextual cues or motivational state, as described earlier (see Fazio 1990). Following this, it might be that, while most patients may actually know that physical activities result in positive health outcomes (their explicit attitudes), they may still hold an alarming attitude toward activity (their implicit attitudes), which keeps on triggering dysfunctional (catastrophic) associations.

5 Patient relapse due to dual attitudes?

The dual attitude hypothesis further states that newly acquired attitudes can override older ones without erasing them. The older attitude remains stored in memory as an implicit attitude, while the newly acquired attitude operates at a conscious, more explicit level (Wilson *et al.* 2000). Thus, habitual implicit attitudes may still exist—even if the explicit components clearly have been renewed (e.g. as a result of treatment or training)—and continue to exert their influence through subsequent automatically triggered responses. It may take little effort to influence one's deliberative evaluation of physical activities by persuading him or her of its beneficial effects with symbolic information in explicit terms, but it probably requires extensive rehearsal and exposure *in vivo* to back-stressing activities to grasp on one's implicit attitudes (Hetts *et al.* 1999; Wilson *et al.* 2000). If not, the newly learned attitude is likely to gradually ebb away while the old residual dysfunctional attitude wins out again (de Jong *et al.* 2003), leading to a possible revival of kinesiophobic responses and, hence, a return of the original avoidance behavior. Thus, the process of (implicit) attitude change may well need much more time and practice of newly acquired insights before a new attitude becomes a habitual and stable construct replacing the prior implicit aversive beliefs (Wilson *et al.* 2000).

Given the pivotal role of dysfunctional implicit beliefs in the process leading to disabling low back pain, researchers and therapists should dispose of appropriate tools in order to study and assess those beliefs in an objective manner (for a critical review, see De Houwer 2002). Relatedly, evaluating treatment success by solely relying on self-reports is likely to result in an over-estimation of the effect. Clearly, then, further research is warranted to determine whether treatment-induced attitude change also comprises attitude change on an implicit level, whether this process of change develops along a different (more extended) time interval (as compared to explicit attitude change), and whether the strength of residual dysfunctional implicit attitudes is predictive of relapse (cf. Wilson *et al.* 2000).

6 The impact of dysfunctional attitudes of health care providers on treatment outcomes

Accumulating evidence suggests that physicians' recommendations concerning advisable levels of activity may exert a substantial impact on clinical outcomes, both in terms of decreasing disability (Burton *et al.* 1999) as in terms of encouraging fear-avoidance and, thereby, increasing disability (e.g. Waddell 1998; Linton *et al.* 2002, also see Chapter 12). Although health care providers are provided with elaborated clinical guidelines describing how to manage back pain on a scientific basis, it appears that their advices still vary widely, and are often restrictive (Di Iorio *et al.* 2000; Rainville *et al.* 2000). In this regard, Houben *et al.* (2004, submitted) demonstrated how clinicians' judgments on the harmfulness of physical activities, and recommendations for return to work or normal activities, related significantly to their treatment orientation (be it biomedical or more biopsychosocial). Clearly, these recommendations might not only be based on patient factors (e.g. pain severity) but also reflect physicians' personal attitudes and beliefs toward pain, which also might be characterized by duality. This possibility was clearly demonstrated by Teachman and colleagues in their studies on weight stigma. Not only did they find evidence for the existence of an implicit antifat bias among a sample of beach tourists (Teachman *et al.* 2003), but equally so among health care professionals who specialize in treating obesity (Teachman and Brownell 2001). Such inconsistency may interfere with treatment focused on acceptance of overweight. These results also show how stigma can survive on a deeply engrained latent level and continue to trigger discrimination despite people's best intentions.

The impact of implicit attitudes can be expected to be especially prominent under time pressure, a condition that is typical for health care situations. Whether attitudinal complexities (implicit versus explicit) in clinicians interact with those of their patients, and have an influence on the process and outcome of treatment, is a virtually unexplored but fascinating area which clearly merits further attention.

7 A model accounting for the implicit and explicit attitudinal components of patients and health care providers

Underlining the complexity of fear-related attitudes in the context of back pain complaints, the available evidence suggests that individuals' implicit and explicit attitudes may independently vary from highly functional to highly dysfunctional. The various combinations between implicit and explicit associations in the context of back pain are integrated in the following heuristic model (see Table 6.1) that allows for some specific predictions.

In line with the reasoning of Fazio (Fazio *et al.* 1995; Dunton and Fazio 1997) and Devine (1989*a*,*b*) concerning "truly unprejudiced" and "truly prejudiced" attitudes toward Blacks, it could be argued that patients for whom implicit as well as explicit attitude estimates hardly give evidence of *any* fear of pain, movement/(re)injury, or work-related activities (and thus apparently truly believe that activity is curative and beneficial for their back) could be entitled as the *true confronter type* (type 1). Indeed, it might be expected that patients with low fear on the explicit as well as on the implicit level are the only ones being predetermined to quick and efficient recovery. Likewise, physicians holding this kind of unambiguous attitudinal component might be those who succeed in convincing their patients that continuing to perform normal activities most probably will speed up the healing process. On the other hand, it could be argued that individuals (patients as well as health care providers) holding an automatically activated negative attitude toward pain and injury, without any explicit tendency to consciously monitor or counter their expression of fear in explicit terms, may be categorized as the *true avoider type* (type 4). Consequently, subjects for whom negative fear-related evaluations are automatically activated, but meanwhile feel motivated to counter the effects of this implicit fear by all means (possibly because they were recommended to get moving by their physician, or, as physicians, were trained to do so) could

Table 6.1 Heuristic typology of back pain patients based on their implicit and explicit back pain relevant attitudes

Implicit level	Explicit level	
	Low fear	**High fear**
Low fear	Type 1— True confronters	Type 2— Dual attitude
High fear	Type 3— Dual attitude	Type 4— True avoiders

be thought of as holding *dual attitudes* (type 3). This pattern is likely to be the case in patients who explicitly report an intention to engage in confrontation in case of back pain, but simultaneously give evidence of a high implicit level of pain-related fear. It appears that this type of patient is able to monitor or mask a latent high level of fear/avoidance beliefs under certain circumstances. Finally, one may intuitively not come up with a type of individual who explicitly reports fear of movement and catastrophic thoughts, while giving evidence of an implicit non-fearful attitude toward back-straining movement (*dual attitudes*, type 2). Nevertheless, based on theoretical assumptions, this kind of dual attitude might also be held by some patients. More research on this matter should clarify this further.

8 Promising experimental paradigms

In the next section, we will successively discuss the most prominent indirect research paradigms and their potential applicability for the study of pain-related fear. We also explain their distinct paradigm-mechanism, merits, and limitations. In accordance with the ideas of De Houwer (2003*b*), we believe that all these measures, to a lesser or a larger extent, do somehow succeed in assessing attitudes indirectly. In this respect, Cunningham *et al.* (2001) were the first to demonstrate convergent validity for implicit attitude measures and the existence of a single "latent attitude." This supports the notion that each measure (in that study) tapped the same construct. To date, a fairly extensive supply of implicit attitude measures are available. However, some recent studies indicate that these implicit attitude assessments might be responsive to changing context or motivational state (Gemar *et al.* 2001; Wittenbrink *et al.* 2001; Huijding *et al.* submitted-*a*; Sherman *et al.* 2003). Thus, they may be measures of specific attitudes with differential predictive power as compared to global attitudes. Although specific studies examining implicit pain-related fear and attitudes in the context of back pain are rather scarce (de Jong and Peters 2002; Goubert *et al.* 2003; Leenders *et al.* 2002), examples of plausible research tracks will be presented whenever applicable.

8.1 Affective Priming Paradigm

A frequently used research paradigm attempting to measure implicit attitudes is the Affective Priming Paradigm (APP; Fazio *et al.* 1986). It measures the extent to which evaluative associations, that are automatically activated by prime stimuli (i.e. positive, negative, or neutral words or pictures as attitude object), have an impact on the speed of classification of subsequently presented target stimuli (i.e. positive or negative adjective). As stated by Fazio (Fazio 1986; Fazio *et al.* 1986), attitudes characterized by a strong association between the attitude object and an attitudinal evaluation can be activated from memory automatically upon mere presentation of the attitude object. In this case, the time needed to evaluate a target as either "positive" or "negative" has been found to be significantly shorter on trials where prime and target share the same valence (affectively congruent prime and target) than on trials involving evaluatively incongruent primes and targets. Furthermore, it has been found that this kind of attitude activation is (1) relatively efficient, (2) difficult to bring under voluntary control, (3) does not depend on a conscious intention to evaluate, and (4) does not depend upon awareness of the activating attitude-object. This is in compliance with the so-called "four horsemen of automaticity" (Bargh 1994; Hermans *et al.* 2000). Automatic attitude activation and the facilitation in affectively congruent trials have been observed in a diversity of studies using this paradigm (Bargh *et al.* 1992; Chaiken and Bargh 1993; Fazio *et al.* 1995; Hermans *et al.* 1998), which attests to the generalizability of this phenomenon (Hermans *et al.* 2000).

Goubert *et al.* (2003) were the first to apply the APP in the context of low back pain, using pictures of back-stressing movements instead of pictures of objects or stimuli. Their first experiment investigated whether back-stressing movements activate an evaluative-negative attitude in healthy volunteers. This study replicated the standard affective priming effect, in that participants were faster to evaluate affectively congruent pairs (picture of high threatening movement—negative target word/picture of low threatening movement—positive target word) than affectively incongruent pairs. This finding casts doubt on the assumption that a negative attitude toward back-stressing activities only develops as a consequence of the experience of chronic pain, but underscores the idea that such negativity might be shaped by cultural myths about back pain or may evolve as a result of acute or recurrent pain. In their second experiment, however, it was found that a chronic low back pain patient sample was faster to evaluate a positive word when it was primed by a picture of a high threatening back-stressing movement than when it was preceded by a picture of a low threatening movement. Accordingly, this would imply that chronic low back pain patients being high in fear of movement/(re)injury at an explicit level, at the same time give evidence of a rather evaluative-positive implicit attitude toward back-stressing movements. Acknowledging that back-stressing activities in patients with chronic low back pain are normally seen as extremely negative, the authors explained this so-called *reverse priming* (first mentioned by Glaser and Banaji 1999 and Glaser 2001) in terms of an over-compensation process. Specifically, these patients may overcompensate when asked to categorize target words, because of the evaluative extremity of the picture primes.

Recently, it has been demonstrated that the APP is sensitive to *context* and *motivational state* (Sherman *et al.* 2003). It was observed that smokers' implicit attitudes were positive toward sensory aspects of smoking (such as a picture of a burning cigarette in an ashtray) but negative toward stimuli depicting brands and packaging of cigarettes (representing possible health outcomes or economic costs of smoking). Meanwhile, the affective evaluation also varied as a function of motivational state (as attained by a manipulation of nicotine deprivation). Following this, and in line with previous suggestions, it might also be interesting to explore differences in explicit/implicit attitudes toward physical activity, as a function of contextual (e.g. home versus clinic) or motivational cues (e.g. acute pain). That is, patients' pain behavior might be ruled by attitudes varying across situational contexts, in that being alone, or being surrounded by colleagues, family, or a therapist most probably will result in different pain or disability outcomes. In addition, it is possible that the behavior of back pain patients (e.g. avoidance or confrontation) has to be understood as a response to a complex attitudinal object (i.e. a certain physical activity to be performed) in which different aspects (e.g. benching, lifting, jumping) might relate to different (aspects of) implicit attitudes. This implies that context-variations may result in dissociations between implicit and explicit attitudes, but also in discrepancies between implicit attitudes themselves.

Furthermore, back pain patients may react differently when triggered by differential motivational states. For instance, varying patients' anticipation of future pain (e.g. whether or not being faced with a certain object that has to be lifted immediately) may result in motivational changes leading to variations in implicit (or explicit) attitudes toward that particular physical activity. Possibly, patients' readiness for change might also be an important factor in selecting an appropriate treatment. Conceivably, the presumed complexity of patients' attitudes toward physical activities when burdened with pain may have serious impact on the development of efficient interventions that seek to change patients' attitudes and pain behavior. One idea that may engender more cost-effective programs, might be stage-matched interventions based on the pain stages of change model (Kerns and Rosenberg 2000).

8.2 Implicit Association Test

The Implicit Association Test (IAT; Greenwald *et al.* 1998) is a computerized categorization task, with the underlying assumption that it should be easier to sort different stimuli into one of four concept categories when two concepts being somehow similar or associated in memory share a single response key (compared to when two unrelated or dissimilar concepts require the same response key). In a first task, one response key represents, for instance, the target concept "flower" along with the attribute concept "positive," whereas the other response key represents "insect" and "negative" (Greenwald and Nosek 2001). Subjects then are instructed to sort stimuli by pressing one of the two keys. In a second task, concept associations (target and attribute) are reversed: Flower names and negative words are assigned to one key, whereas insect names and positive words are assigned to the other. Although the IAT was originally developed to investigate implicit attitudes toward gender and race related issues, the test gradually appeared to prove its usefulness in a diverse area of research fields.

Disorder-specific IATs have been able to differentiate between high versus low socially anxious women (de Jong *et al.* 2001); between high versus low anxiety individuals in terms of differential self-favoring effects (as measured by self-esteem and the general evaluation of others; de Jong 2002); and between formerly depressed and never depressed individuals in terms of a reactivation of negative self-schemata when brought in a negative mood (Gemar *et al.* 2001). These results add to the discriminating power of the IAT.

The IAT appeared also to be applicable to the measurement of attribute-dimensions other than the usual positive–negative valence, as has been highlighted in a study by Wiers *et al.* (2002). In this study, heavy drinkers, compared to light drinkers, did not differ significantly regarding their implicit valence associations toward alcohol but did hold relatively strong implicit associations concerning arousal–sedation. In a similar vein, Teachman *et al.* (2001) successfully used fear, danger, and disgust as the attribute dimensions (in addition to valence) in a study on snake and spider fears. These findings add to the idea that certain attitude objects (such as certain behaviors) may not only trigger a global attitude but may also trigger some more specific associations which may have specific predictive validity.

What renders the IAT an appropriate tool to assess implicit dysfunctional attitudes, next to the usual self-reports of patients' beliefs, has to be found in its specific and additional predictive power (as pointed out previously in Section 3.2). As such, implicit and explicit cognitions uniquely contributed to the prediction of 1-month prospective drinking frequency (Wiers *et al.* 2002) and to the prediction of automatic and strategic fear behaviors (Huijding *et al.* submitted-*a*).

Leenders *et al.* (2002) were the first to develop an IAT to investigate the role of implicit attitudes toward movement and rest in the context of kinesiophobia. They hypothesized that an excessive fear of (re)injury due to physical movement could also affect avoidance of physical activities through a more automatic and unconscious pathway. Therefore, three groups, respectively with high, low, or no fear completed an adapted IAT. It was expected that individuals with a high level of fear of movement would respond more quickly when "threat" and "movement" were paired together on the same response key than when threat and rest were paired together, consequently revealing a more negative association toward movement than toward rest. Conversely, it was expected that individuals with a more positive association toward movement than toward rest, would respond more quickly when safety and movement were paired on the same response key than when safety and rest were paired together. In contrast to these predictions, results revealed that all participants responded faster on "movement–threat"/"rest–safety" combinations than on the reverse response requirement. While the IAT effect was very similar for all three groups, on explicit measures the high fearful group scored significantly different from the low fear and no fear groups. In sum, these results document that not only fearful back pain patients but even low fearful patients or non-phobic volunteers can hold a dual attitude toward physical activity and back-straining movements.

Examining dissociations between implicit and explicit attitudes toward phobic stimuli (i.e. spider cues), de Jong *et al.* (2003) came to comparable findings, in that participants explicitly differing in fear-levels toward spiders displayed very similar negative associations with spiders at the implicit level. In this respect, one could argue that the automatic responding of the non-fearful subjects might rely on the deeply grounded cultural stereotype concerning back pain related movement (as mentioned previously), as this presentation is probably more available in memory than a merely personalized negative association. Indeed, confirming these findings, De Houwer (2002) suggested that IAT effects might sometimes reflect societal views or salience, over and above individualized associations in memory. One may doubt whether the implicit associations *per se* have to be put forward as playing a critical role in kinesiophobia (as in a number of studies results emerged counter to this idea). That is, it might be argued that the implicit attitudes are not responsible for different behavioral outputs in terms of confrontation-avoidance but, rather, it is the extent to which one is capable of masking or monitoring these negative automatic evaluations (cf. de Jong *et al.* 2003). This would imply that non-fearful volunteers and non-fearful back pain patients (showing a dual attitude) are capable of suppressing the automatic negative movement stereotype (which fortunately allows them to keep on functioning), whereas fearful patients do not succeed in overriding their automatically activated fears. As such, the success of suppressing a latent high level of fear/avoidance beliefs will depend on the cognitive resources available at a particular moment, and on motivational and contextual conditions (such as the time pressure burdening the individuals effortful processing) resulting in differential behavioral outcomes (Fazio and Towles-Schwen 1999; Wilson *et al.* 2000).

Addressing some critical notes on the applicability of the IAT, it appears that one of its additional strengths resides in the malleability of IAT effects, which renders this paradigm a useful tool to study context-dependent changes in associations (and conditional beliefs) or changes induced by therapy. However, one of its limitations pertains to the fact that four stimulus categories are supposed to be part of a standard IAT: two target concepts (e.g. "flower" and "insect") and two attribute concepts (e.g. "positive" and "negative"). This points out that—strictly speaking—IAT effects only reveal the *strength* of the associations between the target dimension "flower" and the proposed attribute dimensions *relative* to the strength of the associations between the target concept "insect" and the attribute concepts (De Houwer 2002; de Jong *et al.* 2003). Furthermore, although it has been demonstrated that results of an IAT hardly can be faked or controlled intentionally by participants (which contributes to its feature of implicitness), recent evidence suggests that many participants appear to have some awareness of "what" is being measured and appear to be conscious of their own dispositional or attitudinal attributions in that respect (for more details on this, see De Houwer 2002).

8.3 Affective Simon Paradigma and Extrinsic Affective Simon Test

Another indirect attitude measure, the Affective Simon Paradigma (ASP, De Houwer and Eelen 1998), requires subjects to respond on an arbitrary feature of a stimulus (e.g. color or letter type) while ignoring the valence of the stimulus. Confined by space limitations, we refer to other studies for an in-depth description of its mechanism and broad applicability (e.g. De Houwer and Eelen 1998; De Houwer *et al.* 2001; Fazio 2001; De Houwer 2003*a*; de Jong *et al.* 2003). May it suffice to point immediately to some interesting findings of a study in which high and low fearful chronic low back pain patients carried out a word Simon task to measure the extent to which pain and injury cues are implicitly associated to threat (de Jong and Peters 2002). Participants were explicitly instructed to respond to "a perceptual characteristic of the words" (i.e. to say "Threat" for words in capitals and "Safe" for words in small capitals) and to ignore the "word type" (i.e. neutral words or words referring to pain or injury). High fearful patients were relatively fast when the response requirement for movement-related words was "Threat," and relatively slow when the required response was "Safe." Thus, results indicated that the ASP was capable of differentiating between low and high fearful back pain patients.

Some features of the ASP clearly merit future research. A clear advantage of the ASP over the IAT is that it incorporates the capacity to measure single affective associations instead of relative strengths of automatic pairs of associations (de Jong *et al.* 2003). In addition, because of its power to discriminate, for one, between low and high fearful patients (de Jong and Peters 2002), and because of its resistance to practice effects, the ASP possibly lends itself for use in pre- and post-treatment evaluation or for assessing possible variations in implicit phobia-relevant associations due to experimental manipulations (de Jong *et al.* 2003). This finding, along with the possibility of using pictures (e.g. of back-stressing movements) instead of words, unlocks promising opportunities for using the ASP in the context of chronic low back pain. As such, it would be interesting to determine whether the implicit attitude dimension modifies equally after, for example, an attitude change induction or whether the pace of attitude change deviates (as compared to the explicit dimension). Furthermore, it might be intriguing to unveil whether possible residual dysfunctional implicit associations could function as reliable predictors of future patient relapse (as they might bear the potential to trigger a return of the original dysfunctional explicit cognitions and, as a result, the return of the complaints).

By means of conclusion, we will introduce a recently designed and promising assessment tool (De Houwer 2003*a*)—the Extrinsic Affective Simon Task (EAST). Without going into detail, the EAST has been proposed as a paradigm combining the advantages of the ASP (De Houwer 2003*b*) and the IAT (Greenwald *et al.* 1998), while circumventing the disadvantages of both paradigms. It produces reliable, robust, and considerable effect sizes (De Houwer 2002). Thus far, the EAST has been successfully employed to differentiate between high and low spider fearful individuals (Huijding *et al.* submitted-*b*) and heavy and social drinkers (van den Braak 2002). Because of its capability of measuring single (rather than relative) associations in memory (De Houwer 2002), this tool could be used to assess implicit pain-related fear in the context of back pain problems.

9 Conclusion

As the formation of attitudes essentially helps individuals in structuring their social world (Fazio 2001; Bohner and Wänke 2002), attitudes have clear functional value. As noted earlier, highly accessible attitudes, such as deeply engrained fears, will evoke automatic activation from memory when the object is encountered and, thus, will speed up decision-making on a daily basis. Attitude objects that have been labeled as positive will foster approach behavior, whereas attitude objects that have been defined as negative will prompt avoidance behavior. During the last two decades the issue of automaticity has been studied in a large variety of domains, and has revealed significant implications for both research and applied clinical settings. Considerable progress has recently been made in furthering our knowledge on theoretical and methodological issues regarding attitude strength, attitude structure, implicit attitudes, attitude formation, attitude change, and measurement paradigms (Wilson *et al.* 2000; De Houwer 2003*b*).

For clinicians and therapists, indirect measures might be fruitful for a diversity of reasons. First, it has been suggested that self-reports most probably are clouded with demand characteristics, self-presentational bias, or attributional *a priori* theories. Second, even when patients give no evidence of differences in explicit terms, indirect measures might unveil a significant differentiation between high and low fearful individuals at an implicit level, evidencing the existence of so-called dual attitudes. It is important to note that there may be ambivalence in a person's implicit attitudes (de Jong *et al.* 2002; Sherman *et al.* 2003). That is, back pain patients may hold different implicit attitudes toward different aspects of physical activity at the same time.

In order to study and eventually counter the implicit beliefs underlying kinesiophobia, it is important to develop indirect measures that are suitable to assess the relevant associations that may underlie these specific fears (Vlaeyen and Linton 2000; Vlaeyen *et al.* 2001; Leenders *et al.* 2002). As such, it is not only relevant to find out whether back pain patients fear movement, pain, or work-related activities in general, but also whether they more specifically fear walking, running, lifting weights, or pushing or pulling objects *and* in which particular situation they do so.

Since there is converging evidence that, once established or acquired, attitudes are hard to change, especially when they come to operate automatically (Wilson *et al.* 2000), efforts attempting to promote healthy attitudes toward back pain and coping should start early in life (Goubert *et al.* 2003). Although providing explicit information to alter negatively oriented dysfunctional attitudes is necessary (see Chapter 12), it might be insufficient to alter dysfunctional attitudes at the implicit level. As yet, promising treatment paradigms in this respect are cognitive–behavioral methods, such as graded activity (Vlaeyen *et al.* 2001) and exposure *in vivo* (Vlaeyen *et al.* 2002). The latter not only incorporates a systematic re-activation of the *feared* activities, but also addresses irrational or faulty dysfunctional beliefs via behavioral experiments. Since these treatment modalities are not primarily focused on pain reduction but, rather, on impairment reduction, the modification of attitudes and beliefs play an important role. Importantly, to correct for implicit negative attitudes, repeated exercise with the newly learned attitudes will be needed for the attitude to become habitual, because the modification of attitudes (in chronic low back pain patients) is thought to follow a dynamic and gradual course.

Patients' characteristics and perceptions seem crucial to recovery and, thus, need to be addressed properly in order to avoid relapse. Hence, in order to detect people at risk for chronic pain disability and subsequent prolonged work absence, health care providers should not exclusively rely on self-reports. These can be supplemented using explicit and implicit measures so as to get a more complete attitudinal picture of the patient. This may function as a starting point for selecting a patient-tailored intervention. Furthermore, psychological interventions should address the presumed attitudinal ambivalence in pain-related fear in order to succeed in the desired behavior change; and, clinicians must help patients in making the different aspects of their ambivalent attitude salient (but see Sherman *et al.* 2003). A more comprehensive understanding of the complex processes that shape implicit and explicit attitudes might be of great help to further prevent chronic low back pain and to treat low back pain through specific goal-oriented therapies.

References

Ajzen, I. (1988). *Attitudes, Personality and Behavior.* Milton Keynes: Open University Press.

Ajzen, I. (2001). Nature and operation of attitudes. *Annual Review of Psychology,* **52,** 27–58.

Ajzen, I. and Fishbein, M. (1980). *Understanding Attitudes and Predicting Social Behavior.* Englewood Cliffs, NJ: Prentice-Hall.

Asendorpf, J.B., Bonse, R., and Mücke, D. (2002). Double dissociations between implicit and explicit personality self-concept: The case of shy behavior. *Journal of Personality and Social Psychology,* **83,** 380–93.

Asghari, A. and Nicholas, M.K. (2001). Pain self-efficacy beliefs and pain behaviour. A prospective study. *Pain,* **94,** 85–100.

Banaji, M.R. and Greenwald, A.G. (1994). Implicit stereotyping and prejudice. In M. Zanna and J. Olsen, (eds.), *The psychology of Prejudice: The Ontario Symposium,* pp. 55–76. Hillsdale, NJ: Erlbaum.

Bargh, J.A. (1994). The four horsemen of automaticity: Awareness, intention, efficiency and control in social cognition. In R.S. Wyer and T.K. Srull (eds.), *Handbook of Social Cognition: Vol. 1. Basic Processes,* pp. 1–40. Hillsdale, NJ: Erlbaum.

Bargh, J.A., Chaiken, S., Govender, R., and Pratto, F. (1992). The generality of the automatic attitude activation effect. *Journal of Personality and Social Psychology,* **62,** 893–912.

Bodur, H.O., Brinberg, D., and Coupey, E. (2000). Belief, affect, and attitude: Alternate models of the determinants of attitude. *Journal of Consumer Psychology,* **9,** 17–28.

Bohner, G. and Wänke, M. (2002). *Attitudes and Attitude Change.* East Sussex: Psychology Press.

Braak, A. (2002). Implicit Attitudes Towards Alcohol and Fat: The IAT versus the EAST. Master's Thesis Maastricht University.

Brug, J., Schaalma, H., Kok, G., Meertens, R.M., and van der Molen, H.T. (2000). *Gezondheidsvoorlichting en gedragsverandering. Een planmatige aanpak.* Van Gorcum. Assen.

Burton, A.K., Waddell, G., Tillotson, K.M., and Summerton, N. (1999). Information and advice to patients with back pain can have a positive effect. A randomized controlled trial of a novel educational booklet in primary care. *Spine*, **24**, 2484–91.

Chaiken, S. and Bargh, J.A. (1993). Occurrence versus moderation of the automatic attitude activation effect: Reply to Fazio. *Journal of Personality and Social Psychology*, **64**, 759–65.

Crosby, F., Bromley, S., and Saxe, L. (1980). Recent unobtrusive studies of Black and White discrimination and prejudice: A literature review. *Psychological Bulletin*, **87**, 546–63.

Cunningham, W.A., Preacher, K.J., and Banaji, M.R. (2001). Implicit attitude measures: Consistency, stability and convergent validity. *Psychological Science*, **12**, 163–70.

De Houwer, J. (2002). The Implicit Association Test as a tool for studying dysfunctional associations in psychopathology: Strengths and limitations. *Journal of Behavior Therapy and Experimental Psychiatry*, **33**, 115–33.

De Houwer, J. (2003*a*). The Extrinsic Affective Simon Task. *Experimental Psychology*, **50**, 77–85.

De Houwer, J. (2003*b*). A structural analysis of indirect measures of attitudes. In J. Musch and K.C. Klauer (eds.), *The Psychology of Evaluation: Affective Processes in Cognition and Emotion*, pp. 219–44. Mahwah, NJ: Lawrence Erlbaum.

De Houwer, J. and Eelen, P. (1998). An affective variant of the Simon Paradigma. *Cognition and Emotion*, **12**, 45–61.

De Houwer, J., Crombez, G., Baeyens, F., and Hermans, D. (2001). On the generality of the affective Simon effect. *Cognition and Emotion*, **15**, 189–206.

de Jong, P.J. (2002). Implicit self-esteem and social anxiety: Differential self-favouring effects in high and low anxious individuals. *Behaviour Research and Therapy*, **40**, 501–8.

de Jong, P. and Peters, M. (2002, September). Implicit attitudes toward pain and injury in chronic low back pain patients. Paper presented at the Conference of the European Association of Behavioural and Cognitive Therapies, Maastricht, The Netherlands.

de Jong, P.J., Pasman, W., Kindt, M., and van den Hout, M.A. (2001). A reaction time paradigm to assess (implicit) complaint-specific dysfunctional beliefs. *Behavioral Research Therapie*, **39**, 101–13.

de Jong, P.J., van den Hout, M.A., Rietbroek, H., and Huijding, J. (2003). Dissociations between implicit and explicit attitudes toward phobic stimuli. *Cognition and Emotion*, **17**, 521–46.

Devine, P.G. (1989*a*). Automatic and controlled processes in prejudice: The role of stereotypes and personal beliefs. In A.R. Pratkanis, S.J. Breckler, and A.G. Greenwald (eds.), *Attitude Structure and Function*, pp. 181–212. Hillsdale, NJ: Erlbaum.

Devine, P.G. (1989*b*). Stereotypes and prejudice: Their automatic and controlled components. *Journal of Personality and Social Psychology*, **56**, 5–18.

Di Iorio, D., Henley, E., and Doughty, A. (2000). A survey of primary care physician practice patterns and adherence to acute low back problem guidelines. *Archives of Family Medicine*, **9**, 1015–21.

Dunton, B.C. and Fazio, R.H. (1997). An individual difference measure of motivation to control prejudiced reactions. *Personality and Social Psychology Bulletin*, **23**, 316–26.

Fazio, R.H. (1986). How do attitudes guide behavior? In M.R. Sorrentino and E.T. Higgins (eds.), *The Handbook of Motivation and Cognition: Foundations of Social Behavior*, pp. 204–43. New York, NY: Guilford Press.

Fazio, R.H. (1990). Multiple processes by which attitudes guide behavior. The MODE model as an integrative framework. In M.P. Zanna (ed.), *Advances in Experimental Social Psychology*, pp. 75–109. New York, NY: Academic Press.

Fazio, R.H. (2001). On the automatic activation of associated evaluations: An overview. *Cognition and Emotion*, **15**, 115–41.

Fazio, R.H. and Towles-Schwen, T. (1999). The MODE model of attitude behavior processes. In S. Chaiken and Y. Trope (eds.), *Dual-process Theories in Social Psychology*, pp. 97–116. New York: Guilford.

Fazio, R.H., Sanbonmatsu, D.M., Powell, M.C., and Kardes, F.R. (1986). On the automatic activation of attitudes. *Journal of Personality and Social Psychology*, **50**, 229–38.

Fazio, R.H., Jackson, J.R., Dunton, B.C., and Williams, C.J. (1995). Variability in automatic activation as an unobtrusive measure of racial attitudes: A bona fide pipeline? *Journal of Personality and Social Psychology*, **69**, 1013–27.

Gemar, M.C., Segal, Z.V., Sagrati, S., and Kennedy, S.J. (2001). Mood-induced changes on the Implicit Association Test in recovered depressed patients. *Journal of Abnormal Psychology*, **110**, 282–9.

Glaser, J. (ed.) (2001). *Reverse Priming: Implications for the (Un)conditionality of Automatic Evaluation*. Mahwah, NJ: Erlbaum.

Glaser, J. and Banaji, M.R. (1999). When fair is foul and foul is fair: Reverse priming in automatic evaluation. *Journal of Personality and Social Psychology*, **77**, 669–87.

Goubert, L., Crombez, G., Hermans, D., and Vanderstraeten, G. (2003). Implicit attitude towards pictures of back-stressing activities in pain-free subjects and patients with low back pain: An affective priming study. *European Journal of Pain*, **7**, 33–42.

Greenwald, A.G. and Banaji, M.R. (1995). Implicit social cognition: Attitudes, self-esteem, and stereotypes. *Psychological Review*, **102**, 4–27.

Greenwald, A.G. and Nosek, B.A. (2001). Health of the Implicit Association Test at age 3. *Zeitschrift für Experimentelle Psychologie*, **48**, 85–93.

Greenwald, A.G., McGhee, D.E., and Schwartz, J.L. (1998). Measuring individual differences in implicit cognition: The implicit association test. *Journal of Personality and Social Psychology*, **74**, 1464–80.

Greenwald, A.G., Banaji, M.R., Rudman, L.A., Farnham, S.D., Nosek, B.A., and Mellot, D.S. (2002). A unified theory of implicit attitudes, stereotypes, self-esteem, and self-concept. *Psychological Review*, **109**, 3–25.

Hermans, D., Baeyens, F., and Eelen, P. (1998). Odours as affective processing context for word evaluation: A case of cross-modal affective priming. *Cognition and Emotion*, **12**, 601–13.

Hermans, D., Crombez, G., and Eelen, P. (2000). Automatic attitude activation and efficiency: The fourth horseman of automaticity. *Psychologica Belgica*, **40**, 3–22.

Hetts, J.J., Sakuma, M., and Pelham, B.W. (1999). Two roads to positive regard: Implicit and explicit self-evaluation and culture. *Journal of Experimental Psychology*, **35**, 512–59.

Houben, R.M.A., Ostelo, R.W.J.G., Vlaeyen, J.W.S., Peters, M., Wolters, P.M.J.C., and Stomp-van den Berg, S.G.M. (submitted). Health care providers' orientation towards common low back pain predict perceived harmfulness of physical activities and recommendations regarding return to normal activity. *European Journal of Pain.*

Houben, R.M.A., Vlaeyen, J.W.S., Peters, M., Ostelo, R.W.J.G., Wolters, P.M.J.C., and Stomp-van den Berg, S.G.M. (2004). Health Care Providers' attitudes and beliefs towards common low back pain. Factor structure and psychometric properties of the HC-PAIRS. *The Clinical Journal of Pain*, **20** (1), 37–44.

Huijding, J., Verkooijen, K., and de Jong, P.J. (submitted-*a*). Automatic attitudes toward smoking cues: Influence of context and nicotine.

Huijding, J., ter Hart, L., and de Jong, P.J. (submitted-*b*). Differential predictive power of explicit and implicit measures for controlled vs. automatic behaviors.

Jacoby, L.L. and Kelley, C.M. (1990). An episodic view of motivation. Unconscious influences of memory. In E.T. Higgins and R.M. Sorrentino (eds.), *Handbook of Motivation and Cognition. Foundations of Social Behavior*, pp. 451–81. New York, NY: The Guilford Press.

Keay, K.A., Li, Q.F., and Bandler, R. (2000). Muscle pain activates a direct projection from ventrolateral periaqueductal gray to rostral ventrolateral medulla in rats. *Neuroscience Letters*, **290**, 157–60.

Kerns, R.D. and Rosenberg, R. (2000). Predicting responses to self-management treatments for chronic pain: Application of the pain stages of change model. *Pain*, **84**, 49–55.

Kori, S.H., Miller, R.P., and Todd, D.D. (1990). Kinisophobia: A new view of chronic pain behavior. *Pain Management*, **Jan/Feb,** 35–43.

Leenders, A., de Jong, P., and Peters, M. (2002). De invloed van impliciete attitudes bij kinesiofobie. *Doctoraalscriptie Gezondheidswetenschappen, Universiteit Maastricht.*

Linton, S.J., Vlaeyen, J., and Ostelo, R. (2002). The back pain beliefs of health care providers: Are we fear-avoidant? *Journal of Occupational Rehabilitation*, **12**, 223–32.

McCracken, L.M., Zayfert, C., and Gross, R.T. (1992). The Pain Anxiety Symptoms Scale: Development and validation of a scale to measure fear of pain. *Pain*, **50**, 67–73.

Morgan, M.M. and Carrive, P. (2001). Activation of the ventrolateral periaqueductal gray reduces locomotion but not mean arterial pressure in awake, freely moving rats. *Neuroscience*, **102**, 905–10.

Nisbett, R.E. and Wilson, T.D. (1977). Telling more than we can know: Verbal reports on mental processes. *Psychological Review*, **84**, 231–59.

Oskamp, S. (1977). *Attitudes and Opinions.* Englewood Cliffs, NJ: Prentice Hall Inc.

Ostelo, R.W.J.G., Stomp-van den Berg, S.G.M., Vlaeyen, J.W.S., Wolters, P.M.J.C., and de Vet, H.C.W. (2003). Health care providers' attitudes and beliefs regarding chronic low back pain. *Manual Therapy*, **8**, 214–22.

Rainville, J., Bagnall, D., and Phalen, L. (1995). Health care providers' attitudes and beliefs about functional impairments and chronic back pain. *Clinical Journal of Pain*, **11**, 287–95.

Rainville, J., Carlson, N., Polatin, P., Gatchel, R.J., and Indahl, A. (2000). Exploration of physicians' recommendations for activities in chronic low back pain. *Spine*, **25**, 2210–20.

Sabini, J. (1995). *Social Psychology*, 2nd edn. New York, NY: W.W. Norton & Company.

Sanbonmatsu, D.M. and Fazio, R.H. (1990). The role of attitudes in memory-based decision making. *Journal of Personality and Social Psychology*, **59**, 614–22.

Sarafino, E.P. (1998). *Health Psychology. Biopsychosocial Interactions.* New York, NY: John Wiley & Sons, Inc.

Sherman, S.L., Presson, C.C., Chassin, L., Rose, J.S., and Koch, K. (2003). Implicit and explicit attitudes toward cigarette smoking: The effects of context and motivation. *Journal of Social and Clinical Psychology*, **22**, 13–39.

Spalding, L.R. and Hardin, C.D. (1999). Unconscious unease and self-handicapping: Behavioral consequences of individual differences in implicit and explicit self-esteem. *Psychological Science*, **10**, 535–9.

Sullivan, M.J.L., Bishop, S.R., and Pivik, J. (1995). The Pain Catastrophizing Scale: Development and validation. *Psychological Assessment*, **7**, 523–32.

Tait, R.C. and Chibnall, J.T. (1998). Attitude profiles and clinical status in patients with chronic pain. *Pain*, **78**, 49–57.

Teachman, B.A. and Brownell, K.D. (2001). Implicit anti-fat bias among health professionals: Is anyone immune? *International Journal of Obesity and Related Metabolic Disorders*, **25**, 1525–31.

Teachman, B.A., Gregg, A.P., and Woody, S.R. (2001). Implicit associations for fear-relevant stimuli among individuals with snake and spider fears. *Journal of Abnormal Psychology*, **110**, 226–35.

Teachman, B.A., Gapinski, K.D., Brownell, K.D., Rawlins, M., and Jeyaram, S. (2003). Demonstrations of implicit anti-fat bias: The impact of providing causal information and evoking empathy. *Health Psychology*, **22**, 68–78.

Vlaeyen, J.W.S. and Linton, S.J. (2000). Fear-avoidance and its consequences in chronic musculoskeletal pain: A state of the art. *Pain*, **85**, 317–32.

Vlaeyen, J.W.S., de Jong, J., Geilen, M., Heuts, P.H., and van Breukelen, G. (2001). Graded exposure *in vivo* in the treatment of pain-related fear: A replicated single-case experimental design in four patients with chronic low back pain. *Behavioral Research and Therapy*, **39**, 151–66.

Vlaeyen, J.W.S., de Jong, J., Geilen, M., Heuts, P.H., and van Breukelen, G. (2002). The treatment of fear of movement/(re)injury in chronic low back pain: Further evidence on the effectiveness of exposure *in vivo*. *Clinical Journal of Pain*, **18**, 251–61.

Waddell, G. (1998). *The Back Pain Revolution.* Edinburgh: Churchill Livingstone.

Waddell, G., Newton, M., Henderson, I., Somerville, D., and Main, C.J. (1993). A Fear-Avoidance Beliefs Questionnaire (FABQ) and the role of fear-avoidance beliefs in chronic low back pain and disability. *Pain*, **52**, 157–68.

Wiers, R.W., van Woerden, N., Smulders, F.T.Y., and de Jong, P. (2002). Implicit and explicit alcohol-related cognitions in heavy and light drinkers. *Journal of Abnormal Psychology*, **111**, 648–58.

Wilson, T.D., Lindsey, S., and Schooler, T.Y. (2000). A model of dual attitudes. *Psychological Review*, **107**, 101–26.

Wittenbrink, B., Judd, C.M., and Park, B. (2001). Spontaneous prejudice in context: Variability in automatically activated attitudes. *Journal of Personality and Social Psychology*, **81**, 815–27.

Chapter 7

Disuse and physical deconditioning in chronic low back pain

Jeanine A. Verbunt, Henk A. Seelen, and Johan W.S. Vlaeyen

1 Introduction

In recent years, physical disuse has been presented as one of the perpetuating factors for chronicity in theoretical research models on pain (Hasenbring *et al.* 1994; Vlaeyen *et al.* 1995*a*). Disuse, or a decreased level of physical activity in daily life, would lead to physical deconditioning or an extremely low level of physical fitness. For several decades, physical reconditioning has been proposed in clinical practice as a goal in the treatment of patients with chronic pain, resulting in a variety of rehabilitation programs based on reconditioning. However, inactivity has not only become a topic in chronic pain management, but also in general medicine. About 50 percent of Dutch adults and even more than 60 percent of American adults lead an inactive lifestyle (i.e. performing less than 30 min of moderate-intensity physical activity on 5 days of the week; Pate *et al.* 1995; USDHHS 1996; Hildebrandt *et al.* 1999). This may give rise to the question whether the deconditioning problem in chronic pain exceeds its presence in the general population. The extent of the problem of deconditioning in chronic pain and its specific perpetuating role in chronicity are still unclear. Is physical deconditioning only a result of a decreased physical activity level in pain and is it reversible when pain disappears? Or has deconditioning a perpetuating role for pain itself?

In this chapter, literature on disuse and deconditioning in chronic low back pain will be reviewed. First, the available data on the concepts of disuse and deconditioning will be discussed. Second, the level of physical activity in daily life (PAL) in patients with chronic low back pain will be reviewed. Third, the available data on levels of physical fitness in patients with chronic low back pain is discussed. And finally, future goals in research will be addressed.

2 Defining disuse, deconditioning, and the disuse syndrome

As early as 1199 AD, Maimonides warned of the danger of physical inactivity: "Anyone who lives a sedentary life and does not exercise, even if he eats good foods and takes care of himself according to proper medical principles, all his days will be painful ones and his strength shall wane" (Buschbacher 1996). In the twentieth century, the term "disuse" was introduced. In 1946 Young published "The effects of use and disuse on nerve and muscle," presenting his observations on the inactive human body. He referred to disuse as the process of "not using the musculoskeletal system" in times of physical immobility. Changes in the human body that are the result of long-term immobility are often referred to as deconditioning.

In 1984, Bortz introduced the term *disuse syndrome*. He reviewed the consequences of long-term inactivity and proposed to consider disuse as a syndrome, rather than a symptom. The identifying characteristics of the disuse syndrome, as noted by Bortz, were multidimensional and included cardiovascular vulnerability, obesity, musculoskeletal fragility, depression, and premature aging. The focus was on the physical consequences of inactivity. The psychological consequences were considered to be caused mainly by social deprivation.

In Bortz's concept of the disuse syndrome, the reasons for inactive behavior were not considered. He wrote his paper from a physiological point of view. The main theme of his article was: What will happen to healthy persons if they are extremely inactive? In clinical practice, however, a disuse syndrome will seldom appear as a separate condition. There is almost always a specific reason for depriving oneself from social and physical activities. The causes for such inactive behavior are often of a somatic or a psychological nature. For most people, it is probably a health problem with a great impact on their well-being. The psychological consequences of a health problem confound those of inactivity. Evaluating aspects of the disuse syndrome in healthy persons in an experimental setting is, therefore, easier than evaluating the syndrome in patients suffering from chronic pain. In patients with chronic pain, inactivity can indeed result in psychological problems, according to Bortz's concept. But above all, the impact of pain and the problems in coping with pain seem more likely to provoke psychological distress than inactivity.

In contrast to Bortz's view on the disuse syndrome, which focuses on human (in)activity in general and does not specifically address patients with pain, Mayer and Gatchel (1988) focused on the consequences of long-term inactivity in patients with musculoskeletal pain. They introduced the term "deconditioning syndrome" for patients with pain who also suffer from both physiological and psychological loss of physical fitness. Among the components of physiological deconditioning they included muscle atrophy, decreased cardiovascular endurance, decreased neuromuscular coordination, and a decreased ability to perform complicated repetitive tasks. They referred to psychological deconditioning as a set of behavioral and psychological problems that occur in response to chronic pain and the patient's attempt to cope with that pain. According to Mayer and Gatchel, psychological deconditioning included the response to both pain and inactivity. In the final stage, a deconditioning syndrome is the result of the interaction between physical and psychological deconditioning.

The discrepancy between the concepts of Bortz (1984) and Mayer and Gatchel (1988) is most prominent in the psychological consequences of inactivity. Bortz described the psychological consequences in the syndrome as a *result* of inactivity, whereas Mayer and Gatchel (1988) described psychological deconditioning as a *reaction to* both pain and inactivity and not merely as the result of inactivity.

Clear definitions are a prerequisite for understanding the role of long-term physical inactivity in chronic pain. In this article, three different constructs are proposed: "disuse," "deconditioning," and "disuse syndrome." The term "disuse" can be defined as performing at a reduced level of physical activity in daily life. Disuse refers to a behavioral component leading to physical inactivity. The construct of "physical deconditioning" can best be described as a decreased level of physical fitness with an emphasis on the physical consequences of physical inactivity for the human body. And lastly, the "disuse syndrome" is defined as a result of long-term disuse, which is characterized by both physical and psychosocial effects of inactivity. In this definition, psychosocial consequences of inactivity are reactive to disuse and not reactive to pain itself. Figure 7.1 represents the different constructs and their relations.

Although physical and psychosocial consequences are both important in the disuse syndrome, we focus on the physical consequences in chronic low back pain in this chapter. In a situation of chronic pain, psychosocial consequences, as referred to in the disuse syndrome, are difficult to distinguish from psychosocial consequences of chronic pain. Psychological problems associated with chronic pain are discussed in detail in other chapters of this volume.

3 Models of disuse in chronic low back pain

Why is it so difficult for patients with back pain to return to a normal level of activity after an acute attack of pain? What explains the fact that not every patient with back pain eventually becomes inactive and that only a subgroup

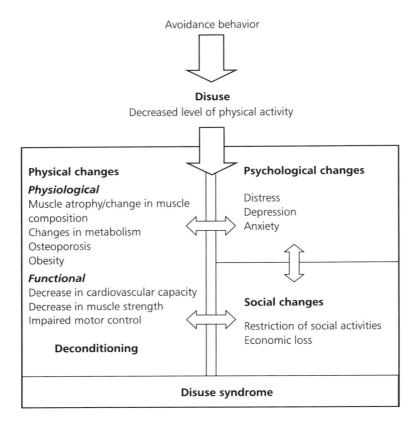

Fig. 7.1 Disuse syndrome: Consequences of long-term inactivity.

of patients develop disuse-related deconditioning? In recent years, several explanatory models have been presented (see, for example, Chapter 1; Hasenbring *et al.* 1994; Vlaeyen *et al.* 1995*a*). They all assume that different strategies in coping with pain play a role in changes in a patient's activity level. Two behavioral coping strategies in particular are mentioned—avoidance behavior and suppressive behavior.

3.1 Avoidance behavior

According to the contemporary fear-avoidance model (see Chapter 1), a sub-group of chronic low back pain patients is afraid of increasing their physical activity level because they fear a reactive increase of their pain or even (re)injury. Their high degree of fear of pain or their expectation of other adverse consequences of increasing movements may be the motivation to restrict movement (Pope *et al.* 1979). In the most extreme situation, the expression "kinesiophobia" is used, referring to an excessive, irrational, and debilitating fear of physical movement and activity resulting from a feeling of vulnerability to painful injury or re-injury (Kori *et al.* 1990; Vlaeyen *et al.* 1995*b*; Crombez *et al.* 1998). According to this model, a state of chronic inactivity, induced by fear of (re)injury, will make it more difficult to return to a normal activity level due to physiological changes of the body system, apart from back pain problems. The physiological changes in this extreme situation of disuse may be equivalent to the deconditioning changes in the disuse syndrome mentioned above.

Fear of movement may result not only in a low activity level, but also in changes in movement patterns. Main and Watson (1996) found a strong relationship between fear-avoidance and guarded movement. Guarded movement is the adaptation of posture in response to pain, which may give a patient short-term alleviation of pain and thus enable him or her to participate in normal activities of daily life. But, after some time, adaptation of posture may result in abnormal motion and a resistant abnormal transfer of loads to other structures of the musculoskeletal system, with further restricted motion. This may contribute to exaggerated illness behavior.

3.2 Suppressive behavior

Hasenbring *et al.* (1994) presented an avoidance-endurance model of pain chronicity. In accordance with the fear-avoidance model, Hasenbring *et al.* refer to a subgroup of patients with low back pain who avoid activities and develop deconditioning and chronic low back pain. But, in addition to this subgroup of patients with avoidance strategies as a coping mechanism, they also identified a second subgroup of patients who have a tendency to cope with pain using endurance strategies. These patients appear to ignore the pain and, by their suppressive behavior, overload their muscles (overuse), leading to muscular hyperactivity. Asmundson *et al.* (1997) have suggested that this subgroup may be those with atypically low and possibly maladaptive levels of fear of pain. Long-term muscular hyperactivity can eventually cause chronic low back pain. According to Hasenbring, both disuse and overuse lead to one-sided and false straining of the muscles, thus enhancing chronification of pain.

The two different ways of coping (i.e. avoidance and suppression) have different effects on the level of physical activity of daily life. According to this model, patients who use avoidance strategies report a low level of physical activities. Patients who apply endurance strategies are likely to report a physical activity level that fluctuates dramatically over time in reaction to pain. They are likely to persevere until increasing pain prevents further activity, then rest completely until the pain subsides or frustration over inactivity stimulates resumption of activity. Subsequently, they persevere again until increasing pain hinders further activity (Harding and Williams 1998). Murphy *et al.* (1997) refer to this as "all or nothing" behavior, representing the so-called "over-activity/under-activity" cycle, which has been observed in many chronic pain patients.

Adequate assessment of the physical activity level over time could provide insight in the way in which a patient tries to cope with the limitations in daily life (Edwards 1986). In the long run, however, both avoidance and suppression coping strategies will, theoretically, result in a low level of physical activity leading to a situation as presented in the disuse syndrome. Also, this low level of physical activity in daily life and its consequences should be measurable in chronic low back pain patients.

4 Disuse in chronic low back pain

Little information exists on the level of physical activity in daily life of patients with chronic low back pain. The results of studies on this subject in chronic low back pain patients are inconclusive. Nielens and Plaghki (2001) found a significantly lower physical activity level in patients with chronic low back pain, which was most pronounced in occupational activities. In recent studies by Protas (1999) and Verbunt *et al.* (2001), the physical activity level of chronic low back pain patients was found to be comparable with that of healthy individuals. A remarkable difference in the studies concerned the percentage of persons with paid jobs. In the Nielens and Plaghki studies, only 20–34 percent of the participants had a paid job, whereas in Verbunt's study 72 percent of patients had a paid job. These different levels of participation in occupational activities could explain the different results of the studies. Persons with chronic low back pain who are still working will have at least a physical activity level that is sufficient to meet the physical demands of their jobs. This could result in a higher general physical activity level when compared to the activity level in a situation in which activities are influenced by pain. It is also important to realize that different assessment methods for PAL were used in the studies. In the studies by Nielens and Protas, the assessment of PAL was based on self-report, whereas assessment in the study by Verbunt *et al.* was based on physiological measurements (i.e. accelerometry, doubly labeled water technique).

To date, the validity of assessment of the level of physical activity in daily life in chronic low back pain by self-report is unclear. A self-report can reflect a difference between how patients actually function and how they believe they function, resulting in a differently reported activity level compared to observed active behavior (Fordyce *et al.* 1984). This will negatively influence the validity of self-report on physical activity in daily life. The discrepancy in reported functioning and actual functioning has been observed before in patients with chronic low back pain. Kremer *et al.* (1981) compared the activity level as reported by patients and as reported by their therapists simultaneously. Patients significantly underestimated their level of activity. In line with this finding, Schmidt (1986) found that patients with chronic low back pain have difficulty in judging their own performance in an experimental setting. Patients were less capable of estimating their physiological level of exertion during a performance test situation than healthy controls. Linton (1985) found a relationship between the level of activity and pain intensity in global interview self-reports, but this relationship gradually disappeared when the measure of physical activity became more overt and objective. This may imply that a patient's perception of his or her activities is biased by other pain-related factors, thus influencing the validity of self-report.

It is surprising that only a few studies on the level of physical activity in patients with chronic low back pain have been performed. The information available does not allow a conclusive statement on the presence of disuse in chronic low back pain. We need new studies on physical activity in daily life in patients with chronic low back pain that make use of valid assessment methods. Behavioral factors, such as avoidance and suppressive behavior, are assumed to play a role in provoking disuse in low back pain. At this point in time, however, insufficient evidence is available to either support or reject the presence of disuse in chronic low back pain. An important component of the level of physical activity in daily life appears to be work status, but this needs to be considered further in future research.

5 Physical activity in daily life: Methods for measurement

Just like in healthy persons, the registration of physical activity in patients with back pain must reflect a mean activity level over more than 1 day in order to represent normal daily life. Gretebeck and Motoye (1992) stated that all methods measuring physical activity in daily life need at least 5 or 6 days of registration to minimize intra-individual variance. Both weekdays and week-end days must be included in the period of measurement. Most methods for measuring physical activity in daily life have been extensively evaluated for validity and reproducibility in a healthy population. However, their psycho-metric properties in a population of patients with chronic low back pain are still unknown. In this section, we will discuss different methods for measuring the level of physical activity in daily life and evaluate their applicability in a population of chronic pain.

5.1 Self-report

Self-report measures, such as questionnaires or diaries, are easy to administer, require little time, and are inexpensive. This makes these measures popular in epidemiological studies featuring large sample studies. Kriska and Caspersen (1997) made a compilation of physical activity questionnaires for health-related research in which they summarized the validity, reliability, and feasibility of the questionnaires. However, as stated in the previous section, it is conceivable that psychometric properties of questionnaires on physical activity are influenced by extraneous factors in a population of patients with chronic pain. Unfortunately, little information on this topic in chronic pain is available, and a difference in discriminative validity has to be considered. Protas (1999) suggested that questionnaires used in a population with chronic low back pain should contain both occupational and leisure time activities, since many individuals with low back pain are still working. An example of a questionnaire that fulfills these criteria is the Baecke questionnaire (Baecke *et al.* 1982).

Examples of questions derived from the Baecke questionnaire are:

- During leisure time I walk . . . never/seldom/sometimes/often/very often
- During leisure time I sport . . . never/seldom/sometimes/often/very often
- At work I lift heavy loads . . . never/seldom/sometimes/often/very often

The test–retest reliability of the Baecke questionnaire in patients with chronic low back pain patients is comparable to that in healthy controls (Jacob *et al.* 2001), while it is easy to administer, inexpensive, and takes little time to analyze.

5.2 Observation

A second technique to evaluate the level of physical activity in daily life is by observation. This may encompass registration of a patient's activities by an observer or by video recording, followed by an interpretation. Observational techniques are generally considered reliable (Bussmann and Stam 1998a), but their administration is costly and time-consuming and, therefore, probably only useful in daily life on a time-sample basis.

5.3 Movement registration

A third possibility is the registration of physical activity in daily life with ambulatory systems, using motion sensors. A variety of systems exist, ranging from pedometers, designed to count steps, to three-dimensional activity monitors, giving more specific data on postures and activities during movement. Most of the motion sensors are small, can register for 1 day up to 4 weeks, and hardly interfere with daily life. In chronic low back pain, research has been done using accelerometry. In a previous study we compared the registration of the level of physical activity in daily life assessed with a tri-axial accelerometer and a registration of physical activity with the doubly labeled water technique (Verbunt *et al.* 2001). The latter is a physiological procedure for which we present detailed information in the next section. The validity of the registration of physical activity during a period of 2 weeks was satisfactory with a correlation coefficient of 0.72. Bussmann *et al.* (1998*b*) reported a good validity of a tri-axial motion sensor, which is based on a combination of accelerometers, in the quantification of behavior (e.g. duration of activities and number of movement transitions) of patients after failed back surgery. Accelerometry makes it possible to measure changes in the quantity of activities and changes in the pattern of physical activities over days. The registration of the level of physical activity in daily life with a tri-axial accelerometer seems applicable in patients with chronic low back pain.

5.4 Physiological measurement

A fourth possibility is the measurement of physiological markers, which is based on the indirect measurement of physiologic responses of the body to exercise. A simple physiology-related method is a 24-h heart rate registration. Heart rate registration hardly interferes with the patient's daily life and its costs are moderate. However, in stress reactions the registration of heart rate as a representation of physical activity can be biased by an increase of the heart rate as a reaction to stress (Raskell *et al.* 1993). Another disadvantage of heart rate registration is the inaccuracy in low-level physical activity (Gretebeck *et al.* 1991). In chronic low back pain, the level of physical activity is probably limited and stress-related problems can be present in coping with pain. Heart rate registration, therefore, seems to be a less than ideal method to measure physical activity in chronic low back pain.

Another physiological technique for physical activity, based on energy expenditure, is the doubly labeled water technique (Westerterp *et al.* 1995). In a healthy population, this technique is generally accepted as the "gold standard" for physical activity assessment in daily life (Bouten *et al.* 1996). It determines the average daily metabolic rate and, together with an estimate of basal energy expenditure, it provides a reliable measure of energy expenditure associated with physical activity in daily life during 1–3 weeks. However, the doubly labeled water technique is expensive and only usable in small sample studies.

6 Deconditioning in chronic low back pain

Disuse leads to deconditioning—a low level of physical fitness. Physical fitness is a multidimensional construct, which includes a combination of physical parameters such as muscle strength, muscle endurance, muscle power, flexibility, cardiovascular capacity, motor control, and body composition. These parameters are negatively affected by a continuous low level of physical activity. If this change in physical parameters is also present in chronic low back pain patients, it would be an indirect sign of the presence of disuse. It is worthwhile to consider a change in physical parameters presented in the disuse model in a population of back pain patients. In the next section, we will discuss research findings that support the physical findings in the disuse model on chronic low back pain. We will successively discuss reported bodily changes due to inactivity in healthy persons and observed changes in patients with chronic low back pain.

6.1 Physiological changes

6.1.1 Muscle atrophy/changes in muscle composition

Inactivity causes changes in all tissues, the most obvious of which are changes in muscle characteristics, such as a decrease in muscle mass (muscle atrophy) and changes in muscle composition. In micro-gravity simulation models, postural muscles that normally counteract the effects of gravity have been reported to become atrophic to a greater extent than fast contracting locomotor muscles (St-Pierre and Gardiner 1987). This implies that muscles situated on the trunk and lower extremities are affected most by deconditioning. This finding has been confirmed in healthy persons in several studies (Berry *et al.* 1993; Greenleaf 1997). In patients with chronic low back pain, muscle atrophy has been reported by Gibbons *et al.* (1997). In patients with more frequent low back pain in the previous year, magnetic resonance imaging (MRI) studies showed a slightly smaller cross-sectional area of the paraspinal muscles and greater signal intensities, possibly due to muscle atrophy.

In healthy subjects, changes in muscle composition, aside from decrease in muscle mass, have been reported (Musacchia 1988). A human muscle contains different muscle fibers, of which fast twitch fibers and slow twitch fibers are the most prevailing. Fast twitch fibers contract fast and are rapidly fatigued, whereas slow twitch fibers contract slowly and can act much longer. In healthy subjects, cessation of normal repetitive low-level activity patterns is supposed to result in transformation of the muscle toward a faster, more fatigable type (St-Pierre and Gardiner 1987; Mannion 1999). In addition to microscopic effects, long-term immobilization can introduce macroscopic anatomic complications, such as a limited range of motion or muscle contractures (Halar and Bel 1988). As a result of infrequent use of the total range of motion of a joint, changes in the connective tissue occur, leading to increased stiffness and contractures. In inactivity, in contrast to immobility, it is hypothesized that contractures may not play such an evident role. The regular use of the arthrogenic range of motion in case of inactivity is supposed to prevent the complication of contractures.

6.1.2 Changes in metabolism

Changes in metabolism result in serious negative effects, such as orthostatic hypotension and reduction of plasma blood volume, leading to dehydration and development of thromboembolic complications. After 30 days of complete bed rest, healthy young men show a decrease in plasma blood volume and red cell volume of 14 and 10 percent, respectively (Greenleaf 1997). Average orthostatic tolerance (during a fast upright movement) was also observed to decrease by 19–43 percent. Since metabolic changes are merely a result of immobility, and not of inactivity, their role in chronic low back pain seems limited.

6.1.3 Osteoporosis

Another problem of deconditioning in immobility is osteoporosis. In a situation of immobility, a lack of muscle pull and gravity on the bones, especially those of the trunk and lower extremity, results in a loss of calcium and leads to osteoporosis (Dittmer and Teasell 1993). Osteoporosis is progressive and may show little or no outward sign until pathological fractures of bone occur. The skeletal calcium loss causes an increased urinary calcium loss. This urinary calcium loss becomes apparent in the first week of bed rest and may continue for months, even after resumption of physical activity (Halar and Bel 1988). Skeletal calcium loss may already occur in a situation of decreased physical activity alone, without actual confinement to bed (Uhthoff and Jaworski 1978). Long-standing disuse osteoporosis is not easily reversed. In a study of primates, immobilized for 7 months, normal bone formation was not seen until 6 months after resumption of activity (Young *et al.* 1986).

6.1.4 Obesity

Deconditioning affects the composition of the body. Lean body mass (i.e. body mass without the mass of fat) decreases during 30 days bed rest, whereas body weight does not change (Greenleaf 1997). This finding suggests that the percentage of body fat will increase as the percentage of muscle mass decreases. Sothmann *et al.* (1991) confirmed this inverse relationship during reconditioning. In a cross-sectional study with three different groups of aerobic fitness levels there was a significant decrease in the percentage of body fat and body weight. In female back pain patients, the percentage of body fat was higher compared to healthy age and gender matched controls (Toda *et al.* 2000). This difference was not present in men. In a previous study in our laboratory, the body fat percentage of patients was comparable to the percentage of healthy controls (Verbunt *et al.* 2001). However, both of the aforementioned studies had a cross-sectional design, making it impossible to provide evidence that an increased body fat percentage is the result of deconditioning in chronic low back pain. It is conceivable that obesity may contribute to the occurrence of back pain and was already present before back pain started.

6.2 Functional changes

6.2.1 Cardiovascular capacity

The most general parameter of physical fitness is cardiovascular capacity, expressed as the maximum oxygen uptake (VO_2max). In healthy individuals confined to bed, VO_2max decreases by 21 percent after 30 days of bed rest (Greenleaf 1997). The gold standard for determining absolute VO_2max is by direct calorimetry. This procedure needs sophisticated equipment to analyze oxygen and carbon dioxide gas and is usually not available in a clinical setting. Therefore, in healthy subjects submaximal test protocols are developed in which VO_2max can be predicted on the basis of the measured heart rate in a steady state. Steady state heart rate is extrapolated to the maximum heart rate on the basis of the known linear increase of heart rate with the increase in oxygen uptake (Astrand and Rohdahl 1977).

Results from studies on cardiovascular capacity in patients with chronic low back pain are unequivocal. Schmidt (1985*b*, 1986), Davis *et al.* (1992), Brennan *et al.* (1987), and Van der Velde and Mierau (2000) found a significantly lower cardiovascular capacity in patients, whereas Battie *et al.* (1989), Hurri *et al.* (1991), Kellet *et al.* (1991), and Wittink *et al.* (2000) found comparable levels for patients and controls. Nielens and Plaghki (1991, 1994, 2001) reported a lower cardiovascular capacity for men, but not for women. When comparing results of different studies on cardiovascular capacity, it is important to consider differences in test procedures. In some studies cardiovascular capacity is measured, based on physiological parameters, as a heart rate and respiratory quotient. Other studies apply exhaustion, as reported by the patient, as reference to calculate total testing time as a measure for cardiovascular capacity. For the interpretation of cardiovascular capacity in patients with chronic pain, it seems better to evaluate physiological parameters. Rates of exhaustion in patients with chronic pain seem to be modified to a larger extent by motivational and cognitive factors as compared to healthy persons (Watson 1999).

6.2.2 The role of work status in cardiovascular capacity

In research on cardiovascular capacity in patients with chronic low back pain, Nielens and Plaghki reported a difference in cardiovascular capacity for men, but not for women (1991, 1994, 2001). They assumed that a reason for this gender discrepancy could be work status. It could be more common for men to lose their jobs as a result of back pain, leading to a loss of their occupational activities. Jobs of male individuals are probably physically more strenuous, resulting in a more explicit change in activity level after job loss compared to women. Since in healthy young men a positive relation was found between heavy physical work and a high level of physical fitness (Tammelin *et al.* 2002), the loss of this work-related activity level in patients will probably result in a more substantial decrease in their physical fitness level. Women, with or without a paid job, on the other hand, are probably more active at home in household tasks and child care, which contributes to keeping them at an activity level that may be considered almost equivalent to that of healthy females in most cases. Again, similar to the interpretation of the activity level, work status is an important factor in interpreting the cardiovascular capacity in patients with chronic low back pain. Unfortunately, information on work status is not available in all studies. Of the studies that do present work status, it is remarkable that in most where no difference in cardiovascular capacity was reported, all persons were still working. Hazard *et al.* (1989) compared the cardiovascular capacity of patients with chronic low back pain who were working and of patients who were not working. They found that patients with a paid job had a better cardiovascular capacity than patients without a job. This underlines the importance of occupational activities in deconditioning in chronic low back pain.

6.2.3 Muscle strength

Immobility is reported to lead to a decrease in muscle strength and endurance, especially in the postural muscles (Dittmer and Teasell 1993; Gogia *et al.* 1988). In healthy persons confined to bed for 4–5 weeks, the maximum isometric peak torque for the quadriceps muscle decreased by 10.3–21 percent (Gogia *et al.* 1988; Dudley *et al.* 1989; Germain *et al.* 1995). Hultman *et al.* (1993), in a cross-sectional design, compared endurance of the lumbar muscles in patients with chronic low back pain and healthy volunteers. The healthy group had significantly longer trunk muscle endurance times than the back pain group. Cassisi *et al.* (1993) confirmed this finding.

Most research on muscle strength in patients with back pain is focused on the lumbar muscles. In the concept of disuse, postural muscles, such as trunk and leg muscles, are also important. Lee *et al.* (1995) reported a decrease in trunk strength combined with a decrease in strength of the knee extensors for patients with chronic low back pain. This finding implies that muscle weakness in chronic low back pain is not just a local problem of the trunk, but a generalized problem, probably due to a lower level of physical activity in daily life.

Again, work status could play a role, since only 31 percent of the patients and 59 percent of the controls reported a job with a heavy physical load, while 28 percent of the patients and 63 percent of the controls regularly participated in sports activities (Lee *et al.* 1995).

6.2.4 Motor control

Motor control is also reported to be affected after a period of bed rest. Immobility decreases coordination and balance (Haines 1974). The impairment of balance appears to be due not so much to muscle weakness, but rather to impaired neural control. Maintaining a high degree of coordination requires frequent performance of an activity under conditions in which the sensory perception of the motor performance can be checked for accuracy and errors may be corrected (Kottke 1966; Dustman *et al.* 1984). Bed rest decreases the amount of proprioceptive stimuli, which are responsible for regulating neuromuscular performance. In chronic low back pain, motor control can be affected too. As mentioned above, guarded movements lead to a change in movement patterns. In a laboratory setting, patients with low back pain had less trunk motion during a specific dynamic task than healthy persons (Rudy *et al.* 1995). The recruitment of stabilizing trunk muscles during motion of the upper limbs appeared to be different in persons with and without back pain. Patients with chronic low back pain showed a delayed onset of contraction of the abdominal muscles, which can be hypothesized to result in inefficient muscular stabilization of the spine (Hodges and Richardson 1996, 1999). The role of pain severity in altered motor control in chronic low back pain must also be considered. In a standardized reach task, postural control in patients with severe pain was poorer than in patients with moderate pain (Luoto *et al.* 1996). With impaired motor control, the problem can either be caused by pain or result from inactivity.

6.2.5 Modifying factors

With functional changes in patients with chronic low back pain it is important to consider factors that may serve to modify physical performance measurement. In assessing physical fitness in patients with chronic low back pain, physical performance is probably modified to a larger extent by motivational and cognitive factors than in healthy persons. Watson (1999) mentioned the importance of evaluating nonphysical contributing factors during performance tests in chronic low back pain. Pain-related variables such as pre-test pain level (Estlander 1999; Schmidt 1986), pain level on exertion (Keller *et al.* 1999), pain threshold (Pope *et al.* 1979) and pain expectancy (Crombez *et al.* 1996) have been shown to correlate with final test results of the different cross-sectional studies. These nonphysiological factors can, therefore, influence performance assessment and indicate that they might bias the validity of the test.

6.3 Psychosocial changes

Distress, depression, and anxiety—the psychosocial variables mentioned in the deconditioning model—have been studied extensively in chronic low back pain. It is beyond the scope of this chapter to review the literature on distress, depression, and anxiety in chronic pain. It is, however, striking that in research findings on persons without pain, these variables seems to be correlated to the level of physical activity. Most research on psychosocial consequences (in persons without low back pain) in deconditioning has been conducted in inactive people instead of in persons during immobility. Thirlaway and Benton (1992) found in 246 healthy men and women that higher levels of physical activity were associated with a better mood. Inactive but fit people reported a poorer mood than inactive and unfit people. These investigators concluded that the positive relation between physical activity and mood state was less mediated by improved physical fitness than performance of physical activity as a social event. Martinson (1990) found that physical work capacity was reduced in depressed people. Crews and Landers (1987), in a review of 34 studies on the relation between physical fitness and stress response, found that aerobically fit people had reduced psychosocial stress responses. In a group of 100 young and healthy police officers after an aerobic training period, which improved physical fitness, Norris *et al.* (1990) found that self-reported stress was reduced and scores for subjective health and well-being were increased. Petruzello *et al.* (1991) conducted a meta-analysis on the anxiety-reducing effects of exercise and found that aerobic, but not anaerobic, exercise was associated with lower anxiety levels. Since deconditioning affects the aerobic energy capacity in particular, anxiety may play a role. Social consequences of long-term immobility can change the person's role in society. Job loss, related economic loss, and restriction of social activities may occur and may have their effects on a person's mood (Waddell 1991). The results of these studies suggest that inactivity is strongly associated with increased emotional distress (and vice versa).

7 Conclusion

Bortz's disuse syndrome is cited frequently in the literature on physical activity and physical fitness in chronic pain. In the studies on chronic low back pain in which a cross-sectional comparison was made between fitness-related parameters in patients and healthy controls, however, results are inconclusive. It is important to realize that disuse, as described in the physiological literature, refers to immobility, whereas, in chronic pain, it refers to a state of inactivity. And, as we cannot judge the magnitude of the decline in fitness-related parameters in chronic low back pain because of the cross-sectional design of most of these studies, a situation of immobility for patients with chronic low back pain probably rarely occurs. Some complications of immobility, such as contractures and dramatic changes in metabolism, are prevented by any activity and will not appear in a state of inactivity. It is, therefore, questionable whether the disuse syndrome, to the extent as reported by Bortz, is applicable as a separate identity in the chronic pain.

Although disuse is not based on immobility, inactivity can still play an important role. It remains important to objectify the level of physical activity in daily life, or its change in patients with low back pain, since the assumption that physical activity decreases with the occurrence of back pain is still the basis of most reconditioning programs. It is remarkable that, in several studies presented in this chapter, no difference could be found between patients and healthy controls in their levels of PAL or physical fitness. Work status is presented as a possible discriminating variable between fit and unfit persons with chronic low back pain. However, this is not exclusively found in persons with back pain. Indeed, only 40–53 percent of the Dutch adults met the target recommendations for physical activity (Hildebrandt *et al.*1999), whereas even less then 40 percent of the American adults do so (USDHHS 1996) Similarly, in a study regarding Australian adults, only 56 percent of the employees of 20 worksites could be classified as physically active (Simpson *et al.* 2000). It could be that disuse or deconditioning is more related to the moment when patients leave their paid jobs, especially in men, than to the moment when back pain appears.

In the evaluation of a decrease in the level of physical activity in daily life, the measurement of intra-individual changes over time in a longitudinal design is preferable. All studies reviewed in this chapter were based on a cross-sectional design in which the levels of physical activity and physical fitness of patients were compared to controls. It also seems important in future research to evaluate changes in work status and associated relationships to changes in physical fitness. If we evaluate physical fitness over time and possible causes of changes in activity levels, such as pain intensity and occupational and sport-related changes, more will be known about their relationships. Finally, the validity of performance tests that measure physical fitness in chronic low back pain has to be taken into account. A multidimensional approach that includes physiological and physical factors influencing the outcome of an exercise test will be useful in future research on chronic low back pain.

In conclusion, the presence of deconditioning and disuse in chronic low back pain as factors contributing to chronicity in chronic pain remains unconfirmed in the literature. In the evaluation of deconditioning and disuse in chronic pain, it is important to consider the psychometric properties of the assessment methods on both PAL and physical fitness. In future research, it may be possible to confirm the assumed relationship between fitness and pain as presented in fear-avoidance.

Acknowledgments

The authors want to thank Andre Knottnerus, Peter Heuts, Kees Pons, Geert van de Heijden, and Eric Bousema for useful suggestions and comments on an earlier draft of this contribution. This work was supported by the Council for Medical and Health Research of the Netherlands (NWO-MW), grant nr. 904-65-090 and Zorgonderzoek Nederland (ZON) grant nr. 96-06-006.

References

Asmundson, G.J.G., Kuperus, J.L., and Norton, G.R. (1997). Do patients with chronic pain selectively attend to pain-related information? Preliminary evidence for the mediating role of fear. *Pain*, **72**, 27–32.

Astrand, P. and Rodahl, K. (1997). *Textbook of Work Physiology, Physiology Bases of Exercise*, 2nd edn, New York, NY: McGraw-Hill.

Baecke, J.A.H., Burema, J., and Frijters, J.E.R. (1982). A short questionnaire for the measurement of habitual physical activity in epidemiological studies. *The American Journal of Clinical Nutrition*, **36**, 936–41.

Battie, M., Bigos, S.J., Fisher, L.D., Hansson, T.H., Nachemson, A.L., Spengler, D.M., Wortley, M.D., and Zeh, J. (1989). A prospective study of the role of cardiovascular risk factors and fitness in industrial back pain complaints. *Spine*, **14**, 141–7.

Berry, P., Berry, M.D., and Manelfe, M.D. (1993). Magnetic resonance imaging evaluation of lower limb muscles during bedrest: A micro gravity simulation model. *Aviation, Space and Environmental Medicine*, **64**, 212–18.

Bortz, W.M. (1984). The disuse syndrome. *The Western Journal of Medicine*, **141**, 691–4.

Bouten, C.V., Verboeket-van de Venne, W.P., Westerterp, K.R., Verduin, M., and Janssen, J.D. (1996). Daily physical activity assessment: Comparison between movement registration and doubly labelled water. *Journal of Applied Physiology*, **81**, 1019–26.

Brennan, G.P., Ruhling, R.O., Hood, R.S., Shultz, B.B., Johnson, S.C., and Andrews, B.C. (1987). Physical characteristics of patients with herniated intervertebral lumbar discs. *Spine*, **12**, 699–702.

Buschbacher, R.M. (1996). Deconditioning, conditioning and the benefits of exercise. In R.L. Braddom (ed.), *Physical Medicine and Rehabilitation*. Philadelphia, PA: W.B. Saunders Company.

Bussmann, J.B.J. and Stam, H.J. (1998a). Techniques for measurement and assessment of mobility in rehabilitation: A theoretical approach. *Clinical Rehabilitation*, **12**, 455–64.

Bussmann, J.B.J., Van de Laar, Y.M., Neeleman, M.P., and Stam, H.J. (1998*b*). Ambulatory accelerometry to quantify motor behaviour in patients after failed back surgery: A validation study. *Pain*, **74**, 153–61.

Cassisi, J.E., Robinson, M.E., O'Conner, P., and MacMillan, M. (1993). Trunk strength and lumbar paraspinal muscle activity during isometric exercise in chronic low-back pain patients and controls. *Spine*, **18**, 245–51.

Crews, D.J. and Landers, D.M. (1987). A meta-analytic review of aerobic fitness and reactivity to psychosocial stressors. *Medicine and Science in Sports and Exercise*, **19**, S114–S120.

Crombez, G., Vervaet, L., Baeyens, F., Lysens, R., and Eelen, P. (1996). Do pain expectancies cause pain in chronic low back patients? A clinical investigation. *Behaviour Research and Therapy*, **34**, 919–25.

Crombez, G., Vervaet, L., Lysens, R., Baeyens, F., and Eelen, P. (1998). Avoidance and confrontation of painful, back straining movements in chronic back pain patients. *Behavior Modification*, **22**, 62–77.

Davis, V.P., Fillingin, R.B., Doleys, D.M., and Davis, M.P. (1992). Assessment of aerobic power in chronic pain patients before and after a multi-disciplinary treatment program. *Archives of Physical Medicine and Rehabilitation*, **73**, 726–9.

Dittmer, D.K. and Teasell, R. (1993). Complications of immobilization and bed rest; part 1: musculoskeletal and cardiovascular complications. *Canadian Family Physician*, **39**, 1428–37.

Dudley, G.A., Gollnick, P.D., Convertino, V.A., and Buchanan, P. (1989). Changes of muscle function and size with bed rest. *Physiologist*, **1**, S65–S66.

Dustman, R.E., Ruhling, R.O., Russell, E.M., Shearer, D.E., Bonekat, H.W., Shigeoka, J.W., Wood, J.S., and Bradford, D.C. (1984). Aerobic exercise training and improved neuropsychological function of older individuals. *Neurobiology of Aging*, **5**, 35–42.

Edwards, R.H.T. (1986). Muscle Fatigue and pain. *Acta Medica Scandinavica*, **711**, 5179–88.

Estlander, A.H., Vanharanta, G.B., Moneta, G.B., and Kaivonto, K. (1999). Anthropometric variables, self-efficacy beliefs, and pain and disability ratings on the isokinetic performance of low back pain patients. *Spine*, **19**, 941–7.

Fordyce, W.E., Lansky, D., Calsyn, D.A., Shelton, J.L., Stolov, W.C., and Rock, D.L. (1984). Pain measurement and pain behaviour. *Pain*, **18**, 53–69.

Germain, P., Guell, A., and Marini, J.F. (1995). Muscle strength during bedrest with and without exercise as a countermeasure. *European Journal of Applied Physiology*, **71**, 342–8.

Gibbons, L.E., Videman, T., and Crites Battié, M. (1997). Isokinetic and psychophysical lifting strength, static back muscle endurance, and magnetic resonance imaging of the paraspinal muscles as predictors of low back pain in men. *Scand Journal of Rehabilitation Medical Supplements*, **29**, 187–91.

Gogia, P.P., Schneider, V.S., LeBlanc, A.D., Krebs, J., Kasson, C., and Pientok, C. (1988). Bed rest effect on extremity muscle torque in healthy men. *Archives of Physical Medicine and Rehabilitation*, **69**, 1029–32.

Greenleaf, J.E. (1997). Intensive exercise training during bed rest attenuates deconditioning. *Medicine and Science in Sports and Exercise*, **29**, 207–15.

Gretebeck, R.J. and Montoye, H.J. (1992). Variability of some objective measures of physical activity. *Medicine and Science in Sports and Exercise*, **24**, 1167–72.

Gretebeck, R.J., Montoye, H.J., Ballor, D., and Montoye, A.P. (1991). Comments on heart rate recording in field studies. *The Journal of Sports Medicine and Physical Fitness*, **31**, 629–31.

Haines, R.J. (1974). Effect of bed rest and exercise on body balance. *Journal of Applied Physiology*, **36**, 323–7.

Halar, E.M. and Bel, K.R. (1988). Contracture and other deleterious effects of immobility. In *Rehabilitation Medicine Principles and Practice*, Delisa J.A. (ed.). J.B. Lippincott, Philadelphia, PA.

Harding, V.R. and Williams, A.C. (1998). Activities Training: Integrating behavioural and cognitive methods with physiotherapy in pain management. *Journal of Occupational Rehabilitation*, **8**, 47–61.

Hasenbring, M., Marienfeld, G., Kuhlendahl, D., and Soyka, D. (1994). Risk factors of chronicity in lumbar disc patients. A prospective investigation of biologic, psychological, and social predictors of therapy outcome. *Spine*, **19**, 2759–65.

Hazard, R.G., Fenwick, J.W., Kalisch, S.M., Redmond, J., Reeves, V., Reid, S., and Frymoyer, J.W. (1989). Functional restoration with behavioral support: A one year prospective study of patients with chronic low back pain. *Spine*, **14**, 157–65.

Hildebrandt, V.H., Urlings, I.J.M., Proper, K.I., Ooijendijk, W.T.M., and Stiggelhout, M. (1999). Are the Dutch still sufficiently physically active? (Bewegen Nederlanders nog wel voldoende?) In V.H. Hildebrandt, W.T.M. Ooijendijk, and M. Stiggelhout (eds.), *Trendrapport Bewegen en Gezondheid 1998–1999*. Lelystad: Koninklijke Vermande.

Hodges, P. and Richardson, C. (1996). Inefficient muscular stabilization of the lumbar spine associated with low back pain. A motor control evaluation of transversus abdominus. *Spine*, **21**, 2640–50.

Hodges, P. and Richardson, C. (1999). Altered trunk muscle recruitment in people with low back pain with upper limb movement at different speeds. *Archives of Physical Medicine and Rehabilitation*, **80**, 1005–12.

Hultman, G., Nordin, M., Saraste, H., and Ohlsen, H. (1993). Body composition, endurance, strength, cross sectional area and density of MM Erector spinae in men with and without low back pain. *Journal of Spinal Disorders & Techniques*, **6**, 114–23.

Hurri, H., Mellin, G., Korhonen, O., Harjula, R., Harkapaa, K., and Luamo, J. (1991). Aerobic capacity among chronic low back pain patients. *Journal of Spinal Disorders & Techniques1*, **4**, 34–8.

Jacob, T., Baras, M., Zeev, A., and Epstein, L. (2001). Low back pain: Reliability on a set of pain measurement tools. *Archives of Physical Medicine and Rehabilitation*, **82**, 735–42.

Keller, A., Johansen, J.G., Hellesnes, J., and Brox, J.I. (1999). Predictors of isokinetic back muscle strength in patients with low back pain. *Spine*, **24**, 275–80.

Kellett, K.M., Kellett, D.A., and Nordholm, L.A. (1991). Effects of an exercise program on sick leave due to back pain. *Physical Therapy*, **71**, 283–90.

Kori, S.H., Miller, R.P., and Todd, D.D. (1990). Kinesiophobia: A new view of chronic pain behavior. *Pain Management*, **3**, 35–43.

Kottke, F.J. (1966). The effects of limitation of activity upon the human body. *JAMA*, **196**, 117–22.

Kremer, E.F., Block, A., and Gaylor, M. (1981). Behavioral approaches to treatment of chronic pain: The inaccuracy of patient self-report measures. *Archives of Physical Medicine and Rehabilitation*, **62**, 188–91.

Kriska, A.M. and Caspersen, C.J. (1997). A collection of physical activity questionnaire for health-related research. *Medicine and Science in Sports and Exercise*, **29**, S3–S201.

Lee, J.H., Ooi, Y., and Nakamura, K. (1995). Measurement of muscle strength of the trunk and the lower extremities in subjects with history of low back. *Spine*, **20**, 1994–6.

Linton, S.J. (1985). The relationship between activity and chronic back pain. *Pain*, **21**, 289–94.

Luoto, S., Taimela, S., Hurri, H., Aalto, H., Pyykko, I., and Alaranta, H. (1996). Psychomotor speed and postural control in chronic low back pain patients. A controlled follow-up study. *Spine*, **15**, 2621–7.

Main, C.J. and Watson, P.J. (1996). Guarded movements: Development of chronicity. *Journal of Musculoskeletal Pain*, **4**, 163–70.

Mannion, A.F. (1999). Fibre type characteristics and function of the human paraspinal muscles: Normal values and changes in association with low back pain. *Journal of Electromyography and Kinesiology*, **9**, 363–77.

Martinsen, E.W. (1990). Benefits of exercise for the treatment of depression. *Sports Medicine*, **9**, 380–9.

Mayer, T.G. and Gatchel, R.J. (1988). Functional restoration for spinal disorders: The sports medicine approach. Lea and Febiger, Philadelphia, PA.

Murphy, D., Lindsay, S., and Williams, A. (1997). Chronic low back pain: Predictions of pain and relationship to anxiety and avoidance. *Behaviour Research and Therapy*, **35**, 231–8.

Musacchia, X.J. (1988). Disuse atrophy of skeletal muscle animal models. *Exercise and Sport Sciences Reviews*, **16**, 61–87.

Nielens, H. and Plaghki, L. (1991). Evaluation of physical adaptation to exercise of chronic pain patients by steptest procedure. *The Pain Clinic*, **4**, 21–5.

Nielens, H. and Plaghki, L. (1994). Perception of pain and exertion during exercise on a cycle ergometer in chronic pain patients. *The Clinical Journal of Pain*, **10**, 204–9.

Nielens, H. and Plaghki, L. (2001). Cardiorespiratory fitness, physical activity level, and chronic pain: Are men more affected than women? *The Clinical Journal of Pain*, **17**, 129–37.

Norris, R., Carroll, D., and Cochrane, R. (1990). The effects of aerobic and anaerobic training on fitness, blood pressure, and psychological stress and well-being. *Journal of Psychosomatic Research*, **34**, 367–75.

Pate, R.R., Pratt, M., and Blair, S.N. (1995). Physical activity and public health: A recommendation from the Centers for Disease Control and Prevention and the American College of Sports. *JAMA*, **273**, 402–7.

Petruzello, S.J., Landers, D.M., Hatfield, B.D., Kubitz, K.A., and Salazar, W. (1991). A meta-analysis on the anxiety-reducing effects of acute and chronic exercise. *Sports Medicine*, **11**, 143–82.

Pinsky, J. and Crue, D.L. (1984). Intensive group psychotherapy, In Wall P.D. and Melzack R. (eds.), *Textbook on Pain*. Edinburgh: Churchill Livingstone.

Pope, M.H., Rosen, J.C., Wilder, D.G., and Frymoyer, J.W. (1979). The relation between biomechanical and psychological factors in patients with low-back pain. *Spine*, **5**, 173–8.

Protas, E.J. (1999). Physical activity and low back pain, In M. Mitchell *et al.* (eds.), *Pain 1999 An Updated Review; Refresher Course Syllabus*, 9th World Congress on Pain. Seattle, WA: IASP press, Seattle.

Raskell, W.L., Yee, M.C., Evans, A., and Irby, P.J. (1993). Simultaneous measurement of heart rate and body motion to quantitate physical activity. *Medicine and Science in Sports and Exercise*, **25**, 109–15.

Rudy, T.E., Boston, J.R., Lieber, S.J., Kubinski, J.A., and Delitto, A. (1995). Body motion patterns during repetitive wheel rotation task. A comparative study of healthy subjects and patients with low back pain. *Spine*, **20**, 2547–54.

Schmidt, A.J. (1985*a*). Cognitive factors in the performance level of chronic low back pain patients. *Journal of Psychosomatic Research*, **29**, 183–9.

Schmidt, A.J. (1985*b*). Performance level of chronic low back pain patients in different treadmill test conditions. *Journal of Psychosomatic Research*, **29**, 639–45.

Schmidt, A.J. (1986). Persistence Behaviour of Chronic Low Back Pain Patients in Treadmill test with False and Adequate Feedback. Thesis, Maastricht University.

Simpson, J.M., Oldenburg, B., Owen, N., Harris, D., Dobbins, T., Salmon, A., Vita, P., Wilson, J., and Saunders, J.B. (2000). The Australian national workplace health project: Design and baseline findings. *Preventive Medicine*, **31**, 249–60.

Sothmann, M.S., Hart B., and Horn, T.S. (1991). Plasma catecholamine response to acute psychological stress in humans: Relation to aerobic fitness and exercise training. *Medicine and Science in Sports and Exercise*, **23**, 860–7.

St-Pierre, D. and Gardiner, P.F. (1987). The effect of immobilization and exercise on muscle function: A review. *Physiotherapy Canada*, **39**, 24–36.

Tammelin, T., Nayha, S., Rintamaki, H., and Zitting, P. (2002). Occupational physical activity is related to physical fitness in young workers. *Medicine and Science in Sports and Exercise*, **34**, 158–65.

Thirlaway, K. and Benton, D. (1992). Participation in physical activity and cardiovascular fitness have different effects on mental health and mood. *Journal of Psychology Research*, **36**, 657–65.

Toda, Y., Segal, N., Toda, T., Morimoto, T., and Ogawa, R. (2000). Lean body mass and body fat distribution in participants with chronic low back pain. *Archives of Internal Medicine*, **160**, 3265–9.

Tulder, M.W., Koes, B.W., and Bouter, L.M. (1995). A cost-of-illness study of back pain in the Netherlands. *Pain*, **62**, 233–40.

Uhthoff, H.K. and Jaworski, Z.F.G. (1978). Bone loss in response to long-term immobilization. *The Journal of Bone and Joint Surgery*, **60**, 420–9.

US Department of Health and Human Services, Physical Activity and Health (1996). A Report of the Surgeon General. Department of Health and Human Services, Centers for Disease Control and Prevention, National Center for Chronic Disease Prevention and Health Promotion, Atlanta.

Velde, G. van der and Mierau, D. (2000). The effect of exercise on percentile rank aerobic capacity, pain, and self-rated disability in patients with chronic low back pain: A retrospective chart review. *Archives of Physical Medicine and Rehabilitation*, **81**, 1457–63.

Verbunt, J.A., Westerterp, K.R., Van der Heijden, G.J., Seelen, H.A., Vlaeyen, J.W., and Knottnerus, J.A. (2001). Physical activity in daily life in patients with chronic low back pain. *Archives of Physical Medicine and Rehabilitation*, **82**, 726–30.

Vlaeyen, J.W.S. and Linton, S.J. (2000). Fear-avoidance and its consequences in chronic musculoskeletal pain: A state of the art. *Pain*, **85**, 317–32.

Vlaeyen, J.W.S., Kole-Snijders, A.M.J., Boeren, R.G.B., and Van Eek, H. (1995a). Fear of movement/(re)injury in chronic low back pain and its relation to behavioral performance. *Pain*, **62**, 363–72.

Vlaeyen, J.W.S., Kole-Snijders, A.M.J., Rotteveel, A., Ruesink, R., and Heuts, P.H.T.G. (1995b). The role of fear of movement/(re)injury in pain disability. *Journal of Occupational Rehabilitation*, **5**, 235–52.

Waddell, G. (1991). Low back disability, a syndrome of western civilization. *Neurosurgery Clinics of North America*, **4**, 719–38.

Watson, P.J. (1999). Non-psychological determinants of physical performance in musculoskeletal pain, In M. Mitchell *et al.* (eds.), *Pain 1999 An Updated Review; Refresher Course Syllabus 9th World Congress on Pain*. Seattle, WA: IASP press.

Westerterp, K.R., Wouters, L., and Van Marken Lichtenbelt, W.D. (1995). The Maastricht Protocol for the measurement of body composition and energy expenditure with labeled water. *Obesity Research*, **3**, 49–57.

Wittink, H., Hoskins Michel, T., Wagner, A., Sukiennik, A., and Rogers, W. (2000). Deconditioning in patients with chronic low back pain. Fact or fiction? *Spine*, **25**, 2221–8.

Young, J.Z. (1946). Effects of use and disuse on nerve and muscle. *The Lancet*, 109–13.

Young, D.R., Niklowitz, W.J., and Jee, W.S.S. (1986). Immobilization associated osteoporosis in primates. *Bone*, **7**, 109–17.

Part II

Assessment

Chapter 8

The object of fear in pain

Stephen Morley and Christopher Eccleston

1 Introduction

Patients with chronic pain fear more than just the continuation of pain. We
have a good understanding of the importance of some of these fears, such as
fear of movement and (re)injury in chronic low back pain. However, outside
of back pain we have advanced very little in our understanding of multiple fears.
Given the chronic and relatively indiscriminate impact of pain on people's lives,
we expect that pain, especially persistent pain, can elicit a wide range of feared
"objects." In some cases the object of fear is likely to be quite specific (e.g.
onset of fugue in migraine). However, our clinical experience has taught us
that patients also report multiple fears, often fears that are abstract and difficult to verbalize, such as the fear of altered identity and diminished self-
respect. Other chapters have documented how to specifically target feared
objects (see, for example, Chapters 1 and 15). In this chapter we outline a formulation of pain with a focus on its ability to threaten core aspects of identity.

   Identity as a concept has a long history in social and clinical psychology,
but has no specific tradition in the study of pain. We introduce a cognitive–
motivational view of identity that emphasizes the dynamic aspect of identity
evolving across a lifespan, and the place of pain in the evolving and adapting
self. Carver and Scheier (1998) offer a useful goal-oriented model of self-
regulation that is briefly reviewed and applied to chronic pain. Our psychology
is unabashedly "normal": We will seek to understand the multiple threats to self
with theory and data from normal experience. We begin with an account of a
clinical case.[1] We then briefly present some data on the "object of fear" in
chronic pain patients before introducing a framework in which to formulate
our argument that has become known as the 3Is—Interruption, Interference,
and Identity. We explore the application of the concepts of goals and self-
regulation to understanding the experience of chronic pain patients. This

---

[1] This case is based on an amalgam of two clinical cases and the details have been altered to
   protect the identity of the individuals concerned.

approach suggests new ways of understanding the personal consequences of chronic pain and new directions in which therapeutic interventions might be developed.

2 **A clinical case**

In his early forties Kevin was an extremely fit man. He worked hard and long hours in the construction industry and was by his own account "a success." He had experienced personal and financial hardship as a child and adolescent. His father was physically and emotionally abusive to his wife and children. Kevin recalled that he and his six siblings banded together to protect each other and their mother. As soon as he could, Kevin left school and started work as a manual laborer. He left home and met and married his first wife. She quickly became pregnant with the first of their five children. Kevin decided that he would not repeat the pattern of behavior shown by his father, but he would provide for his wife and family and whenever possible he would find additional resources for his mother. Over the years Kevin worked hard and provided for his family and bought a small house for his mother. His marriage did not last and he divorced when the youngest child left home. Shortly thereafter he met and married Lucy and had a daughter, Kim, conceived after the accident that brought Kevin to the clinic.

Kevin came to the pain clinic about 4 years after he had injured his back in a work-related accident that required hospitalization. He had been unable to work since the accident. Although his income was reduced, the family still had sufficient money and they had recently moved to a pleasant house in a small town. Clinical assessment showed reduced mobility and activity, but the most marked feature was his distress, reflected in high scores for anxiety and depression on the Hospital Anxiety and Depression scale (Zigmond and Snaith 1983), and a range of strong, negatively valenced emotions. With the aid of a daily diary, and using the cognitive therapy downward arrow technique, he and the therapist were able to construct a descriptive account of his distressing pain episodes as shown in Fig. 8.1.

This analysis revealed a number of features of which Kevin had been unaware. First, he realized that his pain fluctuated in response to various events, over which he had partial control. Second, he found that his immediate interpretation of rising pain levels was one of alarm and danger that led to increased arousal and physical tension. Third, his initial set of thoughts were primarily concerned with the possibility that there might be something physically wrong with him and that continuing his current activity would cause permanent harm. Fourth, he observed that if he allowed his thoughts to continue, they focused upon other distressing and fearful topics. He would think about

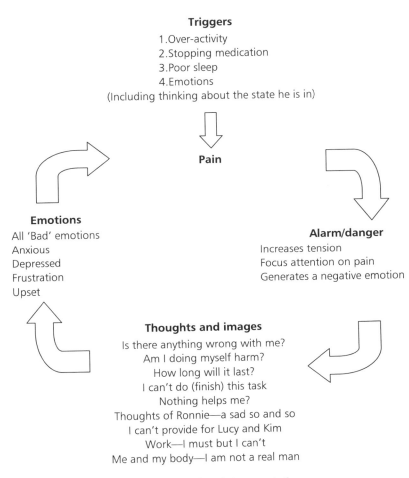

Triggers
1.Over-activity
2.Stopping medication
3.Poor sleep
4.Emotions
(Including thinking about the state he is in)

Pain

Emotions
All 'Bad' emotions
Anxious
Depressed
Frustration
Upset

Alarm/danger
Increases tension
Focus attention on pain
Generates a negative emotion

Thoughts and images
Is there anything wrong with me?
Am I doing myself harm?
How long will it last?
I can't do (finish) this task
Nothing helps me?
Thoughts of Ronnie—a sad so and so
I can't provide for Lucy and Kim
Work—I must but I can't
Me and my body—I am not a real man

Fig. 8.1 Diagrammatic representation of Kevin's presentation.

his performance on the current task and this resulted in a negative appraisal of his expectations of being able to complete the task—a marked downward shift in his self-efficacy. This led him to dwell on the apparent hopelessness of his position, which was accompanied by other thoughts and images. These included thoughts of an ex-work mate, Ronnie, who had chronic pain and had become a shadow of his former self. Kevin admitted that the images of Ronnie scared him because he began to imagine himself in a similar state—a man with a shattered and weak body. He also thought of his responsibility toward Lucy and Kim and his potential inability to provide for them. These thoughts were profoundly distressing and frightening and he was initially reluctant to reveal them; indeed, he recounted how he tried to avoid thinking about them.

Not surprisingly, the thoughts and images generated in response to pain intensified his emotional state. This was experienced as a mélange of anxiety, frustration, and depression, perhaps best described as anxious distress. Finally, Kevin reported a marked reduction in his social activity. He now rarely went out with friends and reduced the amount of contact he had with his immediate family. His reasons for this were that he feared his inability to manage if he experienced an upsurge of pain. Elaboration of this fear suggested a number of facets. He feared that others would not understand his predicament, that others might pity him, and that he would be a burden on them. Kevin found the social consequences of his pain the most distressing and difficult to articulate and understand, and his anxiety and worry about social engagements was marked.

Kevin's presentation illustrates that chronic pain establishes itself in the context of an ongoing and unfolding personal dynamic related to the current stage of a life cycle. Pain will impact on ongoing developmental tasks and particular goals determined by personal concerns and strivings. Clinically, we are able to understand some of the meaning of Kevin's distress and anxiety when we take into account his dominant motivational states and earlier experiences.

3 Objects of fear in pain

Kevin showed a variety of fears. This is a common observation in chronic pain patients. For example, he displayed an understanding and fear about who he would be in the future. Davies (2003) investigated chronic pain patients' future possible selves using a relatively simple question and answer method (Hooker and Kaus 1992). Davies asked participants to think about two aspects of themselves in the future: (1) what they hoped they would be, and (2) what they feared they would be. Table 8.1 shows data from a subsample of 30 participants. Their fears are summarized into five categories.[2] The first category relates to the possible spread of the pain with respect to its continuation, duration, intensity, and extensions to other parts of the body. The second category relates to some of the feared functional consequences of persistent pain, ranging from being more restricted and unable to perform functions to the acquisition of overt signs of disability (e.g. using a wheelchair). The third category concerns future possible health and medical treatment threats. One might expect to observe some of these fears in any population and they are not

---

[2] These categories are not definitive and readers are invited to consider alternative ways of organizing the data.

Table 8.1 Feared-for possible selves from data kindly provided by Dr Caitlin Davies. The numbers in parentheses show the number of times that feared-for self was mentioned

Pain	Functional	Health	Financial	Social and family
Worsening pain (3)	Having no activity	Having a stroke (2)	Having to move house (2)	Not seeing friends
Still having pain when I am old (2)	Unable to plan to do anything	Fear of being reliant on treatment	Financial worries (3)	Not able to communicate
Passing out with the pain	Being more restricted	Having surgery		Children not getting what they should from me
In pain forever	Unable to work	Developing multiple sclerosis		Children leaving me
The pain happening in the other arm	Loosing my job	Having arthritis		Being a burden (2)
	Being immobile (3)	Becoming incontinent		Being left alone (3)
	Being dependent on others (2)	Loosing 'my marbles'		Pushing my husband away
	Being inactive— unable to do housework	Loss of vision and hearing		Family breaking down
	Never being able to walk or dance again	Death		Rejection and discrimination by others
	Becoming wheelchair bound (5)			Loosing my wife and family (3)
				Divorce
				Being left out of the family
	Being old before my time			Note being a fit mother
				Being left alone— starving to death

necessarily related to the presence of persistent pain, but the question arises as to whether the presence of pain is associated with an increased likelihood that one will also fear ill-health in general (Hadjistavropoulos *et al.* 2000, 2001). Also within the third category are fears that appear to be explicitly connected with the presence of pain (e.g. becoming reliant on treatment, staying on morphine). The fourth category relates to the adequacy of financial provision. Although the participants in this study lived in a society (United Kingdom) where there is comprehensive health care (free at the point of delivery) and an extensive social-welfare system, chronic pain still has a considerable impact on a person's financial well-being. The final category contains a large number of items relating to participants' positions in the family and social circumstances. Informal analysis suggests that one superordinate theme is the ultimate loss of all social contacts, leading to complete abandonment and social isolation. Indeed, one participant feared "being left alone and starving to death." Some of the expressed fears concern the consequences of one's own behavior; not being able to fulfill expected social roles (e.g. being a grandparent or a "fit" mother), while others concern the functional consequences of changed behavior (e.g. "My wife is not content—leaving me because I can't dance any more"). The theme of being a burden was common and confirms observations made in an earlier study in which patients described one aim of their communication strategy as not presenting themselves as a burden to their immediate family. One apparent paradox in chronic pain is that a person may express a fear of being isolated and, yet, deliberately avoid or withdraw from social activity in an attempt to reduce the burden on others and to maintain their self-esteem (Morley *et al.* 2000).

These fears have also been observed in some qualitative analyses of chronic pain patients. Although the data has been abstracted at different levels, Table 8.2 summarizes a number of these studies. None of the studies cited in Table 8.2 used a validated quantitative method to assess fears in pain patients but, in their review, Asmundson and his colleagues (Asmundson *et al.* 1999) noted several studies reporting an increase in fear and avoidance in chronic pain patients that was not limited to fear and avoidance of physical activity and subsequent work-related disability. Using a range of standardized questionnaires and formal diagnostic criteria there was evidence of enhanced fear and avoidance of both social activities and health (blood/injury/illness) related issues. The question arises whether the reduction of physical activity associated with chronic pain acts as a mediator and, by reducing access to social opportunities ensures, that fear and avoidance increase as a default, or whether social fear and avoidance is attributable to some other aspect of the experience of chronic pain sufferers?

Table 8.2 Summary of qualitative studies of chronic pain

Study	Sample	Aims	Methods	Themes
Jones (1985)	Unspecified; chronic pain patients	Personal reflection on own work	Not specified	Four threats to selfhood: self in relation to life-contingencies, self in relation to one's own self, self in relation to others, and self in relation to meaning
Hellstrom (2001)	21 (6 M): in patients, heterogenous chronic pain	To explore the temporal aspects of patients conceptions of the self	Empirical phenomenological psychological method	The "body and I"—the distanced foreign body; maintaining the consistency of the past self; the "entrapped" self; projected selves—selves defined by others
Henriksson (1995a, (1995a,b; 1996)	40 F: fibromyalgia in Sweden and USA	To identify factors that can explain and give further understanding to how fibromyalgia influences everday life	Unspecified	Encounters with health care system and others; reactions from others; consequences
Osbourn and Smith (1998)	9 F; low back pain	To explore personal experience	Interpretive phenomenological analysis	Searching for an explanation; comparing self with other selves; not being believed; withdrawing from others
Johansson et al. (1999)	20 F: primary care, undefined musculoskeletal pain	To interpret meaning from a gender perspective	Grounded theory	Lack of control; victim of undiscovered disease; risked identities as capable women
Kugelman (1999)	14 (7 M): inpatients with mostly work related injuries	To examine how the sample describe and experience chronic pain	Hermeneutical–phenomenological from three perspectives	
Jackson (2000)	Various	To experience the lived reality of the chronic pain patient	Participant observation	Identity dissolution; being overwhelmed; being misunderstood
Delgardo et al. (2001)	Study 2—9 (M and F)	To characterize the effect of pain on identity		Pain modifies individual representations and induces fear and a feeling of discomfort linked to self-image and self-ideal

Note: M: males; F: females.

There are some caveats with respect to the literature cited above. Most studies have used small samples of convenience or used sampling methods that are consistent with the (qualitative) study aims but not aimed at representativeness. Most samples are clinic based and this may distort the overall picture obtained—so we must be careful in generalizing to the pain population at large (Crombie *et al.* 1999). The measurement of fear and anxiety also leave something to be desired. The cited studies mainly rely on self-report and unstructured assessments, without extensive descriptive or diagnostic follow through. In addition to verbal reports of subjective and cognitive state, full assessment of fear requires evidence about several components, including behavioral avoidance or escape, and physiological arousal. We should also consider if there are common factors that could explain any association with pain. For example, negative affectivity and anxiety sensitivity are distributed widely in the population and associated with propensity to acquire fear, to report symptoms, and to magnify symptoms (McClure and Lilienfeld 2001; Gatchel and Dersh 2002). Nevertheless, the available evidence suggests that chronic pain patients show an extensive array of objects of fear ranging from fear of pain and disability, fear of specific physical illness to family, and social and existential anxieties.

What unifies this range of fears and why is there variation between people with chronic pain in the extent of their fears? Before attempting to answer these questions, we note that pain, especially chronic pain, is not uniquely associated with anxiety and fear. Arguably, until recently there has been more research on the relationship between chronic pain and depression, much of which has centered on the causal relationship between these and the equivalence of depression in pain and mental health (Turk and Salovey 1984; Romano and Turner 1985; Banks and Kerns 1996; Pincus and Morley 2001). Our view is that, for the most part, depression in chronic pain is a consequence of pain and that this can be understood in terms of a stress–diathesis model in which loss of roles and personal competencies is central. A second emotional complex receiving increased attention is anger and aggression (Burns *et al.* 1998; Okifuji *et al.* 1999; Fernandez 2002). In psychological theory, anger is closely related to frustration of goal-directed efforts and it is, therefore, not surprising that people with chronic pain should experience considerable frustration because of continual interference with daily tasks by pain. What is notable is that in studies by Price and his colleagues (Price *et al.* 1987; Wade *et al.* 1990; Wade *et al.* 1996; Price 1999), where anxiety, depression, frustration, anger, and fear are assessed concurrently, both chronic and acute pain patients appear to indicate that they experience all these emotions in varying quantities; but, the one rated as the most intense is frustration. One issue at stake is to formulate an account of the emotional experience in chronic pain that can accommodate the full range of emotions. Although we will give primary focus to fear, we will try to indicate how the formulation can accommodate other emotional experiences. It is possible to understand these problems if we frame the problem of chronic pain in the context of the sufferers' lives and the extent to which pain impacts on normal psychological processes.

4 Three Is: Interruption, interference, and identity

We suggest that the range of "feared objects" in chronic pain is to be expected because of the overwhelming threat value of pain and its capacity to interrupt, interfere, and, ultimately, impact on a person's identity. In order to understand the anxiety and fear experience of a particular person one needs to be able to consider how the experience of chronic pain impacts upon their life. To do this, one must consider salient motivational states that the pain threatens. What is it about pain that is so distressing and what are the objects of fear in pain? We suggest that chronic pain is a particularly potent elicitor of anxiety, and other negative emotions, because of three disruptive capacities: interruption, interference and identity. As a consequence, there is rarely one "object of fear" in pain. More often there are many potential fears that arise from the capacity of pain to threaten the whole range of a person's existence. We do not claim that only chronic pain has this capacity, because it is clear that many chronic diseases can threaten a person (Contrada and Ashmore 1999); but, we believe that chronic pain is at the extreme end of health threats in its capacity to threaten a person at every level. In the presence of persistent pain, problem-solving needs to occur at each level. We will suggest that, for many individuals, problem-solving becomes fixed or "stuck" at the level of interruption, where the aim of any acceptable solution is the elimination of pain. Our discussion will only briefly review interruption and interference because these receive more extensive treatment elsewhere in this volume. We will focus more on the impact of chronic pain on the third I—identity.

4.1 Interruption

A primary feature of pain is its capacity to interrupt ongoing behavior on a moment-to-moment basis. Pain demands attention to be switched from its current engagement. In laboratory studies the extent of the interruption is a function of not only the stimulus characteristics, such as the novelty and intensity of the pain, but also individual differences in threat perception (catastrophizing) and somatic awareness (Eccleston and Crombez 1999). For the chronic pain patient, this repeated attentional interruption can lead to a heightened or hypervigilance (see Chapter 4). Not only does the immediate experience of the pain interrupt ongoing behavior, but also the cognitive activity elicited by the pain (e.g. thoughts of the possible harm affect the person's cognitive functioning, Grisart and van der Linden 2001). This secondary interruption may be particularly threatening for the chronic pain patient because it leads to the establishment of negative biases. Kevin's account of the initial thoughts of harm seems to fulfill this function and direct his attention away from the current task to an appraisal of his physical state, thereby distracting him from the task.

4.2 Interference

Banks and Kerns (1996) noted the unique capacity of pain "to pervade consciousness and interfere with cognitive functioning" (p. 102). But, it is perhaps the interference and threat of interference with behavior that has the most visible impact on the pain sufferer. The effect of interference in daily life is seen in the frequent reports of frustration made by chronic pain patients. Interference is reflected in the extent of disability assessed in a range of measures from the simple Pain Disability Index (Chibnall and Tait 1994) to the comprehensive Sickness Impact Profile (Follick *et al.* 1985; Jensen *et al.* 1992). Crucial to the treatment of pain patients is the extent to which interference reflects a functional limitation without the influence of psychological factors, such as fear-avoidance and activity–rest cycle. Despite the interruptive capacity of pain, it does not necessarily lead to complete interference of ongoing behavior. Pain may interrupt behavior momentarily; but, it may still be possible to complete a task satisfactorily. For example, Kevin found that pain interrupted his attempts to wash dishes but, on most occasions, he was able to complete this household chore. Initially this had been the source of frustration; this resolved and he came to regard completion of this chore as a valuable social activity that reinforced his sense of self-efficacy.

The repeated experience of pain while executing a task may result in interference either because the sufferer cannot complete the task or because the repeated interruption by the pain degrades performance so much that the person judges it as unsatisfactory when assessed against their implicit standards or another person's real or perceived demands. For example, Dick *et al.* (2002) have recently shown that attentional task-related interference is widespread in chronic pain patients and is related not only to problems in concentration but also to a loss of working memory, making errorless task completion unlikely. For many patients, chronic pain has the capacity to interfere with tasks ranging from seemingly mundane everyday acts of self-care to those that have immense and obvious social and economic consequences (i.e. work). However, interference with even mundane "low-level" everyday tasks is psychologically and socially significant because they put a burden on others and exert pressure on the sufferer to redefine the self.

4.3 Identity

Chronic pain is associated with suffering, but not always. Understanding why there is variation between individuals in their response to chronic pain is a major goal of contemporary research. Leventhal *et al.* (1999) have introduced the cognitive–psychological construct of self-schemata to capture the relatively organized structure of self-referential cognition. For them, the key issue in any threat to identity is whether repeated interference with major goals will impact on the self-schemata and, thereby, on the person's identity. For example, Chapman and Gavrin (1999) note that: "Painful arthritis in the fingers would have a minor impact for most middle aged people, but could be devastating for a professional concert musician because it affects what he or she is and *can hope to be in the future*" (p. 2234; emphasis added).

It is the threat to a person's sense of who they are that generates a range of emotional responses, including fear and anxiety. Identity is complex and dynamically formed, and maintained by a person's interaction with their social and material environment and their reflection and appraisal of that interaction. Kevin's case history illustrates some of the influences on his identity and the challenges that arose when this was threatened. Jackson (2000) argues that this self-altering aspect is not necessarily a specific property of pain, but may be a specific aspect of the lack of choice to experience such a powerful interference in life. She comments:

> All powerful, overwhelming feelings have this property [to alter self]: being profoundly in love, like being in severe pain, requires leaving the everyday lifeworld and thereby transforming the experience of self so the "me" and "not-me" converge in some ways— or at least have different boundaries. The difference is that one usually journeys to the province of passionate love willingly whereas pain animates the sufferer to return to the everyday painless world. (p. 149)

4.3.1 The importance of time in identity

Chronic pain interferes with a person's current tasks, plans, and goals and causes a "biographical disruption" (Bury 1988) that changes the person's perspective of himself or herself both with respect to the past and future. This challenges and threatens the person's sense of self, and requires a response to accommodate or assimilate the challenge (Schmitz *et al.* 1996). In clinical settings, patients often make reference to aspects of their past. It is not unusual to hear the following: "When this (the pain) has finished I'll get back to what I was like."

This may be elaborated with examples of behavior and competencies that a person used to possess. These lost competencies cover the complete gamut of behavior, from walking the dog, doing simple household chores, and gardening to more vigorous exercise. For example, a 45-year-old man with long-standing back pain made a reference to playing competitive soccer in the park on Sunday mornings. The implication behind these expressions is that re-establishing lost competencies will recover an identity that has been suspended (identity suspension). For many patients the "real me" is referenced by the past, but returning to this past state is often neither possible nor age appropriate. Consider the middle-aged man with back pain: When asked about his desire to return to playing soccer it became clear that this past-self was inappropriate—he had stopped playing regularly 10 years ago, before the injury that led to his back pain. The important issue was that playing soccer was an exemplar of his identity as a fit, active man. He appeared to be using anachronistic standards to evaluate his aspirations. A common example of this is the frequent reference by chronic pain patients to disturbed sleep and the expressed desire to be able to sleep as a younger person (i.e. with 7–8 h of undisturbed sleep). Natural age-related changes in sleep cycles mean that normal sleep for middle aged and older adults will include more frequent periods of wakefulness (Horne 1988). It would be mistaken to conclude that sleep should not be a target for intervention (Currie *et al.* 2000) but, rather, that treatment goals need to be set by age appropriate standards and not by reference to past performance.

Perhaps the most salient aspect of biographical disruption is apparent when the future is considered (Hellstrom *et al.* 2000; Hellstrom 2001). Chronic pain essentially disrupts the expected trajectory of development and there are two aspects to this disruption that commonly appear in patients' descriptions of their plight. First is the idea that they have been thrown forward in their developmental time: It is not uncommon to hear this expressed as "I feel old before my time." This is often expressed with reference to slowing and reduced physical performance, and a sense that they have missed the normal experience of gradual age appropriate deterioration in performance competence and reduction of their behavioral repertoire. A second aspect is perhaps more disruptive and difficult to accommodate emotionally. For example, Julia, a woman in her mid-forties acquired sacral nerve damage due to incompetent neurosurgery that had left her with compromised bilateral sensory and motor function. Reflecting on her state she said that "I hadn't expected to be disabled in old age. I had a vision of a slow, graceful decline in which I remained fit and competent, with just ordinary aches and pains … just like my mother." The essential feature of her account is a dislocation in her expected developmental trajectory. It was not just that she recognized that she was "prematurely old" in some sense but that it did not fit with her imagined possible self. Indeed, it was this dislocation and disruption that appeared to enhance her emotional distress. This was expressed as anxiety about her inability to adapt and this inhibited her active problem-solving about her future.

5 Goals and identity

One notable feature of the initial case study is the goal directed and motivational aspects of Kevin's experience. Recall his report that the need to provide for those close to him had been a salient factor in his adult life. He was also motivated to try to preserve a sense of independence and competence and to avoid the expression of pity from others. At a more prosaic level, he reported intense feelings associated with the interference of pain with goals, such as doing the dishes and taking his young daughter for a walk. These and other events provided a challenge to Kevin's sense of identity.

A manifest feature of humans is their goal-directed behavior, their capacity to plan for the future and to organize their behavior to fulfill their plans (Oatley 1992), and their ability to think of self in another context. Planned behavior may be well specified in terms of behavioral acts (go to the supermarket), or rather vaguely described (being a supportive son to an aging and disabled parent), with more or less specific end points and different time frames. The motivational state associated with plans varies considerably. Moreover, plans may be complex and embedded so that their behavioral expression may serve a number of functions. For example, going to the supermarket to buy food may reflect the need to satisfy a current state of hunger, a strategic decision to do the week's personal shopping, and part of the goal of being a supportive son and buying provisions for the disabled parent, or serving the goal of avoiding another aversive requirement. The single act of going to the supermarket may satisfy all four motivational requirements at once.

The conceptualization of goals and motivation is well represented in psychology and there are multiple accounts currently present in the literature, each emphasizing slightly different aspects and nuances (Oatley 1992; Austin and Vancouver 1996; Higgins 1997; Carver *et al.* 1999; Karoly 1999). Nevertheless, there is broad agreement on several issues. First, goals are regarded as internal representations of desired states. Desired states range from biological requirements (including avoiding pain) to relatively transient intra and interpersonal outcomes to themes that may endure for long periods of one's life, such as being successful in one's career. Such a broad definition implies that goals are likely to be represented in a variety of ways, and this is reflected in the variety of levels of analysis encompassed in contemporary research (Austin and Vancouver 1996).

Second, goals can be considered as being organized at several levels, with a certain degree of interdependence between the levels, such that achieving a goal at higher level necessarily depends on the fulfillment of goals at a lower level. Many commentators construe the relationship between goal levels as a hierarchy, although others have expressed concerns about the rigidity and other features implied by such a structure. Carver and Scheier (1998; also see Chapter 3) discuss these issues fully and argue for the retention of a hierarchical organization. Third, humans are construed as having the capacity to pursue multiple goals simultaneously. For theorists this raises issues concerning which goals receive priority at any one time and what factors govern the shifts from goal to goal (Carver and Scheier 1998, 1999). Nevertheless, the main implications of the second and third points are that there may be several pathways to achieving "higher" goals and that a single act may contain several meanings (consider the previous example of shopping at a supermarket). The hierarchical arrangement of goals in which higher goals can be achieved through several routes provides considerable flexibility. Goals that are dependent on just one or two pathways to achieve them are clearly more vulnerable to disruption than goals that have many potential pathways to fulfillment. Goals at higher levels are more likely to have inherent flexibility, but this is not always so. A person may regard a particular concrete action as having great salience in defining the meaning of a higher goal, or they may have a very rigid goal structure in which a particular concrete action is regarded as the only way in achieving the goal.

A fourth issue for goal theories concerns the level of abstraction that best accounts for peoples' action and experience. Studies that ask individuals to list their goals report a range of abstraction, from relatively high levels (e.g. taking care of my family) to more concrete lower levels (e.g. to look good and well turned out) (Emmons and Kaiser 1996). Much behavior is guided by *do* goals concerned with the humdrum of everyday life, such as walking the dog, washing up, making the bed, and shopping. These behaviors often have intrinsic value and are not consciously performed in the pursuit of a higher goal. Nevertheless, the ability to perform these acts may contribute to the maintenance of a higher goal, such as keeping one's marriage intact or *be* goals, such as "being a supportive and nurturing person" (Carver and Scheier 1998). Partners who are unable to fulfill these activities may perceive themselves, and be perceived by their spouse, as not fully sharing the chores of daily life and, thereby, unduly burdening the active partner. As a consequence, they may fear for the repercussions of their inactivity (e.g. ending of the marriage).

There is also marked variation in the way in which goals are articulated. Some may be specific and life long and require dedicated effort over a prolonged period of time. For example, the British politician Michael Hesletine is said to have set himself the goal of becoming Prime Minister and to have planned the intervening goals while he was an undergraduate—he failed. In contrast, a goal may be an implicit emerging expectation that may not be fully articulated until it is challenged, as is often the case in patients with pain or other chronic illnesses. For example, the realization that the capacity to be an active grandparent, or that the grandparent one expected or desired to be is compromised, is a commonly observed cause of distress for chronic pain patients. Goals, whether implicit or explicit, contribute to a person's identity. A critical feature of the hierarchical and abstract nature of goals is the idea that goals at higher levels, which are often *be* goals, are more essential to the individual's sense of self and, thus, to their identity. Lower level, concrete, goals are more meaningful if they are directly linked to a higher goal or if they contribute to the attainment of more than one higher goal.

The fifth feature of goals concerns their valence and the affective consequences of obstructing goal attainment. Theorists conjecture that these two features are important in determining the quality of emotional experience. The fundamental relationships are:

- Goal block—frustration and anger
- Goal disengagement—loss, dejection, depression, relief
- Goal threat—fear, anxiety.

A more complex analysis considers the valence of the goal. Carver and Scheier (1998, 1999), and others, categorize goals as approach or avoidance goals. The distinction is crucial when one considers the direction of movement toward or away from the goal. In Carver and Scheier's analysis, goals are embedded in a feedback loop, individuals monitor the state of their progress to or away from the goal, and they take appropriate corrective action. The crucial distinction is that approach goals require the individual to reduce the discrepancy between their current position and the goal. In contrast, an avoidance goal requires the person to increase the discrepancy between the goal and their current state. The distinction between goal valences is crucial in determining the affective quality. For Carver and Scheier (1998, 1999), attaining an approach goal is characterized by elation and happiness, while non-attainment and loss of the goal is characterized by sadness and depression.[3] Moving away from an avoidance

---

[3] This statement represents a simplification of Carver and Scheier's position in that they propose that the rate of discrepancy reduction or increase contributes to the determining affect.

goal is associated with relief, whereas moving toward an avoidance goal is associated with anxiety and fear. Thus, a consequence of interfering with an individual's attempts to move away from an avoidance goal will generate fear and anxiety. A similar analysis of goals is provided by Higgins (1997), who construes the problem of self-regulation and motivation in terms of an individual's regulatory functions that have "promotion" or "prevention" foci. A crucial point that follows from both Carver and Scheier's and Higgins' analyses is that, whereas individuals often have good knowledge about their proximity to an approach goal, knowing how far they are away from an avoidance goal is inherently a more unstable and unpredictable state. Behavioral analyses of fear and avoidance have often highlighted the role of safety-signals and safety-behavior in determining affect, and this analysis may be extended more generally to avoidance goals.

A major implication of the distinction between approach/avoidance (promotion/prevention) goals is that individuals who are dominated by avoidance goals should be more likely to experience anxiety and fear when these goals are threatened. In other words, when circumstances conspire to prevent a person from keeping the psychological distance between their current state and the avoidance goal, then they will experience anxiety and the goal will be a focus of their fear. In contrast, people whose primary goal state is approach will experience a sense of loss and sadness when their goals are threatened. We suggest that this brief analysis provides a framework for understanding the variety of emotional experience in chronic pain patients. Higgins's (1996, 1997) analysis of the origins of prevention focus suggests that it will be represented by individuals with strong *ought selves* (see next section) and that the content will reflect security needs. The limited amount of data shown in Tables 8.1 and 8.2 appears to be congruent with this prediction. Self-regulation and self-discrepancy theories also suggest that individuals who primarily have approach goals or a promotion focus will experience loss and sadness. As most people will have multiple goals (Oatley 1992), and these could contain a mixture of both approach and avoidance motivations, we would expect people with chronic pain to experience the full gamut of affect in so far as pain interferes with all goal-related activity.

It is arguable that Kevin, whose case introduced this chapter, had organized his life around powerful avoidance goals. He clearly articulated a desire to avoid the poverty and harsh psychological conditions he had experienced as a child. For him, the major perceived consequence of chronic pain was to block his attempts to move away from these goals. The cognitive representation of this goal in his thoughts and vivid images of what he might become were profoundly anxiety provoking. Although anecdotal case studies may provide a starting point for the analysis, we need more compelling systematic evidence and experiments. Initial studies of goal directed behavior and chronic pain, although not designed from the perspective of identity and self-regulation, indicate the potential importance of considering this level of analysis (Karoly and Ruehlman 1996; Affleck *et al.* 1998, 2001).

6 Approaches to studying identity

6.1 Self-discrepancies as a model for investigating pain

A prominent feature of the fears represented in Table 8.1 and in the qualitative studies summarized in Table 8.2 is the presence of social fears seemingly based on a sense of social obligation (i.e. the need to do certain activities to ensure the continuation of social harmony and one's current position). Such obligations might be represented by a rule such as "Unless I do particular things, others will not maintain social proximity to me." The threat of social isolation is profoundly anxiety generating for the majority of people. Within self-discrepancy theory, obligations correspond to the *ought self.* Self-discrepancy theory (Higgins 1987, 1997) posits that the self may be represented in three domains (i.e. *actual, ideal, ought*) and from two standpoints (i.e. *own, significant*). The combination of each domain and standpoint produces six self-state representations. Higgins proposes that different types of self-discrepancies represent different types of negative psychological situations that are associated with different kinds of discomfort. The common method used in self-discrepancy research requires participants to generate a list of descriptors that characterize the various self-aspects (*ideal, ought, actual*). The proximity of aspects to each other is measured by calculating the difference between the numbers of synonyms and antonyms in each pair of aspects.

Although this methodology does not directly assess particular explicit goals, such as maintaining a close relationship with their partner, it captures the essential attributes that a person believes they should possess. These should be congruent with more specific goal-directed activities. An individual might wish to be "kind," both because of the intrinsic value of kindness and also because kindness is perceived as a personal quality that is necessary if he or she is to attain the goal of sustaining a close personal relationship. In this sense, attributes in self-discrepancy tasks may be regarded as a meta-abstraction and representation of a person's motivation and goals. Several studies have confirmed the basic hypothesized relationships between self-discrepancies and experienced affect (Higgins 1987, 1997; Carver and Scheier 1998, 1999) and that people whose self-structure is dominated by *actual–ought* discrepancies are more focused on avoiding negative events (Higgins and Tykocinski 1992;

Higgins *et al.* 1994). As Higgins and colleagues note, their goal is primarily one of safety and one would hypothesize that interfering with this goal will exacerbate anxiety. However, as Carver and colleagues (1999) point out, *ought selves* may contain both approach and avoidance motives. A test of the relationship between avoidance motives and fear in pain patients would need to identify these different components of the *ought self*.

6.2 Future possible selves and self-pain enmeshment

Markus and Nurius (1986) give a temporal perspective to the self. They introduced the concept of possible selves as representations of individuals' ideas about what they might become in the future. Possible selves encompass a person's hopes, fears, goals, and threats that give meaning to a person and provide direction and motivation for behavior. Possible selves provide criteria against which an individual may assess and evaluate the outcomes of their actions. Consistent with self-regulation and self-discrepancy approaches, Markus and Nurius construe possible selves as containing approach and avoidance information.

Chronic pain clearly represents a challenge to an individual's possible selves. Recall Julia, the middle-aged women with compromised lower limb functioning and pain caused by incompetent neurosurgery. Her possible self as an old lady with "normal" aches and pains was completely overturned. Her range of future possible selves now had to incorporate the attributes of "not being mobile" and "increasing reliance on others." This latter attribute was a marked threat to her strongly held identity as a fiercely independent and autonomous person. Despite the challenge to this aspect of her possible self, other aspects of her future self remained intact. She acknowledged that attributes of her current actual self as kind, wise, funny, tolerant, and a listener remained intact and represented attributes of a future possible self that she would be able to sustain and which would enable her to achieve other important personal goals.

We suggest that a critical feature in determining whether chronic pain impacts on a person's identity is the extent to which aspects of the self are enmeshed with the experience of pain. Enmeshment refers to the extent to which aspects of the self are contingent on the presence or absence of pain.[4] Pincus and Morley (2001) outlined a schema model of pain, which hypothesized that a critical feature was the extent to which a chronically activated pain

---

[4] The notion of enmeshment is similar to the notions of entrapment described phenomenologically in qualitative studies of pain patients (Kugelmann 1999; Hellstrom 2001) and has also been noted in studies of chronic mental illness (Rooske and Birchwood 1998; Birchwood *et al.* 2000).

schema become linked with the self-schema. The model was devised to account for a pattern of results observed in tasks that examined information-processing biases. The authors, while acknowledging the potential complexity of the self, simplified their presentation. The previous discussion of goals, self-regulation, and self-discrepancy further delineates important features of the self. The preceding analyses of the motivational qualities of goals suggest that anxiety and fear will be elicited when avoidance goals are enmeshed by pain. If a person's future possible self contains fears, then these fears will become more salient if pain is construed as interfering with the person's avoidance strategies.

Although Pincus and Morley (2001) inferred enmeshment from the experimental data on information processing bias, it is possible to operationalize it and assess its impact directly. Davies (2003) conducted an initial direct test of the self-enmeshment model. Recall that in the first part of her study she asked chronic pain patients to generate hoped-for and feared-for possible selves. Following this, participants generated a list of personal descriptors that characterized these selves and their current *actual* self. Next participants made judgments about the degree of enmeshment between the future selves and pain. An example of a completed task is shown in Table 8.3. Davies used multiple regression analysis to examine the relationships between the proportion of pain contingent hoped-for and feared-for selves and general measures of depression (Beck Depression Inventory; Beck 1978) and anxiety (State-Trait Anxiety Inventory—State form; Spielberger 1983). After adjusting for demographic

Table 8.3 An example of self-description of current-actual, feared-for and hoped-for possible selves

Actual	Feared-for self		Hoped-for self	
Fat	Unable to walk	Y	Fitter	Y
Inactive	Dependent	N	More freedom	Y
Lacking freedom	Bad-tempered	Y	Less lonely	Y
Partly disabled	More restricted	N	Less isolated	Y
Trapped	Miserable	Y	Happier	Y
Isolated	Depressed	Y	Physically active	N
Unable to concentrate	Pessimistic	Y	More mentally able	Y
Despondent	Bed ridden	N	More optimistic	Y
	More stiff	Y		

Note: The participants response to the questions asking them to judge the contingency of each aspect on pain is also shown: Y = yes, N = No. The questions were: Feared-for—"could you be like this *without* pain?" Hoped-for—"could you be like this *with* pain?"

Source: Data kindly provided by Dr Caitlin Davies.

factors, and the level of pain, the proportion of hoped-for self-attributes that were possible with pain predicted the level of depression, and the proportion of pain contingent feared-for attributes predicted anxiety. These results are broadly as expected and suggest one promising approach for elaborating the relationship between the self and pain.

Pain-self enmeshment should be viewed as a normal response to living with a chronic threat of pain and its associated disability. Anthropological studies have examined the extent to which people with chronic pain report a struggle to maintain a separation between pain and self. Patients typically report pain as an aggressor (Good 1992) or an alien attacker (Scarry 1985). Keeping pain as other is a critical aspect of how to cope with an aversive alien attack. Until the meaning of pain can be altered to one that is less aversive, or the patient can understand how pain can be accepted without accepting the negative consequences, then repeated attempts to make pain other than self will persist.

7 Facing threats to the future: Worry and evolving new identities

Chronic pain generates a wide range of fears, not just those relating to pain, injury, and disability but also ones relating to future possible health status and notably those relating to interpersonal relationships. We have suggested that this experience can be understood by considering pain within the three Is framework of interruption, interference, and identity. Pain can generate fear of interruption to current thinking, interference to almost every aspect of daily life, and a threat to identity. Our treatment of identity has been, from the beginning, a dynamic one, focusing on identity as an abstract phenomenon that changes over the lifespan. We have seen that chronic pain is a threat not only to a current concept of self but also to future concepts of self.

7.1 Worry

Recently, Aldrich et al. (2000), interested in the dynamic aspects of worrying, applied the theoretical models of worry and generalized anxiety to an analysis of chronic pain patients. Worry is essentially the cognitive component of anxiety. Quite simply, when we worry we engage in ruminative self-talk (private or public) that is typically about threat to self in the future. Worry is thought to be functional because it maintains a vigilance for a real or perceived threat to self in the future ("I have to keep that in mind") and promotes problem-solving to remove the threat or avoid its consequences ("I must do something about that"). Chronic pain patients, however, report unsurprisingly that they worry more about pain and their health than any other topic, and that they experience these worries as highly intrusive, unpleasant, and difficult to diminish (Eccleston *et al.* 2001). Despite the aversive experience of worry, they find it difficult to stop. Patients report worrying about who they will be in the future and their ability to change the seemingly inevitable consequences of chronic pain.

Worrying about pain may only serve to maintain the prominence of threat to future self. It is hypothesized that worry in chronic pain patients may serve only the function of maintaining a vigilance to threat, but has lost its secondary function, of promoting effective problem-solving. It is early, but there is some evidence that what may characterize chronic pain patients is the extent to which they persevere in unsuccessful attempts to solve insoluble problems (Aldrich *et al.* 2000; van den Hout *et al.* 2003).

7.2 Developing new identity

Chronic pain patients are often faced with the need to reexamine their sense of self. We conjecture that a crucial feature in this is a desire to maintain some sense of continuity and consistency over time. Embedding one's thinking by reference to past aspects of the self initially provides an illusion of consistency and continuity that soon meets the reality of current capacities and the threat that the past may no longer "be achieved." The issues for chronic pain patients are:

◆ How much of their former self can be retained?

◆ What adjustments need to be made to achieve this?

◆ What new aspects need to be developed and how can this be achieved?

◆ Are the new aspects unrelated to prior needs and motivations or do they link with established needs?

Not changing is not an option. In their study of acceptance, Risdon *et al.* (2003) described three core features underpinning varying personal accounts. First, pain sufferers acknowledge the goal of reducing the potential of chronic pain to overpower life. The possibility that pain may dominate, taking precedence at the expense of the rest of one's life, is a realistic fear. The second feature was the acknowledgment that the state of pain is permanent and likely to be for the rest of one's life (McCracken *et al.* 1999) and that, as a consequence, change is necessary. The third feature comprised two important elements relating to self-evaluation. These were resistance to the idea that accepting pain is a sign of personal inferiority (a weak character), and that acceptance does not imply an end to a meaningful life. Or, to phrase this more positively, it is possible to have a meaningful valued life in the presence of persistent pain. Risdon *et al.* (2003) noted that acceptance of chronic pain revolved around the effect of pain on social role functioning and the appraisal of social and self-worth. These themes are also clearly discernable in the thematic qualitative accounts summarized in Table 8.2 and in quantitative studies of anxiety in chronic pain (Asmundson *et al.* 1999). The analysis put forward in this chapter suggests that reducing the capacity of chronic pain to elicit fears will be dependent on understanding and modifying a person's goals, particularly those that have an avoidance component.

8 Conclusion

There are many objects of fear in chronic pain. Some are injury specific, while others are more abstract and affect core psychological processes, such as identity formation and regulation. Chronic pain patients are repeatedly interrupted by pain, making a focus on other life-goals difficult to sustain. For some, this interference in life is easy to manage; for others, it disrupts core aspects of self and threatens not only current identity but also the idea of who one might or can become. For many chronic pain patients, the persistent worry about a failing and unworthy self is a major part of everyday life. Theoretical models and research paradigms for understanding multiple threats and threats to identity by chronic pain are in their infancy, but appear to be promising areas for development.

Acknowledgments

Thanks to Drs Caitlin Davies, Sam Harris, and Stephen Barton for stimulating conversations. We also thank the editors Johan Vlaeyen, Geert Crombez, and Gordon Asmundson for their patience.

References

Aldrich, S., Eccleston, C., and Crombez, G. (2000). Worry about chronic pain: Vigilance to threat and misdirected problem solving. *Behaviour Research and Therapy,* **38**, 457–70.

Affleck, G., Tennen, H., Urrows, S., Higgins, P., Abeles, M., Hall, C., Karoly, P., and Newton, C. (1998). Fibromyalgia and women's pursuit of personal goals: A daily process analysis. *Health Psychology,* **17**, 40–7.

Affleck, G., Tennen, H., Zautra, A., Urrows, S., Abeles, M., and Karoly, P. (2001). Women's pursuit of personal goals in daily life with fibromyalgia: A value-expectancy analysis. *Journal of Consulting & Clinical Psychology,* **69**, 587–96.

Asmundson, G.J.G., Norton, P.J., and Norton, G.R. (1999). Beyond pain: The role of fear and avoidance in chronicity. *Clinical Psychology Review,* **19**, 97–119.

Austin, J.T. and Vancouver, J.B. (1996). Goal constructs in psychology: Structure, process, and content. *Psychological Bulletin,* **120**, 338–75.

Banks, S.M. and Kerns, R.D. (1996). Explaining high rates of depression in chronic pain: A diathesis–stress framework. *Psychological Bulletin,* **119**, 95–110.

Beck, A.T. (1978). *The Beck Depression Inventory.* San Antonio, TX: The Psychological Corporation.

Birchwood, M., Meaden, A., Trower, P., Gilbert, P., and Plaistow, J. (2000). The power and omnipotence of voices: Subordination and entrapment by voices and significant others. *Psychological Medicine*, **30**, 337–44.

Burns, J.W., Johnson, B.J., Devine, J., Mahoney, N., and Pawl, R. (1998). Anger management style and the prediction of treatment outcome among male and female chronic pain patients. *Behaviour Research and Therapy*, **36**, 1051–62.

Bury, M. (1988). Meanings at risk: The experience of arthritis. In R. Anderson and M. Bury (eds.), *Living with Chronic Illness: The Experience of Patients and their Families*, pp. 89–116. London: Unwin Hyman.

Carver, C.S., Lawrence, J.W., and Scheier, M.F. (1999). Self-discrepancies and affect: Incorporating the role of feared selves. *Personality & Social Psychology Bulletin*, **25**, 783–92.

Carver, C.S. and Scheier, M.F. (1998). *On the Self-regulation of Behavior*. Cambridge: Cambridge University Press.

Carver, C.S. and Scheier, M.F. (1999). Themes and issues in self regulation. In R.S. Wyer, Jr. (ed.), *Perspectives on Behavioral Self-regulation*, Vol. XII, pp. 1–105. Mahwah, NJ: Lawrence Erlbaum Associates.

Chapman, C.R. and Gavrin, J. (1999). Suffering: The contributions of persistent pain. *The Lancet*, **353**, 2233–7.

Chibnall, J.T. and Tait, R.C. (1994). The Pain Disability Index: Factor structure and normative data. *Archives of Physical Medicine & Rehabilitation*, **75**, 1082–6.

Contrada, R.J. and Ashmore, R.D. (eds.) (1999). *Self, Social Identity, and Physical Health: Interdisciplinary Explorations*. New York, NY: Oxford University Press.

Crombie, I.K., Croft, P.R., Linton, S.J., LeResche, L., and Von Korff, M. (eds.) (1999). *Epidemiology of Pain*, 1st edn. Seattle, WA: IASP Press.

Currie, S.R., Wilson, K.G., Pontefract, A.J., and deLaplante, L. (2000). Cognitive-behavioral treatment of insomnia secondary to chronic pain. *Journal of Consulting & Clinical Psychology*, **68**, 407–16.

Davies, C. (2003). Self-discrepancy Theory and Chronic Pain. Unpublished Dissertation in Clinical Psycholology, University of Leeds, Leeds.

Dick, B., Eccleston, C., and Crombez, G. (2002) Attentional functioning in fibromyalgia, rheumatoid arthritis and musculoskeletal pain patients. *Arthritis & Rheumatism:Arthritis Care and Research*, **47**, 639–44.

Eccleston, C. and Crombez, G. (1999). Pain demands attention: A cognitive-affective model of the interruptive function of pain. *Psychological Bulletin*, **125**, 356–66.

Eccleston, C., Crombez, G., and Aldrich, S. (2001) Worrying about chronic pain: A description and an exploratory analysis of individual differences. *European Journal of Pain*, **5**, 309–18.

Emmons, R.A. and Kaiser, H.A. (1996). Goal orientation and emotional well-being: Linking goals and affect through the self. In L.L. Martin and A. Tesser (eds.), *Striving and Feeling: Intertactions among Goals, Affect, and Self-regulation*, pp. 79–98. Mahwah, NJ: Lawrence Erlbaum Associates.

Fernandez, E. (2002). *Anxiety, Depression, and Anger in Pain: Research Findings and Clinical Options*, 1st edn. Dallas, TX: Advanced Psychological Resources.

Follick, M.J., Smith, T.W., and Ahern, D.K. (1985). The Sickness Impact Profile: A global measure of disability in chronic low back pain. *Pain*, **21**, 67–76.

Gatchel, R.J. and Dersh, J. (2002). Psychological disorders and chronic pain: Are there cause–effect relationships? In D.C. Turk and R.J. Gatchel (eds.), *Psychological Approaches to Pain Management: A Practitioner's Handbook*, 2nd edn., pp. 30–51. New York, NY: Guilford Press.

Good, B. (1992). A body in pain—the making of a world of chronic pain. In Mary-Jo Delvecchio, B. Good *et al.* (eds.), *Pain as a Human Experience: An Anthropological Perspective*, pp. 29–48. Berkely, CA: University of California Press.

Grisart, J.M. and Van der Linden, M. (2001). Conscious and automatic uses of memory in chronic pain patients. *Pain*, **94**, 305–13.

Hadjistavropoulos, H.D., Hadjistavropoulos, T., and Quine, A. (2000). Health anxiety moderates the effects of distraction versus attention to pain. *Behaviour Research and Therapy*, **38**, 425–38.

Hadjistavropoulos, H.D., Owens, K.M.B., Hadjistavropoulos, T., and Asmundson, G.J.G. (2001). Hypochondriasis and health anxiety among pain patients. In G.J.G. Asmundson, S. Taylor, and B.J. Cox (eds.), *Health Anxiety: Clinical and Research Perspectives on Hypochondriasis and Related Conditions*, pp. 298–323. Chichester: Wiley.

Hellstrom, C. (2001). Temporal dimensions of the self-concept: Entrapped and possible selves in chronic pain. *Psychology and Health*, **16**, 111–24.

Hellstrom, C., Jansson, B., and Carlsson, S.G. (2000). Perceived future in chronic pain: The relationship between outlook on future and empirically derived psychological patient profiles. *European Journal of Pain*, **4**, 283–90.

Hendriksson, C.M. (1995*a*). Living with continuous muscular pain—patient perspectives: I: Encounters and consequences. *Scandinavian Journal of Caring Sciences*, **9**, 67–76.

Hendriksson, C.M. (1995*b*). Living with continuous muscular pain—patient perspectives: II: Strategies for daily life. *Scandinavian Journal of Caring Sciences*, **9**, 77–86.

Hendricksson, C.M. and Burckhardt, C. (1996). Impact of Fibromyalgia on everyday life: A study of women in the USA and Sweden. *Disability and Rehabilitation*, **18**, 241–8.

Higgins, E.T. (1987). Self-discrepancy: A theory relating self and affect. *Psychological Review*, **94**, 319–40.

Higgins, E.T. (1996). *Emotional Experiences: The Pains and Pleasures of Distinct Regulatory Systems*. Hillsdale, NJ: Lawrence Erlbaum Associates.

Higgins, E.T. (1997). Beyond pleasure and pain. *American Psychologist*, **52**, 1280–300.

Higgins, E.T., Roney, C.J.R., Crowe, E., and Hymes, C. (1994). Ideal versus ought predilections for approach and avoidance distinct self-regulatory systems. *Journal of Personality & Social Psychology*, **66**, 276–86.

Higgins, E.T. and Tykocinski, O. (1992). Self-discrepancies and biographical memory: Personality and cognition at the level of psychological situation. *Personality & Social Psychology Bulletin*, **18**, 527–35.

Hooker, K. and Kaus, C.R. (1992). Possible selves and health behaviors in later life. *Journal of Aging & Health*, **4**, 390–411.

Horne, J. (1988). *Why We Sleep: The Functions of Sleep in Humans and Other Mammals*. Oxford: Oxford University Press.

Jackson, J. (2000). *Camp Pain: Talking with Chronic Pain Patients*. Philadelphia, PA: University of Pennsylvania Press.

Jensen, M.P., Strom, S.E., Turner, J.A., and Romano, J.M. (1992). Validity of the Sickness Impact Profile Roland scale as a measure of dysfunction in chronic pain patients. *Pain*, **50**, 157–62.

Jones, L.P. (1985). Anxiety as experienced by chronic pain patients. *Journal of Religion and Health*, **24**, 209–17.

Karoly, P. (1999). A goal systems-self-regulatory perspective on personality, psychopathology, and change. *Review of General Psychology*, **3**, 264–91.

Karoly, P. and Ruehlman, L.S. (1996). Motivational implications of pain: Chronicity, psychological distress, and work goal construal in a national sample of adults. *Health Psychology*, **15**, 383–90.

Kugelmann, R. (1999). Complaining about chronic pain. *Social Science & Medicine*, **49**, 1663–76.

Leventhal, H., Idler, E.L., and Leventhal, E.A. (1999). The impact of chronic illness on the self system. In R.J. Contrada and R.D. Ashmore (eds.), *Self, Social Identity, and Physical Health: Interdisciplinary Explorations. Rutgers Series on Self and Social Identity*, Vol. 2, pp. 185–208. New York, NY: Oxford University Press.

Markus, H. and Nurius, P. (1986). Possible selves. *American Psychologist*, **41**, 954–69.

McClure, E.B. and Lilienfeld, S.O. (2001). Personality traits and health anxiety. In G.J.G. Asmundson, S. Taylor, and B.J. Cox (eds.), *Health Anxiety: Clinical and Research Perpectives on Hypochrondriasis and Related Conditions*, pp. 65–91. Chichester: Wiley.

McCracken, L.M., Spertus, I.L., Janeck, A.S., Sinclair, D., and Wetzel, F.T. (1999). Behavioral dimensions of adjustment in persons with chronic pain: Pain-related anxiety and acceptance. *Pain*, **80**, 283–9.

Morley, S., Doyle, K., and Beese, A. (2000). Talking to others about pain: Suffering in silence. In M. Devor and M.C. Rowbotham, and Z. Wiesenfeld-Hallin (eds.), *Progress in Pain Research and Management*, Vol. 9, pp. 1123–9. Seattle, WA: IASP Press.

Oatley, K. (1992). *Best Laid Schemes: The Psychology of Emotions*. Cambridge: Cambridge University Press.

Okifuji, A., Turk, D.C., and Curran, S.L. (1999). Anger in chronic pain: Investigations of anger targets and intensity. *Journal of Psychosomatic Research*, **47**, 1–12.

Pincus, T. and Morley, S. (2001). Cognitive processing bias in chronic pain: A review and integration. *Psychological Bulletin*, **127**, 599–617.

Price, D.D. (1999). *Psychological Mechanisms of Pain and Analgesia*. Seattle, WA: IASP Press.

Price, D.D., Harkins, S.W., and Baker, C. (1987). Sensory–affective relationships among different types of clinical and experimental pain. *Pain*, **28**, 297–307.

Risdon, A., Eccleston, C., Crombez, G., and McCracken, L. (2003). How can we learn to live with pain? A Q-methodological analysis of the diverse understandings of acceptance of chronic pain. *Social Science & Medicine*, **56**, 375–86.

Romano, J.M. and Turner, J.A. (1985). Chronic pain and depression: Does the evidence support a relationship? *Psychological Bulletin*, **97**, 18–34.

Rooske, O. and Birchwood, M. (1998). Loss, humiliation and entrapment as appraisals of schizophrenic illness: A prospective study of depressed and non-depressed patients. *British Journal of Clinical Psychology*, **37**, 259–68.

Scarry, E. (1985). *The Body in Pain: The Making and Unmaking of the World*. New York, NY: Oxford University Press.

Schmitz, U., Saile, H., and Nilges, P. (1996). Coping with chronic pain: Flexible goal adjustment as an interactive buffer against pain-related distress. *Pain*, **67**, 41–51.

Spielberger, C.D. (1983). *State-trait Anxiety Inventory for Adults*. Redwood City, CA: Mind Garden Inc.

Turk, D.C. and Salovey, P. (1984). "Chronic pain as a variant of depressive disease": A critical reappraisal. *Journal of Nervous & Mental Disease*, **172**, 398–404.

van den Hout, J.H.C., Vlaeyen, J.W.S., Houben, R.M.A., Soeters, A.P.M., and Peters, M.L. (2001). The effects of failure feedback and pain-related fear on pain report, pain tolerance, and pain avoidance in chronic low back pain patients. *Pain*, **92**, 247–57.

van den Hout, J.H.C., Vlaeyen, J., Heuts, P.H., Zijlmena, J.H.L., and Wijnen, J.A.G. (2003). Secondary prevention of work related disability in non-specific low back pain: Does problem solving therapy help? A randomized clinical trial. *Clinical Journal of Pain*, **19**, 87–90.

Wade, J.B., Dougherty, L.M., Archer, C.R., and Price, D.D. (1996). Assessing the stages of pain processing: A multivariate analytical approach. *Pain*, **68**, 157–67.

Wade, J.B., Price, D.D., Hamer, R.M., Schwartz, S.M., and Hart, R.P. (1990). An emotional component analysis of chronic pain. *Pain*, **40**, 303–10.

Zigmond, A.S. and Snaith, R.P. (1983). The Hospital Anxiety and Depression Scale. *Acta Psychiatrica Scandinavica*, **67**, 361–70.

Chapter 9

Assessment of fear and anxiety associated with pain: Conceptualization, methods, and measures

Daniel W. McNeil and Kevin E. Vowles

1 Introduction

This chapter focuses on issues concerning the assessment of fear and anxiety associated with pain, with three major purposes. One intent is to identify and discuss conceptual issues that have implications, including epistemological ones, for our understanding of negative affect that is related to pain. A second point is to discuss methods of measurement and application of these methods to fear of, and anxiety associated with, pain in both acute and chronic populations. Finally, a third aspect of this chapter is a review of major assessments, providing an overview of other available tools as well. In addressing this third point, it is hoped that this work will provide a reference and review of currently available measures of pain-related fear and anxiety for use in clinical and research settings.

In the literature, the words *fear* and *anxiety* have been used to describe negative affective states that include activation in verbal reports (e.g. "I am afraid"), physiology (e.g. increased cardiovascular response), and overt motoric behavior (e.g. avoidance behavior). In spite of accumulating evidence that these constructs are unique, as discussed later in this chapter, the terms fear and anxiety unfortunately are used interchangeably and, in fact, loosely. At times, in this specific area, these descriptors are used inaccurately, suggesting that one or the other of these constructs is being measured when, in fact, there is no evidence supporting that only one of these states is being independently assessed. Nevertheless, anxiety and fear (as well as other emotions) certainly impact, and are affected by, pain, so they will be broadly, and inclusively, considered in this chapter.

2 Conceptual issues

Pain and fear are constructs, rather than being disease or other pathological states in and of themselves. Each of these constructs has been regarded as a "lump" (e.g. Lang 1968), suggesting an amorphous internal state that controls behavior. Nevertheless, from a scientific and clinical perspective, these constructs are best conceptualized as responses, most commonly manifested as a pattern of behavior, broadly defined to include motoric, physiological, and cognitive activity. The issues in assessing (and treating) these constructs, as patterns and series of behavior, have been documented in both the fear (e.g. Lang 1968; see Birbaumer and Ohman 1993) and pain (e.g. Cleeland 1986) literatures. Further complicating the challenge of assessing fear of pain is the issue that each of them often are adaptive, natural, and rational responses to sensory stimuli and environmental events. So, too, can pain-related fear and anxiety be reasonable reactions. Particularly at high levels of intensity, it is only natural that one experiences fear about continuing or anxiety regarding future pain. They also can be adaptive in that they can propel a person to take action to meet the anticipated challenges of acute, time-limited pain, such as when a pregnant woman fearful about labor attends childbirth classes to prepare, or when a dental patient seeks out coping skills training prior to oral surgery. Additionally, persistent (or even chronic) pain, if only of low levels, may be a cue to obtain medical evaluation and treatment, such as when a person with low back pain visits a physician, receives treatment from a physical therapist, and then engages in prescribed exercises. To truly understand pain-related fear and anxiety, therefore, it is necessary to measure both its pathological and normative manifestations.

The meaning of the pain in relation to emotion also is a critical issue. Lang (1985) discusses meaning as one of the critical components, in addition to stimulus and response properties, of information that is a basis for emotional responding. If the pain is symptomatic of a chronic, progressive disease state, such as cancer, fear may be both expected and typical. To not have at least some degree of fear about such pain would perhaps represent a different pathological state, denial.

A further consideration is that there is great similarity in how the constructs of pain and fear of pain, historically and presently, have been assessed, and there is some overlap in conceptualization and treatment (Gross and Collins 1981). For both constructs, there is (over)reliance on self-reports, with some descriptors reflective of each one (e.g. distress). Physiologically, response topographies are alike, generally indicating autonomic activation. Motoric behaviors also are similar, functioning to allow avoidance or escape.

Conceptually, Gross and Collins note that the influence of anxiety (and fear) on pain has been of primary interest, while the opposite relation, pain–impacting anxiety or fear responses, has been less of a focus.

Finally, to understand the assessment of fear of pain, it is essential to identify conceptual and definitional issues about distinctions between fear and anxiety that are only beginning to be clarified. Certainly, it seems likely that pain interacts with fear and anxiety (McNeil and Rainwater 1998), as well as other emotional states such as depression (Robinson and Riley 1999). In the scientific and lay literatures, the constructs of fear and anxiety historically have been overlapping. These terms most often are used interchangeably. Nevertheless, various theoretical models, as well as conceptual and empirical work (McNeil *et al.* 1993) has emphasized that these states are distinct (Craske 1999; Barlow 2002).

In approaching the assessment of pain and negative emotional states it is essential, therefore, to define whether: (1) one seeks to evaluate fear of pain, or (2) anxiety associated with pain. It is important to note that, in an individual, it is possible to be afflicted by a "double anxiety/fear" associated with pain. A person may be anxious about long-term chronic migraine headache pain, as it may affect enjoyment of, or participation in, work and social activities. At the same time, this person may be fearful about the pain involved in dressing change and debridement associated with a severe burn. Such combinations of anxiety and fear are unexplored, and may be synergistic, competitive, or unrelated. (See Bolles and Fanselow 1980 for a theoretical discussion of how acute pain and fear/anxiety may interact. See Chapter 1 for a contemporary model that describes a theoretical model of chronic pain, in which fear of pain, as a defensive motivation, leads to pain-related anxiety, with accompanying preventative motivation.)

It also is imperative to determine whether one is evaluating anxiety or fear that is related to pain, or unrelated to pain (Weisenberg *et al.* 1984). In the first scenario, a patient with recurring headaches might worry about whether there is some potentially lethal organic process going on that is yet undetected by her physician and health care team. This anxiety primarily is cognitive in nature, disrupts the person's life in that there is worry that leads to frequent health care seeking, but does not lead to a flight or fight response with a robust physiological response. The anxiety clearly is related to the pain, and its possible meaning as a signal of some destructive underlying process. In the other case, an individual with low back pain may experience pain when he engages in mild physical exercise (e.g. lifting a bag of groceries) while recovering from a work-related injury. This pain then evokes a fear response in that it is believed to be a signal that the injury is being exacerbated. The fearful response includes physiological activation (e.g. blood pressure increase, muscle tension) and overt behaviors, such as escape (e.g. putting down the grocery bag) and compensation (e.g. holding one's back), along with verbal reports of pain (e.g. "Ow. I can't even lift a grocery bag. How are those doctors ever going to get me back to work?"). Anxiety and/or fear also can be manifested along with pain, even if they are unrelated. For example, a person with Generalized Anxiety Disorder may worry about finances and the safety of family members, but those concerns can be independent of his arthritis. Similarly, an individual may experience Panic Disorder with Agoraphobia, but this fear can be independent of pelvic pain. It should be noted, however, that in some cases, pain and seemingly unrelated anxiety and/or fear may be conceptually and functionally consistent, such as in the case of social phobia (Asmundson *et al.* 1996) or posttraumatic stress disorder (Asmundson *et al.* 2002). Regardless of their relation, it is important to assess pain as well as fear and anxiety, as these later states, even if unrelated, may interfere with one's ability to cope and to respond to the threat of pain.

Given that assessing fear of (and anxiety about) pain primarily involves the intersection of two constructs—pain and fear (and anxiety)—each of which individually can only be imperfectly measured, there is great challenge in this area. In both the pain and fear/anxiety arenas, there is no "gold standard" by which other measures can be compared. Many conceptualizations of these states rely solely on the self-report of patients, neglecting behaviors (e.g. overt motoric, physiological) other than verbal ones. This approach is problematic in that sometimes these behaviors "speak louder than words," such as in the case of a dental phobic individual sitting in a dental chair, tightly grasping the arms of the chair ("white knuckle syndrome") and sweating profusely, all the while not reporting, or even denying, fears, including those about procedure–related pain.

3 Measurement issues and methods

Generally speaking, behavior can be assessed across three broad domains (Cone 1978), including cognitive/affective, overt/motoric, and physiological; these arenas have been documented across the fear and anxiety (Lang 1968; Hugdahl 1981) and pain literatures (Vlaeyen *et al.* 1995*a*). These content areas may be assessed using various methods, including those involving self-report (nonverbal and verbal), observation by others, and instrument/apparatus (Eifert and Wilson 1991). It is easy to fall into the trap of intermixing the content area to be assessed and the method of assessment, but they are best conceptualized as distinct (Eifert and Wilson 1991).

Although the overt motoric behavior and physiological response (Norton and Asmundson 2003) domains should be co-equal with the cognitive/affective one, the latter is the most frequently assessed, likely because it is often the easiest to measure via self-report. Pain, fear, and anxiety most often are assessed in the cognitive/affective domain (content) with verbal reports (method), what an individual indicates as being reflective of his or her current feeling state. These verbal or self-reports can be in the form of spoken words or ratings, paper-and-pencil responses, marks on visual analog scales, and ratings or other responses using a computer. Verbal reports are limited, as there are cognitive processes that take place outside of conscious awareness. Similarly, memory can adversely affect recall, not only in the cognitive/affective domain, but in the overt behavioral and physiological ones as well.

Pain and fear also can be assessed usefully via observation of overt behaviors, including obvious (e.g. using a cane in walking) and more subtle (e.g. facial expressions) ones. There are great logistical constraints in conducting such assessments, particularly in clinical practice. Nevertheless, the roles of avoidance and escape behaviors are extremely important, and are frequently underestimated. Arntz *et al.* (1990), for example, found that anxious individuals expected more dental pain than nonanxious individuals. The anxious individuals expected more pain than they actually experienced but their actual pain experiences were no different than nonanxious individuals. The anxious persons' recollection of the pain of the experience, however, increased over time, returning to the prior expected level. This finding indicates the key role that avoidance behaviors play in fear of pain. Indeed, whether an individual has a confrontation versus an avoidance behavioral style of responding to pain has been found to be a critical issue (Crombez *et al.* 1998).

More specifically focusing on fear and anxiety related to pain, these negative affective states in *chronic* pain have been classified into three dimensions (Vlaeyen *et al.* 1995). First, there is fear of nociceptive stimulation, fear of the pain itself, focusing on its sensory aspects (Lethem *et al.* 1983; Vlaeyen and Linton 2000). Second, there is a fear of pain-causing activities (Waddell *et al.* 1993). Within this same dimension, there also can be fear of activities that could *potentially* cause pain, similar to the fear of fear seen in certain anxiety disorders. Third, and finally, there is a fear of movement/re-injury (i.e. kinesiophobia; Kori *et al.* 1990). Specifically in this domain, the fear of movement and physical activity is related to assumptions by the patient that it will delay healing or cause (re)injury, and that convalescence is the most appropriate strategy to maintain or improve health and functioning.

The best methods of assessment are, of course, multimodal and multimethod. While it sometimes is the only logistical possibility, relying solely on verbal report as a method is limited. While they can be, and in this area, sometimes are used as a *method* to evaluate motoric behavior and physiological response, the reliability of such reports is questionable. As will be seen later in this chapter, however, the current state of the fear of pain literature is such that self-reports typically are the sole assessment method.

4 Pain-related anxiety and fear assessment strategies

As noted, most of the available literature consists of work on self-report of anxiety about pain, or fear of pain, typically focusing on cognitive and affect-ive states. Therefore, the current review will emphasize these self-report measures. In general, there are four major self-report measures that assess fear of pain; each will be discussed in detail. In addition, self-report measures that have not been as widely utilized, but that, nonetheless, are relevant to pain-related fear and anxiety also will be discussed. Finally, consistent with the three-systems model of fear (Lang 1968), the assessment of physiological and overt behavior domains will be covered.

4.1 Measures of cognition and affect

4.1.1 Fear-Avoidance Beliefs Questionnaire

The Fear-Avoidance Beliefs Questionnaire (FABQ; Waddell *et al.* 1993) consists of 16 items and two subscales: (1) beliefs about possible harm result-ing from physical activity (FABQ-Physical; 5 items), and (2) beliefs about pos-sible harm from work-specific activities (FABQ-Work; 11 items). Items are rated on 0–6 Likert-type scales. Sample items from the physical subscale include: "Physical activity might harm my back" and "I should not do physical activities which (might) make my pain worse." Items from the Work subscale include: "My work makes or would make my pain worse" and "My work aggravated my pain." Waddell *et al.* (1993) reported a 48-h test–retest reliabil-ity across items of 0.74, with all items except two showing a concordance of greater than 0.61. It should be noted, however, that the number of participants in these analyses was rather small (i.e. $N = 26$). In the larger normative sam-ple, the internal consistency of the measure was excellent in both chronic and acute pain, Chronbach's $\alpha = 0.82$ and 0.74, respectively (Waddell *et al.* 1993). Crombez *et al.* (1999), however, found that only the Work subscale has accept-able internal consistency, with αs of 0.84 and 0.92 across two samples, while the αs for the Physical subscale were 0.52 and 0.57, which they attributed to the low number of items on that subscale. Finally, Waddell *et al.* (1993) reported that the subscale scores were moderately related to pain intensity and that the Work subscale was more strongly correlated with measures of disabil-ity and work loss, even after pain intensity was controlled.

The two-factor structure of the measure appears to be relatively robust; however, the original principal–components analysis performed by Waddell *et al.* (1993) indicated that some of the subscale items did not significantly contribute to the factors. These items were excluded from the suggested scoring method; therefore, the FABQ-Physical subscale score includes only four items and the FABQ-Work subscale includes seven items. The utility of the items that are excluded from scoring is unclear. Recent investigations have confirmed that the subscales are differentially related to physical- and work-related activities. Specifically, physical performance on tasks assessing flexibility or weight lifting are more strongly related to the FABQ-Physical subscale (Crombez *et al.* 1999; Al-Obaidi *et al.* 2000) and more work-related issues are differentially related to the Work subscale. The latter issues include work loss (Waddell *et al.* 1993), reported disability for work (Ciccone and Just 2001), work restrictions due to pain complaints (Fritz and George 2002), and treatment-related changes in physical ability for work (Vowles and Gross 2003). Although the scores of the two subscales often are significantly correlated (Crombez *et al.* 1999; George *et al.* 2001; Vowles and Gross 2003), they appear to be assessing different constructs. Collectively these findings provide support for the factor structure of the measure.

4.1.2 Fear of Pain Questionnaire-III

Based on the need to assess fear associated with both acute and chronic pain, across a number of different environmental contexts, and potentially developmentally in the case of injury possibly leading to chronic pain, McNeil and Rainwater (1998) designed the Fear of Pain Questionnaire-III (FPQ-III). The measure was developed for use with both clinical and nonclinical populations and the item content reflects this purpose with participants rating how much they fear the pain associated with specific situations on a 1 (not at all) to 5 (extreme) Likert-type scale. The measure consists of 30 items which can be summed to derive a total score and three subscale scores: Fear of Severe Pain (e.g. "having someone slam a heavy car door on your hand"), Minor Pain (e.g. "biting your tongue while eating"), and Medical/Dental Pain (e.g. "having one of your teeth drilled").

The measure has demonstrated good to excellent internal consistency in both clinical (i.e. headache, chronic pain; Hursey and Jacks 1992; Sperry-Clark *et al.* 1999) and nonclinical populations (McNeil and Rainwater 1998) with subscale and total score αs ranging from 0.86 to 0.95. Similarly, scores on the measure are relatively stable over time, with reported 3 week test–retest reliabilities ranging from 0.69 for the Severe Pain subscale to 0.76 the Medical Pain subscale (McNeil and Rainwater 1998). Further, the three-factor structure is stable (McNeil and Rainwater 1998; Osman *et al.* 2002) and correlational analyses indicate that the FPQ-III relates well to other measures of pain-related fear and general negative affect (Osman *et al.* 2002), although these associations are moderate and suggest that the FPQ-III is assessing a construct separate from the one assessed by these other measures. Furthermore, McNeil and colleagues have used the FPQ-III extensively in dental and orofacial populations, where scores on the FPQ-III account for a significant portion of variability in reported dental fear (McNeil *et al.* 2001). Normative data for both orofacial pain and chronic pain patients have been published (McNeil *et al.* 2001; Sperry-Clark *et al.* 1999, respectively). Confirmatory factor analytic data are available, supporting the three-factor structure of the FPQ-III (McKee *et al.* submitted).

In general, scores have been higher in females and lower in males, relative to one another, although there have been some differences in which subscales were elevated, depending on population. With regard to nonclinical samples, McNeil and Rainwater (1998) found that females reported higher levels of fear of pain across all three subscales, Osman *et al.* (2002) found such differences on the Severe and Medical Pain subscales only. Further, in a sample of 200 individuals with chronic pain, Sperry-Clark *et al.* (1999) reported that the Medical Pain subscale was higher in females. As with many other fear and anxiety verbal report instruments, females report lower scores and males higher ones, although the subscale(s) involved in these differences may differ, depending on population.

A 9-item short form has been developed (Kennedy *et al.* 2001). As is the case with the FPQ-III, a total score and three subscale scores, each consisting of 3 items, can be calculated. Preliminary analyses of the shorter version have indicated a strong relation with the FPQ-III, as well as moderate correlations with other measures of pain-related anxiety and dental fear. Furthermore, the short form retains the excellent internal consistency of the longer version (Chronbach's α ranging from 0.74 to 0.86).

4.1.3 Pain Anxiety Symptoms Scale

The Pain Anxiety Symptoms Scale (PASS; McCracken *et al.* 1992) contains 40 items which are designed to assess behaviors related to the fear of pain. Each item is answered on a 0 (never) to 5 (always) point Likert-type scale and a total score, as well as four subscale scores, can be derived. The 10-item subscales assess avoidance of painful activities (e.g. escape/avoidance; "I try to avoid activities that cause pain"), negative and anxious cognitions associated with pain (e.g. cognitive anxiety; "When I hurt I think about pain constantly"), fearful thinking about pain (e.g. fearful appraisal; "I think that if my pain gets too severe, it will never decrease"), and physiological symptoms of anxiety associated with pain (e.g. physiological anxiety; "When I sense pain, I feel dizzy or faint"). The measure was originally normed on chronic pain patients and has been used almost exclusively within this population, although it has also been utilized to some extent in acute pain populations (i.e. headache; Bishop *et al.* 2001) and non-patients (Osman *et al.* 1994). Across studies, the measure has demonstrated good internal consistency, with reported αs ranging from 0.74 to 0.94 (McCracken *et al.* 1992, 1993). Furthermore, repeated administrations, separated by a period of approximately 14 days, have yielded test–retest correlations of r's ≥ 0.93 among the subscales at different time periods, with the exceptions of the escape/avoidance subscale, which had an $r > 0.77$ across administrations (McCracken *et al.* 1993).

The PASS total score has been more frequently utilized than its subscale scores. The total score is positively correlated with measures of general anxiety, pain, and self-reported disability (McCracken *et al.* 1992; McCracken and Gross 1995; Crombez *et al.* 1999), as well as nonspecific physical complaints (McCracken *et al.* 1998). In addition, the total score is associated with actual physical capacity, as indexed by one's ability to lift or carry certain amounts of weight (Burns *et al.* 2000).

McCracken and colleagues also have investigated the utility of the PASS total score in predicting outcomes following interdisciplinary treatment programs for chronic pain (McCracken and Gross 1998; McCracken *et al.* 2002). Their analyses indicate that changes in PASS total score are important components to treatment-related changes in chronic pain, including improvements in pain intensity, affective distress, self-reported activities, and disability. Further, these improvements were shown to be independent of observed changes in depression and physical ability.

Although the four-factor structure of the measure has been supported by both the original authors (McCracken *et al.* 1992, 1993) and others (Osman *et al.* 1994), Larsen *et al.* (1997) found that a five-factor model, consisting of catastrophic thoughts, cognitive interference, coping strategies, escape/avoidance behaviors, and physiological anxiety symptoms, is more appropriate. Based on these findings, a revised questionnaire was constructed, and was found to consist of five somewhat different lower-order factors (i.e. catastrophic thoughts, interference, approach behaviors, monitoring and prevention, and physiological arousal; McWilliams and Asmundson 1998).

Recently, a shorter 20-item version of the PASS has become available (McCracken and Dhingra 2002). This short form, termed the PASS-20, retains the four subscales of the original measure, as well as its psychometric properties. The normative group included 282 individuals with chronic pain; psychometric analyses indicated that the shortened PASS subscales retained their internal consistency (mean $\alpha = 0.81$) and were highly correlated with the subscales of the original measure (mean $r = 0.95$). Finally, the shorter version was significantly related to measures of pain intensity, depression, and self-reported disability, similar to the relation between these scales and the original PASS (McCracken and Dhringa 2002). Another study with 201 patients referred to a physiotherapy clinic suggested the PASS-20 retained its four-factor structure, and its psychometric properties (Coons *et al.* in press).

4.1.4 Tampa Scale of Kinesphobia

Kori *et al.* (1990) coined the term *kinesiophobia* to refer to an excessive and irrational fear of physical activity resulting from a perceived vulnerability to pain or re-injury. They designed the Tampa Scale of Kinesphobia (TSK) to assess this fear of movement. The original version of the measure includes 17 items, which are summed to obtain a single composite score (Kori *et al.* 1990). Sample items include, "Pain always means I have injured my body" and "If I were to try to overcome it, my pain would increase." Participants rate the degree to which the content of each item applies to them on a 1–4 scale. A Dutch translation of the measure has been widely utilized by Crombez, Vlaeyen, and colleagues who have demonstrated the measure's acceptable internal consistency, with reported Cronbach's αs ranging from 0.68 to 0.80, and normally distributed score profiles (Vlaeyen *et al.* 1995; Crombez *et al.* 1999). The TSK total score is positively related to self-reported disability and negatively related to performance on a back flexion and extension task (Crombez *et al.* 1999).

A shortened version of the TSK has also been suggested (Clark *et al.* 1996). This version contains only 13 items as it excludes 4 of the original items that had poor correlations with the total score. The shortened version of the scale has greater internal consistency than the original (Cronbach's $\alpha = 0.86$; Clark *et al.* 1996) and is composed of two lower-order factors that load on a single higher-order factor (Clark *et al.* 1996; Geisser *et al.* 2000). The first subscale, labeled Pathological Somatic Focus, assesses one's belief that the occurrence of pain indicates underlying serious bodily damage and the second, called Activity Avoidance, assesses beliefs that activities which increase pain should be avoided. Alternately, the first subscale can be conceptualized as assessing the more cognitive and emotional aspects of fear of pain and the second the more behavioral aspects. Geisser *et al.* (2000) found that the Activity Avoidance subscale was more strongly related to floor to waist and waist to shoulder lifting ability than the Pathological Somatic Focus subscale.

A confirmatory factor analysis (Goubert *et al.* 2003) of the original TSK, combining data from eight studies of Dutch and Flemish chronic pain patients, also supported a two-factor model of the measure. The two-factor solution is very similar for both the original and shortened versions, and is suggested as a superior model to an earlier proposed four-factor solution (Vlaeyen *et al.* 1995).

4.1.5 Additional self-report measures

Although the FABQ, FPQ-III, PASS, and TSK have been the most widely utilized assessments of pain-related fear in published studies, some additional measures also exist. These tools include the Burn Specific Pain Anxiety Scale (Taal and Faber 1997), a 9-item scale that focuses on worry and fear associated with procedure pain and wound healing. There is a 6-item Fear Self-Statements subscale, specific to sickle cell disease, which was added to the Coping Strategies Questionnaire (Rosenstiel and Keefe 1983) by Gil *et al.* (1989). The Survey of Pain Attitudes (SOPA; Jensen *et al.* 1987) was originally developed to assess patient attitudes along five rationally derived dimensions, including pain control, pain-related disability, medical cures for pain, solicitude of others, and pain medications. Later, a sixth subscale assessing perceived harm from physical activities was added, which was found to be related to self-report disability (Jensen *et al.* 1994). The relation of the Harm scale to other measures of pain-related fear has not yet been evaluated. The 16-item Pain Sensitivity Index (Gross 1992) focuses on cognitions associated with fear related to pain. The 13-item Pain Catastrophizing Scale evaluates thoughts and feelings while pain is being expressed (Sullivan *et al.* 1995). The 10-item Pain Discomfort Scale (Jensen *et al.* 1991) was developed to assess the emotional component of pain, including 1-item relating to fear. Gottlieb (1994) presented the Pain Beliefs Questionnaire (PBQ), which was designed to evaluate four aspects of an individual's beliefs regarding pain, including disability expectations, self-efficacy, depressogenic cognitions, and pain-related anxiety. The limited amount of data regarding Gottlieb's PBQ has supported its factor structure and demonstrated its ability to differentiate between individuals with and without chronic pain (Gottlieb 1986). Further, Mikail *et al.* (1993) found that the pain-related anxiety factor of the PBQ was moderately related to measures of affective distress. Finally, the 26-item Pain Distress Inventory recently was published. In addition to depression, anger, and pain sensitivity factors, there is a somatic anxiety dimension (Osman *et al.* 2003).

There also are two general measures, reviewed briefly here, that have been used to assess pain-related fear and anxiety. The first of these instruments is the McGill Pain Questionnaire (MPQ). The MPQ contains an Affective subscale, consisting of 14 words in five categories (Melzack 1975). Much more utilized in the pain-related fear and anxiety area is the Anxiety Sensitivity Index (ASI; Peterson and Reiss 1992), which is a 16-item questionnaire that measures fear of the negative consequences of anxiety symptoms. The measure has demonstrated acceptable levels of internal consistency (Telch *et al.* 1989) and test–retest reliability (Mailer and Reiss 1992). The ASI also appears to measure a distinct construct from that tapped by measures of state or trait anxiety (McNally 1994; Schmidt and Cook 1999).

With regard to the ASI's relation to pain-related fear and anxiety, Asmundson and colleagues have argued that high levels of anxiety sensitivity may exacerbate the affective distress and avoidance behavior that is commonly observed in highly fearful individuals with chronic pain (Asmundson and Norton 1995; Asmundson and Taylor 1996; Asmundson 1999; Asmundson *et al.* 1999). Further, other research has supported this assertion by indicating that the ASI is a better predictor of total and subscale scores for both the PASS and FPQ-III than measures of pain severity and depression (Zvolensky *et al.* 2001). This finding led the authors to argue that anxiety sensitivity was perhaps one of the most important predictors of pain-related fear and anxiety. In addition, Asmundson and Taylor (1996) used structural equation modeling to illustrate that anxiety sensitivity directly worsens reported fear of pain, but that it does not directly affect pain-related avoidance behaviors. Instead, the effects of anxiety sensitivity on avoidance behaviors occur via its influence of pain-related fear. In sum, these findings have led some to argue that pain-related fear and anxiety are best conceptualized as a manifestation of anxiety sensitivity (Greenburg and Burns 2003), rather than distinct constructs. Existing data, however, are inconsistent with such an idea, as general anxiety and overall psychological distress (McNeil *et al.* 2001; Thornsgaard *et al.* 1992) have only been found to have a low to moderate relation between FPQ-III scores and measures of these constructs.

4.1.6 Measurement of cognition and affect using instrumentation and apparatus

There are cognitive processing tests that have been used experimentally with pain patients, in part assessing emotionality associated with pain. There are several studies that have employed the Stroop color-naming test (e.g. Pearce and Morley 1989). Some studies have found both generalized (i.e. response slowing to all stimuli) and specific (i.e. response slowing to emotional or pain-related stimuli) effects (e.g. Beck *et al.* 2001). Other studies have found only generalized effects (e.g. Duckworth *et al.* 1997; Pincus *et al.* 1998). A related study using the dot probe paradigm suggested the importance of anxiety sensitivity in pain patients' responses to pain and injury-related words (Asmundson *et al.* 1997). These methodologies are in an early stage of development in this area, but have great potential promise in teasing apart the relative effects of pain relative to anxiety and fear. These studies are discussed and reviewed in more detail in Chapter 4.

4.2 **Physiological measures**

The importance of psychophysiological recording has become increasingly recognized in the understanding of psychopathological states, particularly the anxiety disorders (Turpin 1991). This has implications for the understanding of pain-related fear and anxiety. Physiological measures may be particularly important in the teasing apart of fear and anxiety reactions associated with pain, as there is believed to be greater reactivity in the former state and lesser in the latter one (e.g. McNeil *et al.* 1993). In the general pain area, our understanding of psychophysiology is rudimentary (Flor *et al.* 2001). Over the past two decades, however, Flor and her colleagues have maintained an important program of psychophysiological pain research, including both peripheral measures (e.g. electromyography and cardiovascular assessment) and central ones (e.g. electroencephalogram and event-related potentials).

As already noted, the work that has been performed regarding the assessment of fear and anxiety associated with pain has almost exclusively used self-report. Work in our laboratory with nonclinical research participants, however, has included the assessment of heart rate and muscle tension (Carter *et al.* 2002). Assessing pain responsivity in the presence of various emotional states, psychophysiological responding was found to decline over a sequence of pain episodes, and responsivity was affected by gender of participant and experimenter. Consistent with theoretical ideas about the anxiety state included in this experiment, no strong physiological reactivity was noted; fear was not assessed in this paradigm. Rainwater (1989) found suggestions of greater heart rate reactivity in nonclinical participants high in fear of pain, versus those with low scorers on the FPQ. Other work from our research group has included acute pain endodontic patients, and measurement of heart rate reactivity and cortisol responsivity (Gochenour 2003; Sorrell 2003). Certain fear-provoking steps (e.g. injection) elicited strong cardiac response during root canal therapy, while cortisol response was found to be high prior to the procedure, then to decrease, and then to increase back to initial levels immediately after the procedure.

Conceptually, assessment of psychophysiological responding is relatively neglected among the community of researchers in this area, although it is conceptually important. Norton and Asmundson (2003), for example, suggested an amendment to the fear-avoidance model of chronic pain, to include psychophysiological responding. The even more contemporary model that includes both fear and anxiety as separate constructs, also specifically includes autonomic arousal as an important feature (see Chapter 1). Nevertheless, there is little methodological attention paid to psychophysiological measures in this area. For the science to fully progress, consistent with a three-systems understanding of fear, such measures must be included as part of a comprehensive assessment in both clinical and research arenas.

4.3 Overt behavior measures

The general pain literature has paid some attention to body posturing, avoidance and escape behavior, and social behavior relating to pain (e.g. Keefe *et al.* 2001). Additionally, facial expressions associated with pain have generated some interest (e.g. Craig *et al.* 2001). Nevertheless, as with psychophysiological methods, overt behavioral assessment is significantly underdeveloped relative to self-report. Paralleling the general literature, assessment of overt behaviors associated with fear and anxiety relating to pain is in an early developmental stage.

There are, however, numerous studies that have found differences in physical performance among different individuals that can be accounted for by levels of pain-related fear or anxiety. Across studies, self-reported levels of pain-related fear and anxiety are strongly correlated with physical performance; although these correlational designs do not allow evaluation of causation, it appears that fear and anxiety are of critical importance in the determination of physical performance, as noted earlier in this chapter (e.g. Crombez *et al.* 1999).

Measures of physical impairment (e.g. Waddell *et al.* 1992) hold some promise for evaluation in this area, as they can be reflective not only of injury and disease states, but also of pain-related fear and anxiety. Some efforts have directly compared impairment measures with fear-avoidance beliefs (e.g. Fritz *et al.* 2001). Perhaps even more promising a methodology than measures of impairment are the functional capacity evaluations used by physical therapists, as they include more "real world" tasks that may more readily evoke avoidance and escape behaviors. This avenue of research remains to be explored.

Assessment of facial expressions would seem to hold significant promise for this field, given the existing literatures in the areas of pain (Craig *et al.* 2001) and general emotion (Zajonc 1985). Since specific patterns of facial muscle activity have been identified with pain (Craig *et al.* 2001) and emotions such as fear (Zajonc 1985), facial expressions would seem an ideal means for making comparisons of similarity and differences between these states. Such an approach may allow a sophisticated assessment of possible synergistic, competitive, or parallel processes involved in the sequential and/or simultaneous experience of pain with fear or anxiety. Moreover, facial feedback models have the potential to aid in understanding the development of chronic pain (Adelmann and Zajonc 1989).

Although not specifically a method of assessment, it should be noted that Vlaeyen and colleagues have published a series of papers highlighting the utility of direct exposure to physical activities as a treatment for reducing fear of pain (Vlaeyen *et al.* 2002*a,b,c*; also see Chapter 14). In sum, these papers suggest that pain-related fears are reduced only when patients are presented with a set of activities individually tailored to address pain-specific concerns and not when activity is merely increased over time. Therefore, an ideographic approach may be important during the assessment phase of treatment in order to clearly identify activities that provoke fear and/or anxiety for the individual.

Assessment of overt behaviors that are part of the constellation of pain-related fear and anxiety presently is an underdeveloped area. Nevertheless, evolving methodologies in facial expression, functional capacity evaluations, and physical activity/pain exposure present significant opportunities to further our understanding of these states in terms of their development and basic cognitive and emotional structure.

5 Conclusion

No longer in its infancy, the literature on fear of pain is developing and evolving well. The state of the science in assessing fear and anxiety associated with pain is at a stage that can allow exploration of the construct, testing of conceptual models, and evaluating the outcome of clinical treatments, much as a toddler would explore his world once he has learned to walk. Nevertheless, much work remains in the arena of assessment of pain-related fear and anxiety. Future directions include refinement of existing verbal report instruments and development of new ones. Observational methods are needed to tease apart the relative contributions of fear/anxiety and pain to overt behavior (e.g. facial expressions). We echo the sentiments of Vlaeyen and Linton (2000), who note that there is a clear need for further work in the assessment of overt behaviors associated with levels of pain-related fear and anxiety. Experimental and clinical work is needed to include psychophysiological methods, as they, along with overt behavioral measures, have been neglected in this area.

As an observational method, standardization of assessment of physical ability is greatly needed. There are a variety of tasks which have been used to assess physical/functional abilities within chronic pain and the major conclusion has been that fear and anxiety associated with pain generally are strongly related to this physical functioning. However, given the breadth of types of physical tasks that have been utilized, it is difficult to draw conclusions across studies and determine why different facets of pain-related fear and anxiety are differentially related to different behaviors. Examples of physical assessment modalities include chest press, leg lift, and lumbar flexion/extension. One possibility is to use tests already utilized by physical therapists (e.g. functional capacity evaluations.)

It is encouraging to see that this field is beginning to acknowledge differences between fear and anxiety responses associated with pain (McNeil and Rainwater 1998; also see Chapter 1). This growing emphasis follows from conceptual advances in the general anxiety and fear literature. Nevertheless, this evolution should involve related states, such as stress and pain, which has its own, separate literature. Only by ultimately including a variety of emotions (e.g. depression, stress, anxiety, and fear) will this field maximally progress (see Keefe *et al.* 2001).

Test selection remains as an issue, although not too much emphasis should be encouraged here, given the present over-reliance on self-reports to the exclusion of other methods of assessment. Given the comparable findings between the self-report measures reviewed in this chapter, is one measure as good as any other? All appear to have adequate to good psychometric properties and have been utilized in appropriate populations. Each has demonstrated the importance of fear of pain construct in relation to other theoretically or empirically relevant constructs. Although few studies have directly compared the measures with one another, a limited amount of data does exist. First, McCracken *et al.* (1996) correlated the trait form of the State-Trait Anxiety Inventory (STAI; Spielberger *et al.* 1983), FPQ-III, FABQ, and PASS with various self-report measures related to pain severity, perceived disability, and pain behaviors, using a small ($N = 45$) sample of general chronic pain patients. The authors concluded that anxiety- and fear-related responses that are specifically related to pain are more useful than general measures of anxiety in the prediction of pain-related distress. As noted earlier, however, other data suggest the importance of general anxiety proneness (e.g. the ASI) in predicting anxiety and fear associated with pain (Zvolensky *et al.* 2001). In a related study, Crombez *et al.* (1999) utilized the FABQ, TSK, and PASS in order to assess the role of pain-related fear in reported disability across three samples of low back pain patients. Their results suggested that the TSK and FABQ were more strongly associated with self-reported disability and poor behavioral performance than was the PASS. The PASS was more closely related with measures of negative affect and pain catastrophizing. Randall *et al.* (1994) directly compared the FPQ-III and PASS, finding that each scale significantly predicted pain behavior, although they differed in whether it was threshold (i.e. PASS) or tolerance (i.e. FPQ-III). Given these results, there is evidence to suggest that the FABQ and TSK specifically assess the potential for avoidance (or confrontation) of potentially fearful activities in terms of behavioral performance and that the PASS may be more related to psychosocial and emotional aspects of fear or pain

(Crombez *et al.* 1999). As noted above, however, the escape/avoidance subscale of the PASS, which theoretically is supposed to assess potential for avoidance, has yet to be evaluated in relation to avoidance behaviors. In addition, the FPQ-III was originally designed to assess the influence of fear and anxiety about pain across many life domains; thus, it has been argued that it is a more general measure of one's potential to avoid painful, or potentially painful, situations (McNeil and Rainwater 1998), especially those involving acute pain. In fact, available research suggests that the FPQ-III is useful in the assessment of psychosocial distress in headache patients (Hursey and Jacks 1992) and dental/-orofacial pain patients (McNeil *et al.* 2001). As the FPQ-III can assess pain-related fear and anxiety before pain becomes chronic, it may be particularly useful in predicting the development of such syndromes. This issue of test selection is not one of "Which measure is best?" but is a matter of which measure or measures best taps the population or concept under investigation.

Finally, it is important to note the moderate relation between pain intensity and fear across studies (e.g. Waddell *et al.* 1993). This finding suggests that pain intensity, which has historically been regarded as one of the key outcome measures in evaluating the efficacy of chronic pain treatment (see Turk and Okifuji 2002 for a review), may not be as centrally important as previously believed. Others variables that have been shown to predict pain-related distress, disability, physical ability, and treatment outcome—and pain-related fear and anxiety in particular (Vlaeyen *et al.* 1995; McCracken and Gross 1998; Geisser *et al.* 2000; McCracken *et al.* 2002)—may be as or more critical.

It is hoped that comprehensive clinical evaluation of chronic pain patients will, in the future, include assessment of pain-related fear and anxiety. Assessment of highly fearful and/or anxious patients necessarily should include other emotional states, particularly depression. Acute exacerbations of chronic pain may elicit the most fear, and so methodologies should be developed specifically to evaluate such stages. Nevertheless, in order to fully advance this field, pain-related fear and anxiety must be studied not only in people with chronic pain but also in those who are healthy and those with acute pain. This will allow for the further understanding of the etiology, maintenance, and exacerbation of chronic pain.

References

Adelman, P.K. and Zajonc, R.B. (1989). Facial efference and the experience of emotion. *Annual Review of Psychology*, **40**, 249–80.

Al-Obaidi, S.M., Nelson, R.M., Al-Awadhi, S., and Al-Shuwaie, N. (2000). The role of anticipation and fear of pain in the persistence of avoidance behavior in patients with chronic low back pain. *Spine*, **25**, 1126–31.

Arntz, A., van Eek, M., and Heijmans, M. (1990). Predictions of dental pain: The fear of any expected evil is worse than the evil itself. *Behaviour Research and Therapy*, **28**, 29–41.

Asmundson, G.J.G. (1999). Anxiety sensitivity and chronic pain: Empirical findings, clinical implications, and future directions. In S. Taylor (ed.), *Anxiety Sensitivity: Theory, Research, and Treatment of the Fear of Anxiety*. Mahwah, NJ: Erlbaum.

Asmundson, G.J.G. and Norton, G.R. (1995). Anxiety sensitivity in patients with physically unexplained chronic back pain: A preliminary report. *Behaviour Research and Therapy*, **33**, 771–7.

Asmundson, G.J.G. and Taylor, S. (1996). Role of anxiety sensitivity in pain-related fear and avoidance. *Journal of Behavioral Medicine*, **19**, 577–86.

Asmundson, G.J.G., Kuperos, J.L., and Norton, G.R. (1997). Do patients with chronic pain selectively attend to pain-related information?: Preliminary evidence for the mediating role of fear. *Pain*, **72**, 27–32.

Asmundson, G.J.G., Jacobson, S.J., Allerdings, M.D., and Norton, G.R. (1996). Social phobia in disabled workers with chronic musculoskeletal pain. *Behaviour Research and Therapy*, **34**, 939–43.

Asmundson, G.J.G., Norton, P.J., and Norton, G.R. (1999). Beyond pain: The role of fear and avoidance in chronicity. *Clinical Psychology Review*, **19**, 97–119.

Asmundson, G.J.G., Coons, M.J., Taylor, S., and Katz, J. (2002). PTSD and the experience of pain: Research and clinical implications of shared vulnerability and mutual maintenance models. *Canadian Journal of Psychiatry*, **47**, 930–7.

Barlow, D.G. (2002). *Anxiety and its Disorders: The Nature and Treatment of Anxiety and Panic*, 2nd edn. New York, NY: Guilford.

Beck, J.G., Freeman, J.B., Shipherd, J.C., Hamblen, J.L., and Lackner, J.M. (2001). Specificity of Stroop interference in patients with pain and PTSD. *Journal of Abnormal Psychology*, **110**, 536–43.

Birbaumer, N. and Öhman, A. (1993). *The Structure of Emotion*. Seattle, WA: Hogrefe & Huber.

Bishop, K.L., Holm, J.E., Borowiak, D.M., and Wilson, B.A. (2001). Perceptions of pain in women with headache: A laboratory investigation of the influence of pain-related anxiety and fear. *Headache*, **41**, 494–9.

Bolles, R.C. and Fanselow, M.S. (1980). A perceptual-defensive-recuperative model of fear and pain. *Behavioral and Brain Sciences*, **3**, 291–323.

Burns, J.W., Mullen, J.T., Higdon, L.J., Wei, J.M., and Lansky D. (2000). Validity of the Pain Anxiety Symptoms Scale (PASS): Prediction of physical capacity variables. *Pain*, **84**, 247–52.

Carter, L.E., McNeil, D.W., Vowles, K.E., Sorrell, J.T., Turk, C.L., Ries, B.J., and Hopko, D.R. (2002). Effects of emotion on pain reports, tolerance, and physiology. *Pain Research and Management*, **7**, 21–30.

Ciccone, D.S. and Just, N. (2001). Pain expectancy and work disability inpatients with acute and chronic pain: A test of the fear avoidance hypothesis. *The Journal of Pain*, **2**, 181–94.

Clark, M.E., Kori, S.H., and Brockel, J. (1996). Kinesiophobia and chronic pain: Psychometric characteristics and factor analysis of the Tampa Scale. *American Pain Society Abstracts*, **15**, 77.

Cleeland, C.S. (1986). How to treat a "construct". *Journal of Pain and Symptom Management*, **1**, 161–2.

Cone, J.D. (1978). The Behavioral Assessment Grid (BAG): A conceptual framework and a taxonomy. *Behavior Therapy*, **9**, 882–8.

Coons, M.J., Hadjistavropoulos, H.D., and Asmundson, G.J.G. (in press). *Psychometric Properties of the Pain Anxiety Symptoms Scale—20*. European Journal of Pain.

Craig, K.D., Prkachin, K.M., and Grunau, R.V.E. (2001). The facial expression of pain. In D.C. Turk and R. Melzack (eds.), *Handbook of Pain Assessment*, 2nd edn, pp. 153–69. New York, NY: Guilford.

Craske, M.G. (1999). *Anxiety Disorders: Psychological Approaches to Theory and Treatment*. Boulder, CO: Westview Press.

Crombez, G., Vervaet, L., Lysens, R., Baeyens, F., and Eelen, P. (1998). Avoidance and confrontation of painful, back-straining movements in chronic back pain patients. *Behavior Modification*, **22**, 62–77.

Crombez, G., Vlaeyen, J.W.S., Heuts, P.H.T.G., and Lysens, R. (1999). Pain-related fear is more disabling than pain itself: Evidence on the role of pain-related fear in chronic back pain disability. *Pain*, **80**, 329–39.

Duckworth, M.P., Iezzi, A., Adams, H.E., and Hale, D. (1997). Information processing in chronic pain disorder: A preliminary analysis. *Journal of Psychopathology and Behavioral Assessment*, **19**, 239–55.

Eifert, G.H. and Wilson, P.H. (1991). The triple response approach to assessment: A conceptual and methodological reappraisal. *Behaviour Research and Therapy*, **29**, 283–92.

Flor, H., Miltner, W., and Birbaumer, N. (2001). Psychophysiological recording methods. In D.C. Turk and R. Melzack (eds.), *Handbook of Pain Assessment*, 2nd edn., pp. 76–96. New York, NY: Guilford.

Fritz, J.M. and George, S.Z. (2002). Identifying psychosocial variables in patients with acute work-related low back pain: The importance of fear-avoidance beliefs. *Physical Therapy*, **82**, 973–83.

Fritz, J.M., George, S.Z., and Delitto, A. (2001). The role of fear-avoidance beliefs in acute low back pain: Relationships with current and future disability and work status. *Pain*, **94**, 7–15.

Geisser, M.E., Haig, A.J., and Theisen, M.E. (2000). Activity avoidance and function in persons with chronic back pain. *Journal of Occupational Rehabilitation*, **10**, 215–27.

George, S.Z., Fritz, J.M., and Erhard, R.E. (2001). A comparison of fear-avoidance beliefs in patients with lumbar spine pain and cervical spine pain. *Spine*, **26**, 2139–45.

Gil, K.M., Abrams, M.R., Phillips, G., and Keefe, F.J. (1989). Sickle cell disease: Relation of coping strategies to adjustment. *Journal of Consulting and Clinical Psychology*, **57**, 725–31.

Gochenour, L.L. (2003). Cortisol Responsivity: Association with Fear and Pain Related to Root Canal Therapy. Unpublished Master's Thesis, West Virginia University, Morgantown, WV.

Gottlieb, B.S. (1984, November). Development of the Pain Beliefs Questionnaire: A preliminary Report. Paper presented at the meeting of the Association for Advancement of Behavior Therapy, Philadelphia, PA.

Gottlieb, B.S. (1986, August). Predicting Outcome in Pain Programs: A Matter of Cognition. Paper presented at the meeting of the American Psychological Association, Washington, DC.

Goubert, L., Crombez, G., Van Damme, S., Vlaeyen, J.W.S., Bijttebier, P., and Roelofs, J. (2004). Confirmatory factor analysis of the Tampa Scale for Kinesiophobia: Invariant two-factor model across low back pain patients and fibromyalgia patients. *Clinical Journal of Pain*, **20**, 103–10

Greenburg, J. and Burns, J.W. (2003). Pain anxiety among chronic pain patients: Specific phobia or manifestation of anxiety sensitivity? *Behaviour Research and Therapy*, **41**, 223–40.

Gross, P.R. (1992). Is pain sensitivity associated with dental avoidance? *Behaviour Research and Therapy*, **30**, 7–13.

Gross, R.T. and Collins, F.L. Jr. (1981). On the relationship between anxiety and pain: A methodological confounding. *Clinical Psychology Review*, **1**, 375–86.

Hugdahl, K. (1981). The three-systems-model of fear and emotion: A critical examination. *Behaviour Research and Therapy*, **19**, 75–85.

Hursey, K.G. and Jacks, S.D. (1992). Fear of pain in recurrent headache suffers. *Headache*, **32**, 283–6.

Jensen, M.P., Karoly, P., and Huger, R. (1987). The development and preliminary validation of an instrument to assess patients' attitudes toward pain. *Journal of Psychosomatic Research*, **31**, 393–400.

Jensen, M.P., Turner, J.A., Romano, J.A., and Lawler, B.K. (1994). Relationship of pain-specific beliefs to chronic pain adjustment. *Pain*, **57**, 301–9.

Keefe, F.J., Williams, D.A., and Smith, S.J. (2001). Assessment of pain behaviors. In D.C. Turk and R. Melzack (eds.), *Handbook of Pain Assessment*, 2nd edn., pp. 170–87. New York, NY: Guilford.

Keefe, F.J., Lumley, M., Anderson, T., Lynch, T., and Carson, K.L. (2001). Pain and emotion: New research directions. *Journal of Clinical Psychology*, **57**, 587–607.

Kennedy, S.G., McNeil, D.W., Hursey, K.G., Vowles, K.E., Sorrell, J.T., Lawrence, S.M., Patthoff, E.B., Whipkey, D.T., Broadman, L.M., Vaglienti, R.M., and Huber, S.J. (2001). Development of a Short Form of the Fear of Pain Questionnaire. Poster presented at the meeting of the Association for the Advancement of Behavior Therapy, Philadelphia, PA.

Klepac, R.K. (1986). Fear and avoidance of dental treatment in adults. *Annals of Behavioral Medicine*, **8**, 17–22.

Kori, S.H., Miller, R.P., and Todd, D.D. (1990). Kinisophobia: A new view of chronic pain behavior. *Pain Management*, **Jan/Feb**, 35–43.

Lang, P.J. (1968). Fear reduction and fear behavior: Problems in treating a construct. In J.M. Shilien (ed.), *Research in Psychotherapy*, Vol. III. Washington, DC: American Psychological Association.

Lang, P.J. (1985). The cognitive psychophysiology of emotion: Fear and anxiety. In A.H. Tuma and J.D. Maser (eds.), *Anxiety and the Anxiety Disorders*. Hillsdale, NJ: Lawrence Erlbaum.

Larsen, D.K., Taylor, S., and Asmundson, G.J.G. (1997). Exploratory factor analysis of the Pain Anxiety Symptoms Scale in patients with chronic pain complaints. *Pain*, **69**, 27–34.

Lethem, J., Slade, P.D., Troup, J.D.G., and Bentley, G. (1983). Outline of a fear-avoidance model of exaggerated pain perception—I. *Behaviour Research and Therapy*, **21**, 401–8.

Mailer, R.G. and Reiss, S. (1992). Anxiety sensitivity in 1984 and panic attacks in 1987. *Journal of Anxiety Disorders*, **6**, 241–7.

McCracken, L.M. and Dhingra, L. (2002). A short version of the Pain Anxiety Symptoms Scale (PASS-20): Preliminary development and validity. *Pain Research and Management*, **7**, 45–50.

McCracken, L.M. and Gross, R.T. (1995). The Pain Anxiety Symptoms Scale (PASS) and the assessment of emotional responses to pain. In L. VandeCreek, S. Knapp, and T.L. Jackson (eds.), *Innovations in Clinical Practice: A Sourcebook*, Vol. 14, pp. 309–21. Sarasota, FL: Professional Resources Press.

McCracken, L.M. and Gross, R.T. (1998). The role of pain-related anxiety reduction in the outcome of multidisciplinary treatment for chronic low back pain: Preliminary results. *Journal of Occupational Rehabilitation*, **8**, 179–89.

McCracken, L.M., Zayfert, C., and Gross, R.T. (1992). The pain anxiety symptom scale: Development and validation of a scale to measure fear of pain. *Pain*, **50**, 67–73.

McCracken, L.M., Zayfert, C., and Gross, R.T. (1993). The Pain Anxiety Symptoms Scale: A multimodal measure of pain specific anxiety symptoms. *The Behavior Therapist*, **16**, 183–4.

McCracken, L.M., Gross, R.T., Aikens, J., and Carnrike, C.L.M. (1996). The assessment of anxiety and fear in persons with chronic pain: A comparison of instruments. *Behaviour Research and Therapy*, **34**, 927–33.

McCracken, L.M., Faber, S.D., and Janeck, A.S. (1998). Pain-related anxiety predicts non-specific physical complaints in persons with chronic pain. *Behaviour Research and Therapy*, **36**, 621–30.

McCracken, L.M., Gross, R.T., and Eccleston, C. (2002). Multimethod assessment of treatment process in chronic low back pain: Comparison of reported pain-related anxiety with directly measured physical capacity. *Behaviour Research and Therapy*, **40**, 585–94.

McKee, D.R., McNeil, D.W., Zvolensky, M.J., Weaver, B.D., Graves, R.W., and Cohen S.H. (submitted). *Psychometric evaluation of the Fear of Pain Questionnaire—III in oral surgery patients*. Manuscript submitted for publication.

McNally, R.J. (1994). *Panic Disorder: A Critical Analysis*. New York, NY: Guilford.

McNeil, D.W. and Rainwater, A.J. (1998). Development of the Fear of Pain Questionnaire-III. *Journal of Behavioral Medicine*, **21**, 389–409.

McNeil, D.W., Vrana, S.R., Melamed, B.G., Cuthbert, B.N., and Lang, P.J. (1993). Emotional imagery in simple and social phobia: Fear versus anxiety. *Journal of Abnormal Psychology*, **102**, 212–25.

McNeil, D.W., Au, A.R., Zvolensky, M.J., McKee, D.R., Klineberg, I.J., and Ho, C.C.K. (2001). Fear of pain in orofacial pain patients. *Pain*, **89**, 245–52.

McWilliams, L.A. and Asmundson, G.J.G. (1998). Factor structure and validity of a revised pain anxiety symptom scale. *International Journal of Rehabilitation and Health*, **4**, 95–109.

Melzack, R. (1975). The McGill pain Questionnaire: Major properties and scoring methods. *Pain*, **1**, 277–99.

Mikail, S.F., DuBreuil, S., and D'Eon, J.L. (1993). A comparative analysis of measures used in the assessment of chronic pain patients. *Psychological Assessment*, **5**, 117–20.

Norton, P.J., and Asmundson, G.J.G. (2003). Amending the fear-avoidance model of chronic pain: What is the role of physiological arousal. *Behavior Therapy*, **34**, 17–30.

Osman, A., Barrios, F.X., Osman, J.R., Schneekloth, R., and Troutman, J.A. (1994). The Pain Anxiety Symptoms Scale: Psychometric properties in a community sample. *Journal of Behavioral Medicine*, **17**, 511–22.

Osman, A., Breitenstein, J.L., Barrios, F.X., Gutierrez, P.M., and Kopper, B.A. (2002). The Fear of Pain Questionnaire-III: Further reliability and validity with nonclinical samples. *Journal of Behavioral Medicine*, **25**, 155–73.

Osman, A., Barrios, F.X., Gutierrez, P.M., Kopper, B.A., Butler, A., and Bagge, C.L. (2003). The Pain Distress Inventory: Development and initial psychometric properties. *Journal of Clinical Psychology*, **59**, 767–85.

Pearce, S., and Morley, S. (1989). An experimental investigation of the construct validity of the McGill Pain Questionnaire, *Pain*, **39**, 115–21.

Peterson, R.A. and Reiss, S. (1992). *Anxiety Sensitivity Index manual*, 2nd edn., Worthinton, OH: International Diagnostic Systems.

Pincus, T., Fraser, L., and Pearce, S. (1998). Do chronic pain patients "Stroop" on pain stimuli? *British Journal of Clinical Psychology*, **37**, 49–58.

Rainwater, A.J. III. (1989). The role of experienced pain in the assessment of fear of pain: A predictive validity study of the Fear of Pain Questionairre-III. Unpublished doctoral dissertation. Oklahoma State University, Stillwater.

Randall, C.J., McChargue, D.E., Carter, L.E., Kersh, B.C., Porter, C.A., Nealey, J., Ries, B.J., Turk, C.L., Robinson, E.G., and McNeil, D.W. (1994, April). Comparison of Current Verbal Report Measures of Fears about Pain. Poster presented at the meeting of the Southwestern Psychological Association, Tulsa, OK.

Robinson, M.E. and Riley, J.L. III. (1999). The role of emotion in pain. In R.J. Gatchel and D.C. Turk (eds.), *Psychosocial Factors in Pain: Critical Perspectives*. New York, NY: Guilford.

Rosentiel, A.K. and Keefe, F.J. (1983). The use of coping strategies in low back pain patients: Relationship to patient characteristics and current adjustment. *Pain*, **17**, 33–40.

Schmidt, N.B. and Cook, J.H. (1999). Effects of anxiety sensitivity on anxiety and pain during a cold pressor challenge in patients with panic disorder. *Behaviour Research and Therapy*, **37**, 313–23.

Sorrell, J.T. (2003). Effects of Fear of Dental Pain and Information Type on Fear and Pain Responding During Endodontic Treatment. Unpublished Doctoral Dissertation, West Virginia University, Morgantown, WV.

Sperry-Clark, J.A., McNeil, D.W., and Ciano-Federoff, L. (1999). Assessing chronic pain patients: The Fear of Pain Questionnaire-III. In L. VandeCreek and T.L. Jackson (eds.), *Innovations in Clinical Practice: A Source Book*, Vol. 17, pp. 293–305. Sarasota, FL: Professional Resource Press.

Spielberger, C.D., Gorsuch, R.L., Lushene, P.R., Vagg, P.R., and Jacobs, G.A. (1983). *Manual for the State-Trait Anxiety Inventory (Form Y)*. Palo Alto, CA: Consulting Psychologists Press.

Sullivan, M.J.L., Bishop, S.R., and Pirik, J. (1995). The Burn Specific Pain Anxiety Scale: Introduction of a reliable and valid measure. *Burns*, **23**, 147–50.

Taal, L.A. and Faber, A.W. (1997). The burn specific pain anxiety scale: Introduction of reliable and valid measure. *Burn*, **23**, 147–50.

Telch, M.J., Shermis, M.D., and Lucas, J.A. (1989). Anxiety sensitivity: Unitary personality trait or domain specific appraisals? *Journal of Anxiety Disorders*, **3**, 25–32.

Thornsgaard, S., Hursey, K.G., Oliver, K.C., and McGruder, A.K. (1992). The Fear of Pain Questionnaire: Reliability and Validity in Recurrent Tension Headache Sufferers. Poster presented at the meeting of the Association for Advancement of Behavior Therapy, Boston, MA.

Turk, D.C. and OkiFuji, A. (2003). Psychological factors in chronic pain: Evolution and revolution. *Journal of Consulting and Clinical Psychology*, **70**, 78–90.

Turpin, G. (1991). The psychophysiological assessment of anxiety disorders: Three-systems measurement and beyond. *Psychological Assessment*, **3**, 366–75.

Vlaeyen, J.W.S. and Linton, S.J. (2000). Fear-avoidance and its consequences in chronic musculoskeletal pain: A state of the art. *Pain*, **85**, 317–32.

Vlaeyen, J.W.S., Kole-Snijders, A.M.J., Boeren, R.G.B., and van Eek, H. (1995*a*). Fear of movement/(re)injury in chronic low back pain and its relation to behavioral performance. *Pain*, **62**, 363–72.

Vlaeyen, J.W.S., Kole-Snijders, A.M.J., Rotteveel, A.M., Ruesink, R., and Heuts, P.H.T.G. (1995*b*). The role of fear of movement/(re)injury in pain disability. *Journal of Occupational Rehabilitation*, **5**, 235–52.

Vlaeyen, J.W.S., de Jong, J., Sieben, J., and Crombez, G. (2002*a*). Graded exposure *in vivo* for pain-related fear. In C. Turk and R.J. Gatchel (eds.), *Psychological Approaches to Pain Management: A Practitioner's Handbook*, 2nd edn. New York, NY: Guilford Press.

Vlaeyen, J.W.S., de Jong, J., Geilen, M., Heuts, P.H.T.G., and van Breukelen, G. (2002*b*). The treatment of fear of movement/(re)injury in chronic low back pain: Further evidence on the effectiveness of exposure *in vivo*. *Clinical Journal of Pain*, **18**, 251–61.

Vlaeyen, J.W.S., de Jong, J.R., Onghena, P., Kerckhoffs-Hanssen, M., and Kole-Snijders, A.M.J. (2002*c*). Can pain-related fear be reduced? The application of cognitivie–behavioural exposure *in vivo*. *Pain Research and Management*, **7**, 144–53.

Vowles, K.E. and Gross, R.T. (2003). Work-related beliefs about injury and physical capability for work in individuals with chronic pain. *Pain*, **101**, 291–8.

Waddell, G., Somerville, D., Henderson, I., and Newton, M. (1992). Objective clinical evaluation of physical impairment in chronic low back pain. *Spine*, **17**, 617–28.

Waddell, G., Newton, M., Henderson, I., Somerville, D., and Main, C. (1993). A Fear-Avoidance Beliefs Questionnaire (FABQ) and the role of fear-avoidance in chronic low back pain and disability. *Pain*, **52**, 157–68.

Weisenberg, M., Aviram, O., Wolf, Y., and Raphaeli, N. (1984). Relevant and irrelevant anxiety in the reaction to pain. *Pain*, **20**, 371–83.

Zajonc, R.B. (1985). Emotion and facial efference: A theory reclaimed. *Science*, **228**, 15–21.

Zvolensky, M.J., Goodie, J.L., McNeil, D.W., Sperry, J.S., and Sorrell, J.T. (2001). Anxiety sensitivity in the prediction of pain-related fear and anxiety in a heterogeneous chronic pain population. *Behaviour Research and Therapy*, **39**, 683–96.

Chapter 10

The role of fear-avoidance in the early identification of patients risking the development of disability

Steven J. Linton and Katja Boersma

1 Introduction

Because fear-avoidance beliefs are strongly related to chronic pain, it appears logical that fear-avoidance might be used to predict which patients will develop long-term pain and disability. Indeed, as only a small percentage of the large numbers of patients suffering an acute bout of back pain actually go on to develop chronic problems, early identification is essential for determining who should receive early, preventive interventions. The purpose of this chapter is twofold. First, we will consider the possible use of fear-avoidance, in relation to other psychological factors, in the early identification of patients with spinal pain who risk developing persistent pain and disability. To accomplish this, we will appraise the literature on the fear-avoidance model asking the question of whether these concepts and variables may be used to predict future disability. Second, we will contemplate how clinical screening procedures might best be employed. Rather than simply using a cut-off point to determine high versus low risk, we argue that combining psychological variables, with fear-avoidance in the forefront, provides a unique opportunity for priming a behavioral analysis, developing appropriate targets, and enhancing communication with the patient.

Since the term *fear-avoidance* is used to mean various things, it is important to note that in this chapter we refer to the fear-avoidance model (Vlaeyen *et al.* 1995) and use it as a frame of reference. Therefore, when we refer to fear-avoidance we mean the entire concept, featuring beliefs, catastrophizing, fear and avoidance as opposed to a score on a particular questionnaire. This is an important distinction since there are a relatively large number of instruments that measure one specific aspect of fear-avoidance (see Chapter 9), although the model encompasses many factors. If we are to employ the concept of fear-avoidance in screening, it is imperative that we are clear as to which variables we are dealing with.

Indeed, there is a clear need for the early identification of patients who are at risk of developing persistent pain and disability. Although up to 85 percent of the population at some time may seek care for spinal pain, only 5–10 percent actually develop chronic problems. Treating every patient seeking care for back pain with a secondary preventive intervention would therefore require enormous resources. However, it also appears that initiating a proper intervention early on is essential for preventing long-term problems (Marhold *et al.* 2001). Thus, early identification is needed so that appropriate interventions may be initiated at the proper point in time.

Early identification normally involves screening procedures. Screening is simply a rough assessment to narrow down the number of patients who need to be assessed in more detail. As such, it serves the noble cause of allowing clinicians to concentrate their limited resources on those patients most in need.

Another reason that screening tools may be necessary is that primary health care services, where patients ordinarily enter the system, are often poorly equipped to assess these variables. Such services may lack personnel who have sufficient training and/or the time to conduct a full assessment. Further, a large number of psychological variables have been identified as risk factors, making interview assessments cumbersome and time consuming. Finally, interview techniques are subject to a number of biases and their predictive ability is not yet known (Linton and Halldén 1997, 1998). Thus, a screening instrument to provide a first assessment of these factors is desirable. At best it would be a simple routine that provides a good estimate of risk as well as guidance on how to proceed with the assessment and/or intervention.

To be successful, however, the screening procedure must meet several difficult requirements. Not only must the measure be valid and reliable, but it must also prove its worth clinically. A particular requirement is predictive power; a screening instrument must be able to accurately predict who will develop problems. While screening is by definition a gross assessment, it must still be considerably better than guessing. Moreover, it should do this in an economical way. That is, the method must be practical. It should be easy to administer, provide considerable information, and cost little. Taken together, these criteria are some of the most stringent in clinical practice, and yet they are necessary if early identification is to be helpful.

Screening is not just the *identification* of those "at risk"; it also entails taking action. Therefore, in this chapter we focus on yet another issue: the usefulness of screening in developing the assessment and targeting intervention goals. Let us suppose that an instrument were available that correctly identified patients who will develop long-term pain and disability problems within the next year. How would the clinician best deal with this situation? With no other information than the prediction, the clinician would be left in the dark. Indeed, although it is well known that psychological factors influence the development of long-term disability (Burton *et al.* 1995; Turk 1997; Waddell 1998; Burton *et al.* 1999), it is still common to only provide medical treatments (Vingård *et al.* 2002). Moreover, if these fail, there appears to be a tendency to provide "more of the same" (e.g. more physical therapy, higher doses of pain killers, longer sick leave) rather than to explore more psychologically focused interventions. Thus, a screening procedure that provided information to guide the initial assessment process and help to focus on the most important risk factors would be beneficial. Consequently, we will also consider the use of the screening procedure as a starting point in conducting an initial behavioral analysis of the problem.

In developing a screening instrument it is of interest to examine the literature on psychological risk factors as a background for which constructs might be included. A vast literature on the relationship between various psychological factors and back pain is available. In our recent review, over 900 articles were identified (Linton 2000*b*). Unfortunately, there have been considerable methodological difficulties in studying psychological processes (Turk 1997; Linton 2000*b*) and therefore we focused on prospective studies where the psychological variable was first measured and participants were then followed over time to determine the effect on future pain problems. We located 37 such studies (Linton 2000*a,b*). Of specific interest were the 26 studies that actually examined the development of a back pain problem where outcome was defined as either a new onset or the further development of a problem after acute onset. Psychological factors were unfailingly associated with the onset and development of back pain problems.

In the above review, significant risk factors embodied cognitive, emotional, and behavioral variables. As an illustration, stress, distress/anxiety were linked to back pain in all of the studies investigating it. Moreover, mood and depression were constantly reported to be substantial risk factors. With regard to fear-avoidance, cognitive variables such as beliefs about the pain and catastrophizing were stable features having a particularly significant relationship with the development of dysfunction. Behavioral aspects included coping strategies where passive strategies demonstrated poorer outcomes. Finally, high levels of pain behavior and dysfunction were a risk factor for future back pain problems. In another review of 21 prospective studies, we have also found that psychological factors at work (e.g. job satisfaction, monotonous tasks, work relations, stress) are clearly linked to future pain and disability (Linton 2001).

Thus, various psychological factors including fear-avoidance are related to future back pain problems and might be utilized in a screening instrument.

Fortunately, several attempts have been made at putting these factors into a screening instrument that can predict future pain and disability problems (Waddell *et al.* 2003). For example, Main and colleagues (Main *et al.* 1992; Main and Watson 1995) developed an instrument based on a measure of depression and distress and showed that it helped identify patients seeking orthopedic care who were at risk of a poor outcome. In an exciting development since it entails a method for use in primary care settings, Gatchel *et al.* (1995) employed a personality inventory, questionnaires, and a clinical diagnostic interview to assess patients seeking care for acute back pain. Scores on several psychological factors correctly classified 87 percent of the patients' work status 6 months later. The Vermont Screening Questionnaire (Hazard *et al.* 1996) consists of only 11 items, but is designed as an aid for predicting future compensation among people filing an injury report. They showed that the instrument was a good predictor with 94 percent sensitivity and 84 percent specificity. However, the study only covered those filing an injury claim and suffered from a substantial dropout and refusal rate.

2 Örebro musculoskeletal pain screening questionnaire

We developed the Örebro Musculoskeletal Pain Screening Questionnaire as a tool for clinicians in the early identification of problem cases (Linton and Halldén 1998; Boersma and Linton 2002). In this chapter, we use this screening questionnaire as a platform from which to examine the possible role of fear-avoidance in the early identification of patients at risk for developing chronic disability. It is a clinical instrument designed to complement medical examinations and provide information concerning the likelihood that a patient will develop disability. It consists of 25 items focusing on psychological factors shown in Table 10.1. As seen in the table, it provides information about various aspects of the problem including fear-avoidance beliefs, function, experienced pain, beliefs about the future, stress, mood, work, and coping. The items contain statements or assertions that patients rate on Likert scales ranging from 0 to 10. The instrument is self-administered and most patients complete it within 7 or 8 min; a trained health care provider can score and evaluate it in a couple of minutes; and, it provides an overall score from which risk may be roughly judged as well as ratings on each item. The latter may be used in discussing and communicating with the patient. Several studies have shown that this questionnaire is reliable and valid (Linton and Halldén 1998;

Table 10.1 An overview of the items in the Örebro Musculoskeletal
Pain Screening Questionnaire

Question	Variable name
1. What year were you born?	Age
2. Are you male or female?	Gender
3. Were you born in Sweden?	Nationality
4. What is your current employment status?	Employed
5. Where do you have pain?	Pain site
6. How many days of work have you missed (sick leave) because of pain during the past 12 months?	Sick leave
7. How long have you had your current pain problem?	Pain duration
8. Is your work heavy or monotonous?	Heavy work
9. How would you rate the pain you have had during the past week?	Current pain
10. In the past 3 months, on the average, how intense was your pain?	Average pain
11. How often would you say that you have experienced pain episodes, on the average during the past 3 months?	Pain frequency
12. Based on all the things you do to cope, or deal with your pain, on an average day, how much are you able to decrease it?	Coping
13. How tense or anxious have you felt in the past week?	Stress
14. How much have you been bothered by feeling depressed in the past week?	Depression
15. In your view, how large is the risk that your current pain may become persistent?	Expected outcome
16. In your estimation, what are the chances that you will be able to work in 6 months?	Expected outcome
17. If you take into consideration your work routines, management, salary, promotion possibilities, and workmates, how satisfied are you with your job?	Job satisfaction
18. Physical activity makes my pain worse.	Fear-Avoidance Belief; FABQ
19. An increase in pain is an indication that I should stop what I am doing until the pain decreases.	Fear-Avoidance Belief; PAIRS
20. I should not do my normal work with my present pain	Fear-Avoidance Belief; FABQ
21. I can do light work for an hour	Function: Work
22. I can walk for an hour	Function: Walk
23. I can do ordinary household chores	Function: Household work
24. I can do the weekly shopping	Function: Shopping
25. I can sleep at night	Function: Sleep

PAIRS, Pain and Impairment Relationship Scale.

FABQ, Fear Avoidance Beliefs Questionnaire.

Hurley *et al.* 2000, 2001; Ektor-Andersen *et al.* 2002; Boersma and Linton 2002; Linton and Boersma 2003).

3 Fear-avoidance as a risk factor for developing chronic problems

In this section we will examine whether fear-avoidance is applicable for predicting long-term pain and disability. The fear-avoidance model is one intriguing explanation for the development of persistent disability. Consequently, several authors suggest that pain-related fear is more strongly related to functional problems than the pain itself (Vlaeyen *et al.* 1995*b*; Waddell 1996, 1998; Crombez *et al.* 1999), refuting the earlier notion that disability is simply caused by the pain (Vlaeyen and Linton 2002). Evidence from cross-sectional studies shows that one of the most powerful predictors of observable physical performance and self-reported disability levels is, in fact, pain-related fear (Vlaeyen and Linton 2002). A salient illustration of this is presented in a study by Mannion *et al.* (2001). In a multivariate analysis, they demonstrated that while pain accounted for about 20 percent of the variance in disability, psychological factors (distress, fear-avoidance, coping) accounted for 36 percent. In this case, the fear of pain might be said to be more disabling than the pain itself. This suggests that fear-avoidance is a unique risk factor.

Although there is good evidence that fear-avoidance is associated with disability in patients with chronic pain (Linton 2000*b*; Vlaeyen and Linton 2002), certain criteria must be met if fear-avoidance is to be employed as a predictor. First, the fear-avoidance must precede the chronicity; that is, we must be able to measure the fear-avoidance in the acute/subacute stage of the pain problem. Second, the fear-avoidance must be related to the development of the pain and disability problem; that is, it should predict who will develop a problem. Let us begin by examining whether (*a*) fear-avoidance actually occurs early on, and (*b*) if fear-avoidance predicts future pain and disability.

3.1 Can fear-avoidance predict future disability?

Some information does suggest that fear-avoidance beliefs may be present early on and long before a chronic disability problem has been noted. In a study of 917 people in the general population, our research group found evidence to support the idea that some people do harbor fear-avoidance beliefs and catastrophizing (Buer and Linton 2002). Participants completed questions taken from the Fear Avoidance Beliefs Questionnaire (FABQ) and the Pain Catastrophizing Scale (PCS) that were slightly reworded so that people in the general population could answer them. Although the scores were much lower than in a clinical population, a normal distribution was found. The results showed that fear-avoidance beliefs as well as catastrophizing occurred in the general population of non-patients. And, some participants obtained the maximum score possible! Moreover, a relationship was reported between fear-avoidance beliefs and current activity levels and between catastrophizing and current pain. Similarly, in a cross-sectional study comparing samples of patients with acute and chronic pain, it was found that fear-avoidance was present in both samples (Ciccone and Just 2001). Moreover, fear-avoidance was strongly related to disability, explaining about 40 percent of the variance.

Several other investigations indicate that fear-avoidance beliefs are present in some patients seeking care for acute back pain (Fritz *et al.* 2001; Sieben *et al.* 2002; Buer *et al.* submitted). These studies typically have assessed patients as part of a broader investigation and, as such, various measurements have been employed. Two studies from the United Kingdom, for example, assessed relatively large numbers of patients presenting with low back pain at a primary care centre (Burton *et al.* 1995; Klenerman *et al.* 1995). In both studies, fear-avoidance beliefs were found to be present among the patients. In a similar setting in the United States it was found that fear-avoidance, measured as worry, was a central feature of those seeking primary care for acute low back pain (von Korff 1999). In our own work we have found fear-avoidance beliefs to be clearly present in two samples of people complaining of acute back problems (Linton and Andersson 2000; Linton and Ryberg 2001). Although levels were lower than in reports for chronic pain patients, these participants nevertheless rated significant levels of these beliefs. Collectively, then, there is evidence that fear-avoidance beliefs occur before a persistent disability. The next question is whether fear-avoidance is related to the development of disability.

To determine whether fear-avoidance might predict functional problems, we compared data from samples ranging from a very mild to a chronic pain problem. If fear-avoidance predicts function, then there should be a relationship between the level of fear-avoidance and the level of dysfunction. We compared four samples of participants representing different stages in the development of a chronic back pain problem. Two groups were selected from the general population and they were not seeking care. However, they did report (on a 0–10 scale) some back pain over the past 3 months and were thus labeled the *mild pain* group (mean pain = 2.0, $n = 227$), and the *moderate pain* group (mean pain = 3.6, $n = 265$). The remaining two groups were from clinical populations seeking help for back pain. The *acute health care* group was seeking care at a primary care facility (mean pain = 5.1, $n = 107$), while the *chronic health care* included patients with long-term back pain problems ($n = 30$). The four groups are thought to represent different stages in the

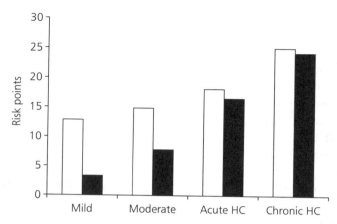

Fig. 10.1 The relationship between fear-avoidance beliefs (white bars) and physical dysfunction (black bars) in four groups of people with musculoskeletal pain. The Mild and Moderate groups were selected from the general population, while the Acute and Chronic groups consists of patients seeking health care. Note that the absolute values increase with chronicity as does the relationship.

development of a chronic pain problem from a very mild problem to a persistent one.

Figure 10.1 shows the results with regard to fear-avoidance beliefs and self-rated function for these four groups. To obtain the data, we summed the scores on the three fear-avoidance items in the Örebro Musculoskeletal Pain Screening Questionnaire (max = 30) and the four items on the dysfunction subscale (max = 40) so that higher scores indicate higher levels of fear-avoidance beliefs and dysfunction.

The figure illustrates several things. First, fear-avoidance beliefs, as measured by the three questions in the screening questionnaire, are present in all four groups. Second, as the pain problem *progresses* from the mild group to the chronic group, the fear-avoidance scores increase, as do functional problems. This suggests that fear-avoidance is strongly related to function. Third, note that fear-avoidance and physical dysfunction seem to become more closely associated as the problem becomes more persistent.

These data illustrate that the acute phase may be a crucial point for screening. While the general population groups with mild and moderate pain show some fear-avoidance and some dysfunction, the levels are relatively low. However, as the problem progresses, both fear-avoidance beliefs and dysfunction increase. Fear-avoidance, then, may be a potent factor for predicting future disability. Keep in mind, however, that these data sets are of cross-sectional nature and therefore they do not necessarily tell us whether fear-avoidance is actually related to future disability. Longitudinal studies are needed to determine the true predictive value of fear-avoidance.

To obtain prospective data, we selected 415 people from the general population who reported no spinal pain during the previous year. These people were asked to complete a questionnaire assessing fear-avoidance beliefs and pain catastrophizing (Linton *et al.* 2000). Subsequently, we followed these people for 1 year to determine who suffered an episode of back pain during the following year. We found that those with high scores on the fear-avoidance scale had twice the risk of suffering an episode of back pain and 1.7 times higher risk of lowered physical function. Moreover, catastrophizing was also related to increasing the risk for pain or lower function by 1.5 times. Thus, we were able to show that fear-avoidance was related to the future inception of back pain and associated functional problems. We concluded that fear-avoidance beliefs might thereby be useful in screening.

In a study of 300 primary care patients seeking help for acute low back pain, fear-avoidance was found to predict future disability (Klenerman *et al.* 1995). Patients were examined and psychological and physiological data were collected. The participants were then followed for 1 year and the Roland and Morris Disability Questionnaire was used to determine functional problems. The fear-avoidance variables were found to be the best predictors of outcome, clearly underscoring that the fear-avoidance was a precursor rather than a consequence of the disability. Based on these results, fear-avoidance appears to be important in the early identification of patients at risk of developing persistent disability problems.

A similar study of 250 patients with low back pain seeking primary care had somewhat different results (Burton *et al.* 1995). Data were collected at the time the patient sought care and participants were followed 1 year to determine outcome according to the Roland and Morris Disability Questionnaire. Similar to Klenerman *et al.* (1995) results showed that the psychological variables (e.g. catastrophizing and distress) were the best predictors of future disability. However, even though the FABQ was used, the final model did not specifically include it. This may be because the Fear-Avoidance Behavior Questionnaire is related to other psychological variables, like the catastrophizing scale on the Coping Strategies Questionnaire, or it may suggest that fear-avoidance is not as important as other psychological variables.

A study from the United States provides additional evidence indicating that fear-avoidance early on is a significant predictor of the development of pain and disability (Fritz *et al.* 2001). To examine the predictive value of fear-avoidance beliefs, 78 participants with work-related low back pain of significant magnitude to require modification of duties were followed over the course of 4 weeks.

The participants were evaluated an average of 5.5 days after injury and they completed a battery of tests including the FABQ. The Oswestry Disability Scale was used as one measure of outcome while unrestricted return to work was another. The results showed that fear-avoidance beliefs were significant predictors of future disability problems, even when initial levels of pain intensity, impairment, and disability were controlled. Indeed, the authors conclude that: "The potential for the FABQ work subscale score measured at the initial examination to assist in the identification of patients at risk for work restrictions extending beyond four weeks could be important for clinicians attempting to make the most effective use of resources to prevent long-term disability" (Fritz *et al.* 2001: 13).

A particularly useful study has examined how pain-related fear develops during a new episode of acute back pain (Sieben *et al.* 2002). In this study, 44 patients seeking care for acute back pain completed daily dairies during a 2-week period. Follow-ups were conducted at 3 and 12 months. Interestingly, these patients had about the same level of pain-related fear as compared to groups in the literature with subacute or chronic problems. These results are intriguing. First, pain-related fear was found to develop in three distinct patterns. During the 2-week period, 39 percent of the patients had a self-rated descending level, while 35 percent had a relatively stable level. On the other hand, 30 percent had an increasing level of pain-related fear during this 2-week period. Importantly, the group with an increasing level during the first 2-week period demonstrated significantly more disability and pain at the follow-up. Consequently, the authors concluded that those with an increasing pain-related fear pattern were at risk for developing disability problems.

A similar result was found in a recent study of patients seeking acute care for fractures (Buer *et al.* submitted). Within 24 h of a wrist or ankle fracture, participants completed a battery of questionnaires including a modified version of the FABQ and the PCS. Patients were followed at 3 and 9 months post-fracture to ascertain how well they had recovered in terms of sick leave, strength, range of motion, pain intensity, and self-rated degree of recovery. Consistent with the previously described study, the results demonstrated different patterns in the development of fear-avoidance. Four groups were identified in terms of their scores at the baseline and 3-month follow-up, producing two groups with "high" scores at the 3-month follow-up (low to high; high to high) and two groups with "low" scores at the 3-month follow-up (high to low; low to low). Comparisons suggested that those with higher levels of fear-avoidance beliefs at the 3-month follow-up (low to high; high to high) were more likely to have a poor outcome at the 9-month follow-up. In fact, for those high on fear-avoidance at the 3-month follow up had a 3.5 fold increase in the risk of having more pain at the 9-month follow-up.

Taken together, the Sieben *et al.* (2002) and Buer *et al.* (submitted) studies provide some evidence that the absolute level of fear-avoidance at the time of injury is not as important as the *development* of fear-avoidance beliefs and behaviors after the injury. Those initially reporting high levels, but where the level subsides, appear to do well, whereas those reporting low levels initially, but experiencing increases, develop complications.

3.2 Evidence from the Örebro Musculoskeletal Pain Screening Questionnaire

Data from the Örebro Musculoskeletal Pain Screening Questionnaire provides some insight into the role of fear-avoidance, as compared to other psychosocial factors, as a clinical tool for predicting future disability and sick leave. Scores on this instrument are related to future sick leave as well as function and correctly identifies approximately 80 percent of those who will have future work disability. As an example, Fig. 10.2 shows the average total score at baseline for participants divided into three categories of sick leave at the 6-month follow-up (Linton and Boersma 2003). The figure illustrates a statistically significant difference in the screening score between the three categories of sick leave. Therefore, the total score reflects the amount of sick leave 6 months later. An important question for this chapter is the contribution of fear-avoidance to this relationship.

We have reported on two distinct studies of the validity of the screening questionnaire and both have shown that fear-avoidance beliefs are strongly correlated with future disability (Linton and Halldén 1998; Linton and Boersma 2003). However, this relationship seems to be moderated by other

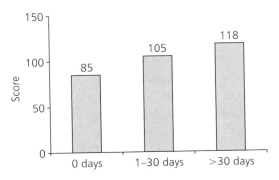

Fig. 10.2 The mean score on the Örebro Musculoskeletal Pain Screening Questionnaire for three groups of patients. Groups were formed on the basis of the number of days off work because of back pain during the past 6 months. The difference in scores is statistically significant.

factors, as discriminant analyses have produced different models in the two studies. In the first study (Linton and Halldén 1998), a set of five variables was found to contribute significantly to the explanation of sickleave 6 months later. These five items were: (1) the belief that one should not work with current pain levels (fear-avoidance), (2) low perceived chance of being able to work in 6 months (expectation), (3) reported difficulties doing light work (function), (4) high perceived stress, and (5) the previous number of sick leave days. As seen, the fear-avoidance item was the strongest predictor in this model, but four other items also contributed to the final model. In the second validity study (Linton and Boersma 2003), we replicated the predictive validity of the questionnaire, but the final model—based on discriminative analyses—included somewhat different items. The three items most strongly related to future sick leave were: (1) gender, (2) previous sick leave, and (3) difficulties in doing shopping (function). For the outcome variable of function 6 months later, four significant items were isolated: (1) poor sleep (function), (2) previous sick leave, (3) pain site (pain), and (4) chance working (expectations). Consequently, although fear-avoidance items were significantly related to outcome at the 6-month follow-up, none of these items were included in the final statistical model (Linton and Boersma 2003). While our clinical judgment is that fear-avoidance is an important determinant of future function and work, these results underscore the idea that several other psychological variables are also important (Linton 2002*b*).

To study the relative importance of the fear-avoidance construct we conducted a cluster analysis on 185 patients who had completed the screening questionnaire and were subsequently followed to ascertain future disability (Boersma and Linton, in press). To focus on the fear-avoidance model, we included the items on pain intensity, mood, fear-avoidance beliefs (sum of three items), and function (sum of four items). The first analysis produced nine clusters! This demonstrates that there are many different profiles associated with pain, underscoring that there are several mechanism involved (Linton 2002*b*). Of the 185 included in this analysis, only seven people had high scores on all four of the variables and the number in any one cluster was a maximum of 40. However, when we examined the relationship between the clusters and future sick leave, we found that the four clusters with the highest levels of sick leave all included high scores on fear-avoidance beliefs.

To simplify interpretation we reduced the number of clusters to four, as shown in Fig. 10.3. The means on pain intensity, mood, fear-avoidance beliefs, and function are displayed in the figure. The subgroups characterize a *low risk* group ($n = 83$) with low scores on all four variables. A *distressed fear-avoidant* group is also seen ($n = 29$) with relatively high scores on all four variables.

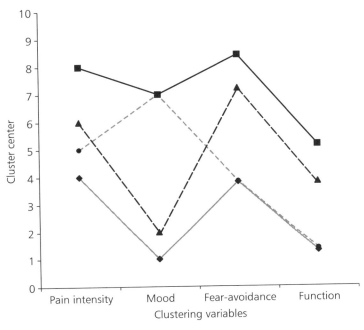

Fig. 10.3 The cluster profiles of patients (N = 185) based on self-rated pain intensity, mood, fear-avoidance, and function. The analysis was designed to produce four clusters: Low risk (solid gray line), Low risk depressed (dashed gray line), Distressed fear-avoidant (solid black line), and Fear-avoidant (dashed black line).

In between these groups are a *fear-avoidant* group ($n = 45$), with high scores on pain, fear-avoidance, and function, but low on mood, as well as a *low risk-depressed mood* group ($N = 28$), with high scores on pain and depressed mood.

3.3 Recapitulation

Fear-avoidance appears to be a potentially important factor in the development of persistent disability and is a predictor for identifying those in danger of such development. We have seen that fear-avoidance in the form of beliefs, catastrophizing, negative expectancies, avoidance, and the like often precede the functional problem. Moreover, the literature to date demonstrates a relationship between fear-avoidance and future disability. Finally, fear-avoidance has often been found to be among the most powerful predictors of future pain and disability and, therefore, appears to be ideal for screening. However, reviews of the literature also underscore the multifactor nature of the relationship between psychological variables and the development of chronic pain and disability. Consequently, other psychological factors may also be good predictors. In fact, one conception of the development of persistent problems maintains that a variety of factors may be important for any one individual; the road to chronic problems is unique to the individual (Linton 2002*b*). Our cluster analysis underscored this fact by showing that there are many different combinations of psychological variables that are relevant. This points to the need for being able to analyze and work with the relationship between variables in order to identify patients "at risk" as well as avenues for secondary prevention.

4 Screening as identification versus an action plan

Screening may be used to simply identify patients "at risk" or it may aim to enhance an action plan. In many medical settings, identification is the main goal since the intervention is then clear. For those risking an infection, for example, a vaccination would be the clear intervention. Likewise, identifying those at risk for cancer would activate a routine for further, in-depth examinations. However, in some situations, identification has no direct consequence for assessment or treatment. In the case of musculoskeletal pain, there is no clear plan of action for those identified as at risk of developing persistent pain and disability. There are guidelines (Koes *et al.* 2001) giving general recommendations, but there is no clear plan for dealing with individual patients. Screening only seems to make sense if it enhances the development of an action plan (i.e. if it promotes a more effective way of proceeding with the case).

Using fear-avoidance and other psychological variables to simply *identify* patients at risk would seem to be a waste of important information. Certainly, going a step further and using the information to develop ideas about goals for intervention as well as factors maintaining the problem would utilize the information more wisely and enhance the assessment. Identifying a patient at risk where fear-avoidance is an issue seems useless if we cannot exploit this information to develop an effective intervention plan for the patient.

To develop an action plan, we argue that the clinician needs to use the screening material as the *starting point* for an analysis. This would focus on possible targets for intervention as well as probable maintaining factors that, in turn, would help in tailoring the intervention to the individual's needs.

5 Screening and behavioral analysis

To be effective, the clinical screening procedure must not stop at assessing risk; it should enhance our communication with the patient and provide targets and ideas for further intervention. It may be argued that the most important

Table 10.2 An overview of possible screening results and how patients at different levels of risk may be dealt within the clinic. Note that the implementation of psychological factors is important in tailoring preventive interventions for those at high risk

Risk level	Assess	Intervention	Likely result	If patient does not improve
Low	Medical only	Usual care: Focus on cure	Patient tends to get better	More of the same
Medium	Medical only	Usual care: Focus on cure	Poor	More of the same
High	Medical and psychological	Targeted behavioral intervention: Focus on prevention	Improvement and prevention	Further behavioral analysis

purpose of screening is to enhance the detailed assessment of those individuals who are at risk of developing long-term problems. In a nutshell, we need to know how to proceed with those at risk. We argue that the screening instrument may be employed as a tool in initiating a behavioral analysis that will generate targets and ideas about what may be maintaining the problem that will be important in selecting effective treatment.

Table 10.2 shows some possible results of screening and underscores the problem of a physiological focus encountered in many medical settings. As the table illustrates, patients with low risk would be expected to recover and, therefore, might be given minimal "usual" treatments (e.g. analgesics and advice). However, for those at high risk there is a real challenge to pinpoint important problems and provide interventions to address them. Typically, patients identified as *at risk* are serviced in the usual medical way. This is a natural tendency since primary care facilities are designed to provide such care. Still, recent evidence shows that while this is the usual treatment, it is not the most effective tactic (Vingård *et al.* 2002). Logically, if a problem is exacerbated by psychological factors, then usual medical treatments would be expected to have disappointing results. Moreover, patients returning for continuing difficulties with their problem may receive more of the previous treatments, but in larger doses, rather than a new analysis or intervention strategy.

Perhaps the greatest clinical utility of screening is its use in a tentative behavioral analysis of the problem. Here we determine the overall risk but also begin to focus on the details of the problem. To do this, we need to know (1) potential risk factors, (2) which targets for intervention have highest priority, as well as (3) what is maintaining or catalyzing the problem. Although a proper assessment of this for chronic pain patients ordinarily takes considerable time, a *mini* behavioral analysis may be conducted for patients early on with the help of the screening questionnaire. An advantage is that interventions may be provided that address the risk factors that are maintaining the development of the problem.

5.1 Determining risk

The overall risk is easily estimated with the help of screening instruments. The Örebro Musculoskeletal Pain Screening Questionnaire, for example, has cut-off points for use in primary care settings. These provide a gross estimation of the probability of the patient being on sick benefits 6 months later. A basic cut-off of 105 was recommended based on the results of the first study (Linton and Halldén 1998), which was later also employed in the New Zealand guidelines (Kendall *et al.* 1998). However, others have found that a higher score was more effective for patients with a longer history of a problem (Hurley *et al.* 2000; Ektor-Andersen *et al.* 2002). Although influenced by the clinical population, cut-off scores are easy to apply to estimate high, medium, and low risk. However, the most important question then arises: how to proceed with the case.

5.2 Identifying potential risk factors

A screening questionnaire provides the advantage of including a number of important potential psychological risk factors for chronic disability. While fear-avoidance is an important psychological factor, we have seen above that it is not the only risk factor. Other variables such as coping, self-perceptions of health and recovery, work conditions, mood, anxiety, stress, and the pain itself are all examples of risk factors. Consequently, the road to chronic disability may be very different for specific individuals. It is, therefore, of essence to determine pertinent psychological factors for each patient.

We recommend that screening procedures be used to identify potential risk factors, including fear-avoidance. One way of accomplishing this is to employ a screening questionnaire that covers many basic and probable factors. In our own work, we examine the answers provided on the Örebro Musculoskeletal Pain Screening Questionnaire to identify high ratings on individual items. Thus, we do not simply look at the total score to estimate risk; we also examine the profile to identify potential targets and maintaining factors.

In the clinical situation, answers to the items on the questionnaire are used as a basis for discussion with the patient. After reinforcing positive behaviors, we ask open-ended questions about items that have atypical responses. Areas of concern, such as a high score on the fear-avoidance items or a high score on the depression item, can in this way be identified and assessed. For example, we may ask, "I see that you have rated your mood with an 8, could you tell me more about this?" This creates an opportunity to assess and understand the patient's beliefs about their problem and probable recovery.

As we proceed through the various items on the questionnaire, a picture begins to emerge concerning potential targets. The patient's conception of the problem becomes clearer. Moreover, barriers to recovery (e.g. workplace factors or fear) become apparent. The patient's goals come to the forefront. In short, the patient and practitioner develop a shared understanding of the problem and what the focus of treatment should be.

A mini behavioral analysis may be conducted to generate information on factors that are causing or maintaining problems. This typically involves combining items on the questionnaire to get a picture of antecedents, behaviors, thoughts, and beliefs, as well as consequences. For example, anticipated problems for a return to work may be enhanced by fear-avoidance beliefs. Specifically, the patient may believe that their work is harmful and should be avoided until after full physical recovery. Or, fear-avoidance beliefs may be at the forefront although some activities, such as walking, are not affected, while others like household chores are. The analysis might then attempt to identify why the patient can walk, but not do household chores. The patient may believe that certain movements (e.g. bending, twisting, lifting) are harmful. Thus, the screening setting offers an opportunity for initiating a behavioral analysis.

Finally, after targeting problems and identifying important maintaining factors, potential interventions may emerge and be discussed. At this point, the clinician may need to employ his or her own problem-solving skills to make decisions with the patient on what might be done and how to proceed. Having established a shared understanding of the cause of the problem and the targets for intervention, it should be easier to establish an alliance with the patient to enhance cooperation. Certain action may be warranted. This may simply involve further, proper assessment. It may also involve advice, information, education, or training skills. Fortunately, many patients may not need additional treatment as information and advice may be sufficient to enhance their own self-care skills.

Sometimes, however, specific interventions designed to prevent the development of long-term pain and disability will be called for. In this case we recommend considering one of two options. The first is a more general one designed to address the broad range of psychological risk factors. In our clinic, we offer a six-session cognitive–behavioral group intervention aimed at teaching participants how to apply a number of relevant coping skills (Linton 2002a). Participants develop their own coping program during the treatment by selecting the coping skills best suited to their problem. Thus, the groups offer a broad approach where patients tailor the program to their own needs. Compared to usual primary care treatment, these cognitive–behavioral groups significantly reduce the risk of developing long-term disability (Linton and Andersson 2000; Linton and Ryberg 2001; Linton *et al.* in press).

The second option is to design a treatment plan based on the findings of the mini behavioral analysis. Depending on the results of this analysis, the various treatment plans could be quite different. However, a common feature, in our experience, and according to the cluster analysis above (Boersma and Linton in press) is fear-avoidance. A common finding is that the patient scores high on the fear-avoidance beliefs items and low on the items about function. If additional questioning reveals that pain-related fear is associated with the low function, then treatment should address this issue. If the problem is in the acute stage, we recommend beginning by examining how well the pain intensity is being controlled. Analgesics and non-pharmacological methods may help the patient to reduce the pain and thereby reduce the fear and functional difficulties. Unfortunately, the problem has often developed beyond the acute stage and a more psychologically oriented treatment may be needed. We suggest considering either graded activity (Lindström *et al.* 1992; Linton 1993) or exposure treatment (Vlaeyen *et al.* 2001). Graded activity appears to be helpful and may be used to help patients gain confidence in increasing their activity and mobility levels. By bringing the patient into contact with feared movements, it may also reduce the fear. Those patients with very high levels of fear-avoidance should be assessed more thoroughly with a fear-avoidance beliefs questionnaire and with some sort of behavioral assessment. In the more extreme cases, exposure training might be recommended. This technique is described in other chapters, but briefly is a systematic method of gradually exposing the patient to feared movements in order to reduce the fear. Although much work remains to be done, initial studies of this technique have shown real promise (Vlaeyen *et al.* 2001; Linton *et al.* 2002; Boersma *et al.* 2004).

6 **Conclusion**

Our review has shown that fear-avoidance is important in the development of future pain and disability problems. Fear-avoidance is often evident at a very early point in the problem and is clearly related to future disability. Therefore, it is also a central risk factor included in screening procedures. Features of fear-avoidance are, in fact, among the best predictors of future problems. However, at the same time, we note that many other psychological factors may influence the development of chronic disability and need to be included in screening procedures as well. Consequently, it is too early to rely solely on fear-avoidance for identifying patients at risk of developing chronic pain problems.

The fact that several psychosocial variables are related to the development of persistent pain makes drawing causal conclusions about the causes of chronicity very difficult. In addition, we know little about how psychological processes relate to the physiological changes taking place during the development of persistent pain. We may ponder whether some sort of general process such as "distress" is the true variable as opposed to the more specific concept of fear avoidance. Indeed, various studies underscore different psychological factors as the most important. In addition, replications, such as of our screening questionnaire above, may not produce models that are exactly alike. Yet, we believe that fear-avoidance is an important predictive variable. Whether it reflects a broader process is difficult to determine at this point. However, fear-avoidance is consistently related to future disability in a wide range of studies. Furthermore, when fear-avoidance is identified, this information provides valuable guidance for planning the treatment. While more work is truly justified, we conclude that the evidence to date clearly shows that fear-avoidance is a central risk factor for the development of chronic disability.

Although screening may focus mainly on identification, we have argued that a screening procedure should also focus on a plan of action. In other words, screening may be used to identify those at risk but, above all, to develop a plan of action that includes psychological aspects. We have argued that the typical medical approach to managing back pain works relatively well for low risk patients. However, for high-risk patients, the treatment is likely to be "usual treatment" and, when this is not effective, "more of the same" will be offered. This in itself may increase the risk for chronicity. Screening provides an ideal opportunity to incorporate psychological aspects that may guide the development of how we proceed.

Screening can be an excellent starting point for a mini behavioral analysis. This entails identifying targets for intervention, determining which factors are maintaining the problem, establishing rapport and partner alliance with the patient, providing information and education, and testing the potential of possible interventions. We have outlined methods for conducting a mini behavioral analysis by using a screening questionnaire as a basis for conducting a focused interview with the patient. This should result in considerable information that may be used in making decisions about how to proceed with the case. Fear-avoidance may frequently be a central element in this process. However, considerable work remains in order to develop and evaluate screening procedures that will help us to prevent the development of persistent pain and disability.

References

Boersma, K. and Linton, S.J. (2002). Early assessment of psychological factors: The Örebro Screening Questionnaire for Pain. In S.J. Linton (ed.), *New Avenues for the Prevention of Pain*, Vol. 1, pp. 205–13. Amsterdam: Elsevier.

Boersma, K. and Linton, S.J. (in press). Early identification of psychological factors: Possibilities for preventive intervention. *Clinical Journal of Pain.*

Boersma, K., Linton, S.J., Overmeer, T., and Janson, M. (2004). Lowering fear-avoidance and enhancing function through exposure in vivo: A multiple baseline study across six patients with back pain. *Pain*, **108**, 8–16.

Buer, N. and Linton, S.J. (2002). Fear-avoidance beliefs and catastrophizing—occurrence and risk factor in back pain and ADL in the general population. *Pain*, **99**(3), 485–91.

Buer, N., Linton, S.J., Samuelsson, L., and Harms-Ringdahl, K. (submitted). The role of fear-avoidance beliefs and catastrophizing in patients with fractures.

Burton, A.K., Battié M.C., and Main, C.J. (1999). The relative importance of biomechanical and psychosocial factors in low back injuries. In W. Karwowski and W. Marras (eds.), *The Occupational Ergonomics Handbook*, pp. 1127–38. Boca Raton, FL: CRC Press.

Burton, A.K., Tillotson, K.M., Main, C.J., and Hollis, S. (1995). Psychosocial predictors of outcome in acute and subchronic low back trouble. *Spine*, *20*(6), 722–8.

Ciccone, D.S. and Just, N. (2001). Pain expectancy and work disability in patients with acute and chronic pain: A test of the fear avoidance hypothesis. *The Journal of Pain: Official Journal of the American Pain Society*, **2**(3), 181–94.

Crombez, G., Vlaeyen, J.W.S., Heuts, P.H., and Lysens, R. (1999). Pain-related fear is more disabling than pain itself: Evidence on the role of pain-related fear in chronic back pain disability. *Pain*, **80**, 329–39.

Ektor-Andersen, J., Örbaek, P., Ingvarsson, E., and Kullendorff, M. (2002). Prediction of Vocational Dysfunction due to Muskuloskeletal Symptoms by Screening for Psychosocial Factors at the Social Insurance Office. Paper presented at the 10th World Congress on Pain, San Diego, CA.

Fritz, J.M., George, S.Z., and Delitto, A. (2001). The role of fear-avoidance beliefs in acute low back pain: Relationships with current and future disability and work status. *Pain*, **94**, 7–15.

Gatchel, R.J., Polatin, P.B., and Kinney, R.K. (1995). Predicting outcome of chronic back pain using clinical predictors of psychopathology: a Prospective analysis. *Health Psychology*, **14**(5), 415–20.

Hazard, R.G., Haugh, L.D., Reid, S., Preble, J.B., and MacDonald, L. (1996). Early prediction of chronic disability after occupational low back injury. *Spine*, *21*(8), 945–51.

Hurley, D., Dusoir, T., McDonough, S., Moore, A., and Baxter, G. (2001). How effective is the Acute Low BAck Pain Screening Questionnaire for predicting 1-year follow-up in patients with low back pain? *The Clinical Journal of Pain*, **17**, 256–63.

Hurley, D., Dusoir, T., McDonough, S., Moore, A., Linton, S.J., and Baxter, G. (2000). Biopsychosocial screening questionnaire for patients with low back pain: Preliminary report of utility in physiotherapy practice in Northern Ireland. *Clinical Journal of Pain*, **16**(3), 214–28.

Kendall, N.A.S., Linton, S.J., and Main, C. (1998). Psychosocial yellow flags for acute low back pain: "Yellow Flags" as an analogue to "Red Flags". *European Journal of Pain*, **2**(1), 87–9.

Klenerman, L., Slade, P.D., Stanley, I.M., Pennie, B., Reilly, J.P., Atchison, L.E., Troup, J.D., and Rose, M.J. (1995). The prediction of chronicity in patients with an acute attack of low back pain in a general practice setting. *Spine*, **20**(4), 478–84.

Koes, B.W., van Tulder, M.W., Ostelo, R., Burton, A.K., and Waddell, G. (2001). Clinical guidelines for the management of low back pain in primary care. *Spine*, **26**(22), 2504–14.

Lindström, I., Öhlund, C., Eek, C., Wallin, L., Peterson, L.E., Fordyce, W.E., and Nachemson, A.L. (1992). The effect of graded activity on patients with subacute low back pain: A randomized prospective clinical study with an operant-conditioning behavioral approach. *Physical Therapy*, **72**, 279–93.

Linton, S.J. (1993). *Psychological Interventions for Patients With Chronic Back Pain.* Geneva: World Health Organization.

Linton, S.J. (2000*a*). Psychologic risk factors for neck and back pain. In A. Nachemsom and E. Jonsson (eds.), *Neck and Back Pain: The Scientific Evidence of Causes, Diagnosis, and Treatment*, pp. 57–78. Philadelphia, PA: Lippincott Williams and Wilkins.

Linton, S.J. (2000*b*). A review of psychological risk factors in back and neck pain. *Spine*, **25**(9), 1148–56.

Linton, S.J. (2001). Occupational psychological factors increase the risk for back pain: A systematic review. *Journal of Occupational Rehabilitation*, **11**(1), 53–66.

Linton, S.J. (2002*a*). Cognitive behavioral therapy in the prevention of musculoskeletal pain: Description of a program. In S.J. Linton (ed.), *New Avenues for the Prevention of Chronic Musculoskeletal Pain and Disability*, Vol. 1, pp. 269–76. Amsterdam: Elsevier.

Linton, S.J. (2002*b*). Why does chronic pain develop? A behavioral approach. In S.J. Linton (ed.), *New Avenues for the Prevention of Chronic Musculoskeletal Pain and Disability*, pp. 67–82. Amsterdam: Elsevier Science.

Linton, S.J. and Andersson, T. (2000). Can chronic disability be prevented? A randomized trial of a cognitive-behavior intervention and two forms of information for patients with spinal pain. *Spine*, **25**(21), 2825–31.

Linton, S.J. and Boersma, K. (2003). Early identification of patients at risk of developing a persistent back problem: The predictive validity of the Örebro Musculoskeletal Pain Questionnaire. *The Clinical Journal of Pain*, **19**, 80–6.

Linton, S.J. and Halldén, K. (1997). Risk factors and the natural course of acute and recurrent musculoskeletal pain: Developing a screening instrument. In T.S. Jensen and J.A. Turner, and Z. Wiesenfeld-Hallin (eds.), *Proceedings of the 8th World Congress on Pain: Progress in Pain Research and Management* Vol. 8, pp. 527–36. Seattle, WA: IASP Press.

Linton, S.J. and Halldén, K. (1998). Can we screen for problematic back pain? A screening questionnaire for predicting outcome in acute and subacute back pain. *The Clinical Journal of Pain*, **14**(3), 209–15.

Linton, S.J. and Ryberg, M. (2001). A cognitive–behavioral group intervention as prevention for persistent neck and back pain in a non-patient population: A randomized controlled trial. *Pain*, **90**, 83–90.

Linton, S.J., Buer, N., Vlaeyen, J., and Hellsing, A.L. (2000). Are fear-avoidance beliefs related to a new episode of back pain? A prospective study. *Psychology and Health*, **14**, 1051–9.

Linton, S.J., Overmeer, T., Janson, M., Vlaeyen J.W.S, and de Jong, J.R. (2002). Graded *in-vivo* exposure treatment for fear-avoidant pain patients with function disability: A case study. *Cognitive Behavior Therapy*, **31**(2), 49–58.

Linton, S.J., Boersma, K., Jansson, M., Svärd, L., and Botvalde, M. (in press). The effects of cognitive-behavioral and physical therapy preventive interventions on pain-related sick leave: A randomized controlled trial. *Clinical Journal of Pain*.

Main, C.J. and Watson, P.J. (1995). Screening for patients at risk of developing chronic incapacity. *Journal of Occupational Rehabilitation*, **5**, 207–17.

Main, C.J., Wood P.L.R, Hollis, S., Spanswick, C.C., and Waddell, G. (1992). The distress and risk assessment method: A simple patient classification to identify distress and evaluate the risk of poor outcome. *Spine*, **17**, 42–52.

Mannion, A.F., Junge, A., Taimela, S., Müntener, M., Lorenzo, K., and Dvorak, J. (2001). Active therapy for chronic low back pain. Part 3 Factors influencing self-rated disability and its change following therapy. *Spine*, **26**(8), 920–9.

Marhold, C., Linton, S.J., and Melin, L. (2001). Cognitive behavioral return-to-work program: Effects on pain patients with a history of long-term versus short-term sick leave. *Pain*, **91**, 155–63.

Sieben, J.M., Vlaeyen, J.W.S., Tuerlinckx, S., and Portegijs, P.J.M. (2002). Pain-related fear in acute low back pain: The first two weeks of a new episode. *European Journal of Pain*, **6**, 229–37.

Turk, D.C. (1997). The role of demographic and psychosocial factors in transition from acute to chronic pain. In T.S. Jensen, J.A. Turner, and Z. Wiesenfeld-Hallin (eds.), *Proceedings of the 8th World Congress on Pain, progress in Pain Research and Management*, Vol. 8, pp. 185–213. Seattle, WA: IASP Press.

Waddell, G. (1996). Low back pain: A twentieth century health care enigma. *Spine*, **21**(24), 2820–5.

Waddell, G. (1998). *The Back Pain Revolution*. Edinburgh: Churchill Livingstone.

Waddell, G., Burton, A.K., and Main, C.J. (2003). Screening of clients for risk of long-term incapacity: A conceptual and scientific review. London: Royal Society of Medicine Press Ltd.

Vingård, E., Mortimer, M., Wiktorin, C., Pernold, G., Fredriksson, K., Németh, G., and Alfredsson, L. (2002). Seeking care for low back pain in the general population. *Spine*, **27**(19), 2159–65.

Vlaeyen, J.W.S. and Linton, S.J. (2002). Pain-related fear and its consequences in chronic musculoskeletal pain. In S.J. Linton (ed.), *New Avenues for the Prevention of Chronic Musculoskeletal Pain and Disability*, pp. 81–103. Amsterdam: Elsevier Science.

Vlaeyen, J.W.S., Kole-Snijders, A.M.J., Boeren, R.G.B., and van Eek, H. (1995*a*). Fear of movement/(re)injury in chronic low back pain and its relation to behavioral performance. *Pain*, **62**, 363–72.

Vlaeyen, J.W.S., Kole-Snijders, A.M.J., Rotteveel, A., Ruesink, R., and Heuts, P.H.T.G. (1995*b*). The role of fear of movement/(re)injury in pain disability. *Journal of Occupational Rehabilitation*, **5**, 235–52.

Vlaeyen, J.W.S., de Jong, J., Geilen, M., Heuts, P.H.T.G., and van Breukelen, G. (2001). Graded exposure *in vivo* in the treatment of pain-related fear: A replicated single-case experimental design in four patients with chronic low back pain. *Behavior Research and Therapy*, **39**, 151–66.

Vlaeyen, J.W.S., de Jong, J., Geilen, M., Heuts PHTG, and van Breukelen, G. (2002). The treatment of fear of movement/(re)injury in chronic low back pain: Further evidence of the effectiveness of exposure *in vivo*. *Clinical Journal of Pain*, **18**, 251–61.

von Korff, M. (1999). Pain management in primary care: An individualized stepped/care approach. In R.J. Gatchel and D.C. Turk (eds.), *Psychosocial Factors in Pain*, 1st edn., pp. 360–73. New York, NY: Guilford Press.

Chapter 11

Patient–therapist relationships among patients with pain-related fear

Heather D. Hadjistavropoulos and
Kristine M. Kowalyk

1 Introduction

As evidenced by this volume, pain-related fear has become an important and widely researched topic within the field of psychology and pain. The importance of helping patients overcome pain-related fear cannot be overemphasized. Successful treatment for chronic pain consistently shows that resolution of fear is key to success and reductions in pain-related fear predict improved treatment outcomes (McCracken and Gross 1998).

Despite the increasing amount of research on the topic of pain-related fear, relatively little attention has been given to the patient–therapist relationship among patients faced with significant pain-related fear. In fact, in the chronic pain literature as a whole, the relationship between patient and therapist has received only modest consideration (e.g. Burns *et al.* 1999). As discussed below, there is substantial research evidence to suggest that the relationship between patient and therapist is important and affects factors such as treatment outcome and adherence to treatment recommendations. Review of the pain-related fear field leads us to hypothesize that pain-related fear has the potential to complicate the formation of a strong working relationship with the patient. Lack of a solid relationship between patient and therapist, in turn, presents a challenge to assisting patients in making short-term and long-term treatment gains. Although development and maintenance of a relationship presents a challenge, a number of strategies are available to the psychologist when attempting to establish relationships with patients who express significant pain-related fears.

This chapter, while primarily focused on psychologists, also addresses and is relevant to other providers, such as physicians and physiotherapists. Review of the literature suggests that, as compared to psychologists, the role of physicians and other physically based providers are more often viewed as consultants than collaborators (Chew-Graham and May 2000). But, this also varies depending on the context of the relationship. Within multidisciplinary teams, for instance, with both physicians and other physically based health professionals, collaboration rather than consultation is emphasized (Feuerstein and Zastowny 1996) and, as such, the formation of a strong relationship between provider and patient becomes central. Physician interest in the present chapter would certainly be consistent with increasing attention in the medical literature given to the provision of patient-centered care—taking a biopsychosocial perspective, treating the patient as a person, including them in decision-making, forming a therapeutic alliance, and also recognizing one's own limits as a professional (Mead and Bower 2000). Recent research within the field of physiotherapy has likewise distinguished traditional and nontraditional physiotherapists (Kumlin and Kroksmark 1992; Thornquist 1992). The more traditional style views the patient as an information recipient seeking appropriate methods of managing physical difficulties and the physiotherapist as a provider of expertise regarding the patient's body (Galley and Foster 1987). In the non-traditional style, patients are viewed as providers of important information about themselves and emphasis is placed on fostering the patient–therapist relationship (Thornquist 1992).

2 Importance of the patient–therapist relationship

The majority of research on the patient–provider relationship is found in the psychological literature. Typically, therapy is viewed as consisting of both a relationship component that is common across many approaches, and a technical component that is unique to the therapeutic approach (Gelso and Hayes 1998). In the present chapter we focus on the relationship component of therapy, and, in particular, the relationship that is formed with the chronic pain patient in the context of therapy that is based in cognitive–behavioral principles (for a brief review of this area see Hadjistavropoulos and Williams, 2004). Within this approach, psychologists and patients view themselves as collaborative scientists or co-investigators who mutually set goals, generate hypotheses, gather data, examine evidence, and formulate conclusions (Beck and Weishaar 1995).

Intuitively, we believe that a strong collaborative relationship will facilitate the outcome of therapy and a poor relationship will undermine it. Based on clinical observations of the therapeutic process, the belief has emerged that building a strong relationship in therapy is especially important in the early stages because faith and willingness to participate in therapy and receptiveness to therapeutic techniques and interventions is highly dependent upon the relationship (Morris and Magrath 1983). Maintaining the relationship is also perceived to be imperative as it provides leverage when therapy becomes demanding and challenging. The relationship thereby enhances the efficacy of techniques in that patients are more likely to be responsive if they trust and have a good relationship with the therapist (Butler and Strupp 1986; Henry *et al.* 1986). As noted by Safran and Segal (1990), in cognitive–behavioral therapy in particular, the quality of the therapeutic relationship mediates the patient's ability to explore his or her thoughts and to change behavior. Beck *et al.* (1990) hold that the more complex and chronic the problem, the greater the need for a positive therapeutic relationship. Stability in the relationship is viewed as important for another reason; the more the patient struggles with the relationship, the more the patient and therapist will attend to the dynamics of the relationship rather than the patient's concerns and dilemmas (Lazarus 1989). Interestingly, it also appears that patients similarly agree that the relationship with the provider is critical. Patients, for instance, emphasize the importance of the therapeutic relationship rather than specific techniques when asked about what is most helpful or useful about therapy (Lambert and Bergin 1994).

Beyond clinical observations, research evidence also supports contentions that the relationship between therapist and patient is crucial to understanding therapeutic outcomes. After reviewing the empirical literature, Orlinski *et al.* (1994) concluded that a positive therapeutic relationship is consistently associated with positive treatment outcomes. The patient's view of the therapist as warm and empathetic as well as their interpretation of the relationship as representing a positive bond is found to be strongly associated with therapeutic change (Lambert and Bergin 1994; Orlinski *et al.* 1994). In a meta-analytic review of 24 treatment studies, Horvath and Symonds (1991) drew attention to the fact that the alliance measured in the first few sessions predicted outcome just as accurately as the alliance measured later in therapy. They also emphasized that the patient's perception of the working alliance is of utmost importance in predicting treatment outcome as compared with the therapist's view of that alliance or other factors, such as the length of therapy.

In addition to assisting with treatment outcome, the therapeutic relationship may also be predictive of dropout rates and treatment satisfaction, although empirical findings are inconsistent in this regard. Some researchers examining what are thought to be core aspects of the therapeutic alliance have failed to find a relationship between dropout and strength of the alliance (e.g. Kokotovic and Tracey 1990). On the other hand, others have found that patient perceptions of therapists' expertness, attractiveness, and trustworthiness, which most likely reflect the quality of the relationship between patient and therapist, are inversely related to patient's likelihood to terminate therapy and report dissatisfaction (McNeill *et al.* 1987). Furthermore, McNeill *et al.* (1987) reported a significant positive correlation between level of satisfaction and number of sessions attended among premature terminators, suggesting that those attending more sessions were more satisfied, and those terminating therapy early were less satisfied.

Consistent with the above research concerning patients and psychologists, there are numerous studies that suggest that satisfaction with the patient–physcian relationship is also associated with better outcomes, such as patient adherence and satisfaction with treatment (Mead and Bower 2000). Satisfaction with the relationship is found to be associated with a lower likelihood of changing physicians (Marquis *et al.* 1983), and with improved health behaviors, such as lower utilization and improved medication adherence (e.g. Pascoe 1983; Thomas and Penchansky 1984). In the context of pain, McCracken *et al.* (1997) reported that treatment satisfaction with a pain clinic, which included satisfaction with the patient–physician relationship, was associated with fewer consultations and fewer visits in the 12 months following treatment. Further, among a sample of low back pain patients, it was found that patients who were satisfied with their medical care emphasized the importance of physician's communication skills (i.e. the physician gave the patient the opportunity to relay concerns and listened) in combination with a complete assessment (Skelton *et al.* 1996). The positive impact of the patient–physician relationship also appears to extend to physiotherapists. Sluijis, *et al.* (1993) describe research suggesting that physiotherapists who attend to relationship factors, such as providing positive feedback to patients, attending to patient needs, and brain storming with patients regarding barriers to compliance, perform better in terms of garnering patient compliance with the treatment regimen.

In sum, there is little debate that a positive relationship between patient and provider serves to improve patient care and outcomes. Below we review how pain-related fear presents a barrier to the formation of a strong patient–therapist relationship. Furthermore, we outline potential strategies for improving the relationship. Tools for monitoring the relationship are outlined in the Appendix.

3 Pain-related fear as a barrier to the patient–therapist relationship

The question of how pain-related fear interferes with the formation of a strong patient–provider relationship is complex. There are a number of factors that have the potential to interfere with this relationship. Some of these are related to the nature of pain-related fear, while others are related to the therapist and the mistakes that can be made with patients who are challenging (e.g. showing a lapse in empathy, providing insufficient education). The following example serves to illustrate a challenging exchange between therapist and patient (note that case examples are based on hypothetical patients drawn from practice).

Barriers to therapeutic alliance	Positive response	Case description
Patient complexity		Paula was a 30-year old nurse's aide who had experienced chronic back pain for the past 2 years. The pain initially occurred when she was transferring a heavy elderly client from a commode to bed, and immediately resulted in lower back and mid-thoracic pain. She was off work for approximately 6 months and received a combination of physiotherapy and massage therapy. She then returned to work, but was re-injured after approximately 1 month, again while transferring a patient. During the transfer she noticed severe low back and thoracic pain much like when she was first injured, but also became both nauseous and dizzy. In order to regain composure, she used cold face cloths and was provided with oxygen by her co-workers. She then attended the Emergency Room where she was referred for physiotherapy, and provided with a prescription of NSAIDs and muscle relaxants. Her physiotherapist diagnosed grade I mechanical thoracic pain and treated her back conservatively three times a week with interferential current therapy, stretching, and mobilizations. Her family physician reviewed her progress on a monthly basis, and arranged for a referral to a specialist at Paula's request. When this consultation did not produce significant findings Paula was referred to a tertiary level treatment program involving medical care, physiotherapy, exercise therapy, occupational

(Continued)

Barriers to therapeutic alliance	Positive response	Case description
		therapy, and psychological services. Upon meeting with the therapist, Paula shuffled slowly and laboriously into the office and lowered herself with enormous care into the chair. She frequently adjusted her position throughout the meeting and on numerous occasions stood up to stretch.Upon rising she was highly guarded in her posture.
Varying perspectives (medical view of pain and injury) Varying treatment goals		She described having little understanding of why she needed to see a psychologist as part of her care, and could not foresee this being beneficial. She related how she had been injured, how her injury had progressed, and the treatment that she had received with vivid detail. She reported being concerned that the specialist had not spent enough time with her and that an MRI had not been performed. Paula further described how she had spent considerable time on the Internet in an attempt to understand her concerns. She reported a significant degree of disability including not only an inability to work but also engage in many leisure activities. She described no significant difficulties in her relationship, and reported that her husband had been quite helpful and supportive. With respect to work, she described missing her work as well as her co-workers, and admitted to concerns that she would never be able to return to her position.
Readiness for treatment (negative perception of providers)	Clarification or role	*Therapist:* Paula do you know why you were asked to see me? *Paula:* I guess it is routine. You'll see though, I don't need any help with my "mind." I think the physiotherapy will be beneficial, but I really don't need anyone to talk to. I know that everyone thinks I am depressed, but if I could just figure out what is going on with my back, I would feel great. I also don't see how they expect me to participate in the exercise program or the work hardening unit. I think the providers are the one's who are out of their mind.

(Continued)

Barriers to therapeutic alliance	Positive response	Case description
	Acknowledge feelings and educate	*Therapist:* You are right about the referral to me being "routine". Many patients don't quite understand what this is all about. Part of my role is to help you understand your injury better, and the factors that may be contributing to increased pain, such as muscle tension, under-activity, poor sleep, stress, or even worry. I'm also here to help you to find new ways to deal with the injury and its consequences; things that maybe you have not tried yet.
Low self-efficacy		*Paula:* Yes. I understand. That is likely quite helpful for some of the patients that I have seen receiving treatment here. What I really need though is to go home and go to bed. I am exhausted. There is really nothing I can do once the pain gets bad like it is today . . . other than sleeping. Medication doesn't even help.
Requirement for participation	Empathy	*Therapist:* I can see that you are tired today. It sounds like coming here and meeting with everyone is quite a bit more than you normally do. *Paula:* It sure is.
	Education Assessment	*Therapist:* Well I don't want to keep you long today. What I'd like to do, however, is set up a time to talk to you further about your injury. It is important for me to obtain a really good understanding of your pain and how it has affected your life. This will help me to help you better. I have a number of questionnaires that I'd actually like you to complete that will assess things like pain severity, and ability to engage in activity. Some measures will also ask about the impact of your pain on your mood, relationships, and vocational plans. *Paula:* I don't mind completing questionnaires. I think that would help you understand where I am coming from. I don't think my file is very accurate.

3.1 **Patient dissatisfaction with care**

It is often in the context of general dissatisfaction with health care that the psychologist attempts to form a relationship with a patient. Evidence collected by our group suggests, for instance, that pain-related fear negatively affects the patient–physician relationship (Hadjistavropoulos *et al.* submitted). Patients with higher pain-related fear report lower levels of satisfaction with the information provided by their physician, the support they receive from their physician, as well as their own ability to initiate communication with the provider. It appears that fear of pain is associated with a deteriorated patient–physician relationship. From the outset the psychologist is in a difficult position. For many chronic pain patients, especially those who have pain-related fear, it is not uncommon for them to have experienced numerous diagnostic tests, and have had contact with multiple providers from a variety of disciplines. Rhodes *et al.* (1999) carried out interviews with patients and found that when physicians are unable to identify a problem or express reservations about whether a solution is available, patients feel alienated and also may feel delegitimized. As noted aptly by Hanlon *et al.* (1987), over time

> Continued medical consultations falling short begin to diminish the trust and hope that remains. Anger and pessimism with the health care systems grows, but no other options are evident so the patient continues to search for successful treatment . . . What the provider confronts then is an exhausted, distrustful, defensive, dysphoric, angry, hopeless . . . patient . . . who hold on to yet one more glimmer of hope that the health care provider can find 'the cure'. (pp. 40–1)

It is in this context that the psychologist attempts to form a positive working relationship.

3.2 **Varying perspectives**

Perhaps one of the most significant barriers to the relationship is the wide gap in how pain is likely to be understood by the patient and therapist. It is common for patients with chronic pain to be seeking medical management, rather than self-management for their condition. They are typically in search of a biomedical explanation and treatment approach (Turk 1996), and can become disgruntled if referred for psychological services (Kerns *et al.* 1999). With any chronic pain patient, not only those with pain-related fear, forming a strong relationship can be challenging when it requires patient acceptance of a self-management approach to treatment as compared to medical management, which patients hope will offer complete relief (Kerns *et al.* 1999). Exacerbating the situation, patients with pain-related fear have a lower acceptance of pain (McCracken 1998), meaning they are more likely to engage in unproductive attempts to control pain or to assume pain implies disability. Lower acceptance of pain will unquestionably make the formation of a relationship with the therapist arduous. The extent to which patients have varying views of pain may, in part, be related to the provider from whom they have been receiving care. Physiotherapists, for instance, who take a biomedical treatment orientation, have been found to be more likely to view daily activities as more harmful to the patient and to be inclined to advise patients to limit daily activity (Houben *et al.* submitted).

3.3 Varying goals

Related to different understandings of pain, the patient and therapist may have different goals for therapy. The typical theory held by patients is that if the pain could be relieved, anxiety would no longer be a problem. The idea that anxiety reduction could improve pain and functioning is time and again seen as foreign. The patient's goal is to avoid pain; they are reluctant to engage in exercise and activity because of fear (Kerns *et al.* 1999). The therapist's goal, on the other hand, is to encourage patients to engage in activities that may provoke sensations of pain. This provides patients with the opportunity to learn that feared consequences will not occur or correct false estimations of the degree of pain present. The quality of the relationship is extremely important when techniques are used that require trust and cooperation and where patients are asked to carry out those activities that they fear will increase pain, disability, and injury. Yet, it is these requests themselves that may serve as the largest threat to feelings of trust and interest in forming a working alliance. When patients are not necessarily in agreement with goals, numerous behaviors may become apparent that will interfere with the relationship, such as missing appointments, arriving late, not participating in discussions, and not carrying out the assigned homework.

3.4 Low readiness for treatment

Notwithstanding the difficulties encountered as a result of varying perspectives and goals, patients with pain-related fear also vary in the degree to which they are ready to engage in a new way of approaching pain. Researchers suggest that the patient–therapist relationship is exceptionally difficult to form with patients who demonstrate low treatment readiness (Keijsers *et al.* 1999). This is in keeping with observations and research by Prochaska and Di Clemente (1982) who found preliminary support for the idea that patients move through various stages of change when attempting to alter problematic behavior. These stages are described as pre-contemplation (no consideration given to changing), contemplation (thinking about changing), preparation (preparing to change), action (actively modifying approach to problem), maintenance (maintaining new approach), and relapse (return to a previous stage). Patients with pain-related fear are predicted to be in the very early stages of change, not quite ready to confront pain-related fear as part of the problem (pre-contemplation or contemplation), and instead are still focused on pain relief. Additionally, due to the nature of chronic pain, which can often be episodic in nature, motivation to engage in a therapeutic relationship may not be static, but may vary considerably over time. Patients with chronic pain may also be particularly passive and reluctant to engage in therapy because of many previous treatment failures (Kerns *et al.* 1999).

3.5 Requirement for participation

Because there is a high degree of effort and participation required in the treatment of pain-related fear, this may present a barrier to forming a positive working relationship. Many patients come to therapy with the expectation that something will be done to them, and are bewildered with the degree of effort, planning, and participation that is required on their part for treatment to be effective. As treatment becomes more complex, intense, and long term, adherence has been found to be low (Kerns *et al.* 1999) and, consequently, the relationship is threatened.

3.6 Low self-efficacy

Low self-efficacy may also be a contributing factor to the formation of a poor working relationship for patients with pain-related fear. When patients have particularly low self-efficacy, they typically experience low confidence in their ability to succeed in treatment. As a result, trust in the therapist and confidence in treatment suggestions are eroded. Among a sample of pain patients attending a work rehabilitation program, those who failed to complete the program had previously expressed significantly lower expectations regarding the likelihood that they would be able to return to work following program completion (Carosella *et al.* 1994). Comorbid with these lowered expectations, patients who drop out of a program also report higher pain intensity and somatic preoccupation ratings as well as perceive themselves to be significantly more disabled than patients who complete a program, even though both groups have similar physical impairments.

3.7 Patient complexity

In general, the patient with pain-related fear does not fit the mold of an ideal patient, and this likely does little to enhance the relationship with the provider. Smith (1985) described the perfect patient as one "who presents with a clear-cut and treatable organic disease, follows directions, makes no demands upon the provider, gets well, and expresses appreciation" (p. 300). Similarly, Finn (1986) describes the endearing patient as one who is concise, arrives on time, presents an organized story of their illness, and complies with recommendations. The patient with pain-related fear has few, if any, of the above characteristics. Research by McCracken *et al.* (1993) suggests that patients who experience pain-related fear have inflated expectations of pain and also demonstrate reduced range of motion during physical activity. They have also been found to have more days of work loss (Waddell *et al.* 1993) and are more likely to report non-specific physical complaints (McCracken *et al.* 1998) that can serve to consume time and effort during a medical evaluation. McCracken *et al.* (1998) have found evidence to suggest that pain-related fear is the greatest predictor of general physical symptoms and that these symptoms arise as a direct result of distressing events related to pain. These non-specific physical complaints add complexity to the presentation.

Patients who experience pain-related fear are also consistently found to have elevated scores on other constructs, such as trait anxiety (McCracken *et al.* 1993), anxiety sensitivity (Asmundson and Norton 1995; Asmundson *et al.* 1999), health anxiety (Hadjistavropoulos *et al.* 2001) as well as depression (McCracken *et al.* 1992). Beyond pain-related fear, these other patient characteristics that co-occur with pain-related fear may add complexity to the development of strong rapport and a working alliance. Supporting this, for instance, is evidence indicating that depressed people are more often rejected by those they interact with (Hammen and Peters 1978) and that anxious patients have difficulty forming a relationship with their therapist (Mallinckrodt *et al.* 1995).

3.8 Therapist frustration

Clinical observations suggest that therapist frustration with patients who present with pain-related fear is a significant problem that impacts on the formation of a strong working alliance. This frustration interferes with therapist ability to maintain rapport with patients, and, thus, perhaps to secure patient participation in treatment. As noted by McCracken, *et al.* (1997) "lack of success in treatment . . . may be unpleasant and frustrating to treatment personnel; this may be unintentionally communicated to the patient, which can compromise the patient's perception of care" (p. 293). Interestingly, review of the psychological literature in general suggests empathic failures are a larger threat to the relationship than technical errors (Safran *et al.* 1990). Psychologists are not alone in experiencing frustration. Burns *et al.* (1999) hypothesized that negative interactions with patients may lead the physician to feel alienated from or critical of the patient, which would then undermine the formation of a positive working relationship. This group found support for this in that physicians in a work-hardening program reported the poorest alliances with patients who were both depressed and angry.

4 Strategies for improving the relationship between therapist and patient

Although many health care providers view the relationship with the patient as important, relatively little attention has been given to how to develop and nurture this relationship, especially among complex patients such as those experiencing pain-related fear. Below we will outline some concrete recommendations for consideration by providers in improving interactions with patients. To our knowledge there are no recommendations that exist in the literature regarding how to form the best relationship with patients with pain-related fear, although many therapists and researchers have written on strategies for relationship building and engaging patients in treatment (e.g. Rothstein and Robinson 1990; Shiang *et al.* 1997; Gelso and Hayes 1998). From this work we have made some recommendations that seem especially pertinent to patients with pain-related fear. It should be emphasized, however, that the information below is based primarily on unsystematic, extended clinical observations. We hope that it will be enlightening and constructive advice for clinicians, but also serve as a stimulus for further research, which would clearly be desirable both in terms of expanding our knowledge and improving practice. We found chapters by Jensen (1996) and Kerns *et al.* (1999) on enhancing motivation for treatment with pain patients to be particularly valuable in writing this section as well as chapters by Eimer (1989) and Miller (1991). The Appendix contains a checklist for therapists to review following sessions as a tool for identifying characteristics that may be contributing to a poor relationship as well as strategies that are worthy of further reflection if the relationship is viewed to be strained.

4.1 Attention to the relationship

First and foremost, therapists must recognize that the therapeutic alliance is vulnerable and needs to be monitored and cultivated on an ongoing basis. Despite the evidence demonstrating how important the relationship is between therapist and patient, there is very little evidence in the literature to suggest that the relationship is nurtured to the degree that is required for therapy to be effective. Although both patient and provider contribute to the relationship, the therapist needs to take primary responsibility for the relationship. This is certainly not easy. As noted by Shiang *et al.* (1997), being a therapist can be likened to driving a car: "It's not clear when to put on the brakes and when to accelerate, whether to take this street or this boulevard—sometimes we're not even sure there is a destination" (p. 85). The relationship is not necessarily stable over time and it cannot be assumed that, once formed, it will not falter (Safran and Segal 1990). Health care providers need to take steps to monitor and assess the nature of the relationship, nurture this relationship, and confront problems when they emerge. Finn (1986) noted that tension in the relationship requires exploration, as does a passive stoic patient. Patients may be reluctant to discuss concerns based on past experiences and, thus, need to be encouraged to talk and communicate.

4.2 Empathy

Empathy is crucial in all therapeutic relationships, but is especially important for consideration with patients with pain-related fear. As noted by Safran and Segal (1990), it is essential to continually make an effort to understand how patients construct reality, which then helps in the tailoring of interventions. As aptly worded by Jensen (1996), empathy involves communicating respect, active reflective listening in order to accurately understand the patient's perspective, and reflecting that understanding back to the patient. It is theorized that feeling understood and accepted by the therapist allows the patient to consider their future options instead of protecting their current mode of operating (Jensen 1996). Empathy can also be critical for improving readiness for treatment (Jensen 1996). In the case example presented above, the therapist's responses to Paula serve to demonstrate how the therapist can respond with empathy and warmth while still attempting to engage the patient in therapy and explore a new perspective. Empathic listening and reflection are highlighted in the following dialogue:

Paula: It's so hard to go through the day being constantly worried about what could happen to my back with just one wrong move. It is impossible to keep my mind on other things when I am constantly worried that my pain will get out of control if I don't pay attention.

Therapist: I can see that this is very upsetting for you and that your worry about pain or the possibility of further injury is having a huge impact on your life. It must be very frustrating not to fully get involved in things because you are worried?

Paula: I also think everyone believes that this is all in my head, but I know from past experience that it can "pop out" in just a second.

Therapist: Many patients tell me that they fear that others think they are imagining their pain. I imagine that is also something you worry about a lot and causes you distress. I want to let you know that I believe that your pain is real and that it is influencing your life. I know you are in a lot of distress and this is why I want to work with you and see if we can find some ways for you to manage your pain and your anxiety.

4.3 Comprehensive assessment

Beyond a working alliance and empathy, a comprehensive assessment is also vital to the relationship. It serves to ensure patients that their circumstances are fully understood prior to treatment and communicates to them that treatment will be tailored to their condition. Without a comprehensive assessment patients often doubt that their special and unique circumstances will be understood and that treatment will be appropriate for them. Without the comprehensive assessment, patients, rather than participating in therapy, will often revert to providing historical information to the therapist in an effort to be understood (Eimer 1989). For further background on assessment, the reader is encouraged to review Chapters 9 through 11.

One of the greatest challenges in the assessment interview is facilitating patient disclosure of relevant information. Patients are usually reasonably able to answer questions about how their injury occurred, how disabled they are, and what treatment they received, but have more significant difficulty describing the social and emotional consequences of their situation. Psychosocial issues do not need to become the focus of attention in the first session, but by the second or third session patients need to be asked questions about pain-related fear. Beginning with a leading question can be helpful in this regard: "Often times when people experience pain for significant periods of time, they become anxious about whether and when they will recover. Have you experienced this?" "Given what you have been telling me about your concerns, I wonder how worried or anxious you are about your condition?" Once disclosure begins, more specific questions can be asked: "What things tend to make you anxious?" "What do you tend to do when you become anxious?" "How do you feel physically, when you begin to become anxious about your pain. Do you experience palpitations, sweating, trembling, shortness of breath, choking, nausea, dizzy, light-headed, or fear of losing control?" "What types of thoughts run through your mind about the pain?" "Do you have strategies for dealing with the anxiety?" "What helps the most?" "What makes it worse?" "When you are anxious is it hard to sleep?" "Is it difficult to concentrate?" "Do you feel more irritable when you are anxious?" "Are you restless?" "Do you feel fatigued?" "Do you notice significant muscle tension?"

Part of the comprehensive assessment that can assist with the relationship involves self-report questionnaires as described in Chapter 9. We have found it helpful to spend some time introducing the questionnaires, including how they will be useful for understanding current problems but also for measuring change over time. It is not uncommon for patients to experience a certain degree of frustration in rating their concerns using Likert ratings scales. Furthermore, the number of questions that are often asked of them can be overwhelming and serve to place a strain on the relationship. As a result, special attention to questionnaires is required to ensure that tools that are meant to be useful do not jeopardize the therapeutic relationship.

4.4 Family involvement

Involvement of family or significant others in therapy can often enhance the therapeutic relationship. Our experience is that patients feel a greater sense of being understood when family members are involved in treatment. Thus, by increasing knowledge of the individual and his or her family life and social context, the therapeutic relationship is enhanced. Furthermore, family members can often facilitate therapy by encouraging the patient to engage in the therapeutic relationship (Sanders 1996). Involvement of family often begins at the time of assessment with questions such as: "How has your spouse reacted to your condition?" "Is your spouse anxious about your condition?" "Does your spouse have suggestions for how to deal with the pain?" "Does your spouse have suggestions for how to deal with the anxiety?" Patients should be asked directly if the spouse or other family members want to be involved in treatment.

4.5 Education

Provision of adequate information regarding the biopsychosocial view of pain and the treatment approach is essential to the formation of the relationship and ensuring readiness for treatment. Without adequate attention to the rationale for treatment, patient concerns about why they are seeing a psychologist can remain for long periods and interfere with the establishment of a therapeutic relationship. As noted by Eimer (1989), ensuring that the patient is socialized to the model assists with the formation of a solid therapeutic relationship. Deyo and Diehl (1986) have noted that the most frequently cited source of dissatisfaction among patients with low back pain is failure to receive adequate information or explanation of their back pain. It is essential that therapists provide patients with education about psychology and the treatment of pain-related fear early on so this does not impede progress. In Chapters 13, 14, and 15 the authors provide excellent information on how to introduce psychological treatment to the patient. Taking time following the provision of the education to ask patients if they have questions or ask how they feel about seeing a therapist is also vital.

Specific to patients who are anxious about their health, which includes pain-related fear, Warwick (1992) emphasizes education as crucial to the relationship, and, in particular, recommends that education be delivered in such a way that health care providers: (1) listen to the patient so that he or she feels understood; (2) examine fears that the patient has and answer specific questions; (3) use simple terminology and explanations; (4) provide consistent statements; (5) provide clear explanations of symptoms, and ensure that information is understood; and (6) maintain interest and a positive attitude.

4.6 Collaborative goal setting

Perhaps the most discussed component of the patient–therapist relationship is the development of a "working" or "therapeutic" alliance. This refers to the idea that the therapist and patient work together with the purpose of assisting the patient with some problem (Gelso and Hayes 1998). Bordin (1979) defines the working alliance as the affective bond between patient and therapist and an agreement between the two on the tasks to be undertaken within sessions and the goals and likely outcomes of therapy. There are several reliable, valid, and convenient measures of the working alliance, including the Working Alliance Inventory (Horvath and Greenberg 1989), the Penn Helping Alliance Questionnaire (Alexander and Luborsky 1986), and the California Psychotherapy Alliance Scales (Gaston 1991).

Turk and Rudy (1991) take the position that engaging patients as collaborators to customize their treatment will go a long way to improve adherence and treatment outcomes. This means that the therapist is a disseminator of information as well as a facilitator and that the therapist and patient collaboratively set observable and measurable, mutually agreed upon goals (Hanlon et al. 1987). This can be an immense challenge in many situations since the patient and therapist can have vastly different views on pain and ideas about the components of treatment. Jensen (1996) suggests that to motivate patients in exploring new views and trying new approaches to treatment it is helpful to probe the patient to recognize discrepancies between behaviors (e.g. avoidance) and goals (e.g. working, engaging in leisure activities). Communication should be characterized by negotiation rather than confrontation (Hanlon et al. 1987). It is critical that the therapist avoid arguing with the patient, which has the paradoxical effect of having patients argue against an adaptive behavior change and can damage the working alliance. The importance of collaborative goal setting is especially evident when one considers research findings that demonstrate that patients who take an active role in their own care have better outcomes, experience feelings of self-efficacy, and are more satisfied with their caregivers than passive patients (Brody et al. 1989). The following example serves to illustrate an example of collaborative goal setting:

Paula: I am so frustrated with getting so little done in a day. I'd really like to have my old life back where I could just get up and "go go go."

Therapist: You mentioned several times now about not meeting your personal goals. I can see how you find this frustrating.

Paula: Yeah. It is very frustrating.

Therapist: I think this may be a good time for us to talk about how perhaps we could work together to help you get closer to being able to "go go go." I believe it will take some time, but I have some ideas about how you may be able to increase your activities and do some of the things you used to enjoy. Is this something you would like to explore?

4.7 Expression of affect

Relationships are often enhanced when patients are able to express and exhibit affect in therapy (McCullough *et al.* 1991). When patients open up in therapy, they will most likely feel increasingly connected to the therapist. McCullough *et al.* (1991) found that emotional responses in therapy are predictive of a positive outcome, whereas "shutting down" predicts a poor outcome. Given the complexity of emotion among patients with pain-related fear, creation of an environment where patients can express emotion is extremely important. For instance, one technique often used in cognitive–behavioral therapy to overcome anxiety is systematic exposure to what one fears (see other chapters in Section 3 of this volume). To have this technique work effectively, the patient must be able to accurately express his or her emotions in order for the therapist to be able to appropriately construct treatment. In the example above, the therapist could have explored further expression of affect with Paula, which may have served to increase the readiness for collaborative goal setting. For example, if the therapist does not feel that the patient is ready to move into goal setting, further attention could be given to expressing and acknowledging affect, which may have heightened readiness to collaborate.

Therapist: You mentioned several times now about not meeting your personal goals. Can you tell me more about what you're missing out on.

Paula: Everything I used to love doing . . . walking, jogging, biking, rollerblading, swimming, going to movies, visiting with friends, dancing.

Therapist: That is a lot of things you used to do. It sounds like you were very active and social before.

Paula: I was . . . I don't feel like myself anymore.

Therapist: Do you tend to keep those feelings of loss to yourself?

Paula: Yeah . . . I don't want to bother other people with my sadness . . . I try not to think about it much myself, but it is hard.

4.8 Highlighting self-efficacy

Discussion and expression of emotion can be beneficial. Therapists, at the same time, need to be aware that they also must help the patient discover feelings of self-efficacy. This too can be beneficial to the relationship and to outcome. Bandura (1977) has long held that one of the most important factors in enhancing the therapist–patient relationship involves helping the patient feel efficacious rather than helpless. Self-efficacy refers to the patient's belief in his or her ability to perform a specific behavior (Bandura 1977). Fear of failure may contribute to lack of collaboration. Therefore, it is important for the therapist to openly discuss with the patient, the patient's fears regarding his or her ability to successfully cope with anxiety and pain and attain future goals, such as return to work. If the therapist does not acknowledge these fears, the underlying cognitions will likely not be challenged and treatment progress may be slowed or terminated.

Therapist: I have an idea for helping you to get back into your normal routine. This is the first step. It won't result in you doing everything you did before right away, but it will help you get on track. Are you up for it?

Paula: I'd say so!

Therapist: What has worked with other patients, and I think would be a good place to start, is this. Get up each day this week as if you were actually going to be going to work. Basically, what you will do is do what you would normally do—shower, eat, read the paper—just as if you were going to be going to work. Then once you are ready for work, what I'd like to suggest is that you stretch and walk as recommended by your therapist. After this, I'd like to suggest that you plan in some other activities for the day—things that you used to enjoy before you were injured. What do you think?

Paula: I think I could do that.

Therapist: Do you have any concerns about this?

Paula: Well what if I overdo it? What if I end up straining my back and then end up doing even less than I do now?

Therapist: I am so glad that you shared those fears with me. It is important that we are on the same page. Why don't we talk about what the day is likely to consist of and make sure that you feel comfortable and plan things that you feel you can do now. We can then work on increasing activity later.

4.9 **Technical competence**

Techniques also play an important role in the development of the relationship. That is, although the relationship is typically viewed as separate from the techniques used by the therapist, it is highly likely that the relationship will affect the nature and choice of techniques, and the techniques, in turn, will influence the nature of the relationship (Gelso and Hayes 1998). Succinctly stated, "the therapy relationship and therapeutic technique are not separate domains, but rather integrated aspects of a single process" (Wright and Davis 1994: 29). Recent research demonstrates that, when considered in combination, interventions, the therapeutic alliance, and fit of the intervention to the patient collectively explain a much greater proportion of the variance in treatment outcome (conservatively estimated at 60 percent) than any variable alone (Beutler and Harwood 2002). Beutler and Harwood (2002) specifically note that interventions account for modest variance in treatment outcome, namely 5–10 percent, and that similarly the therapeutic relationship accounts for somewhere between 7 and 9 percent of variance in treatment outcome. Techniques clearly interact with other aspects of therapy, such as the relationship, to produce a treatment outcome. Technical errors, such as poorly planned exposure or cognitive restructuring can damage the relationship, in particular reducing patient confidence in therapy. What this translates into for therapists is the need to adequately plan techniques and tailor them to the patient. As previously mentioned, one method of ensuring that one appropriately tailors their technique is through comprehensive assessment of the patient and also frequently reviewing how patients are feeling about techniques as you proceed. Chapters 13, 14, and 15 can be used to review techniques associated with pain-related fear. Ensuring adequate time prior to each session to plan and contemplate the techniques as they apply to your patient is recommended. Consultation with colleagues is also highly recommended if in doubt; other providers can often assist with technical competence by providing further insight into core cognitions that may require discussion or assisting in planning exposure exercises.

4.10 **Assignment of homework**

Homework assignments are an essential component of therapy with pain-related fear, but require special attention. Homework can help the relationship in that it serves to communicate recognition of life beyond therapy. At the same time, if not well implemented or reviewed in following sessions, homework assignments can place a strain on the relationship. Ensuring that homework assignments are designed collaboratively, are not too threatening, are simple, fit with daily routine, and are easy to understand will limit the negative effect that homework can potentially have on the relationship. Providing written instructions on the assignment and preparing for obstacles can help prevent failure and, thus, help avoid strain on the relationship. Jensen (1996) recommends that, when patients demonstrate resistance to homework (e.g. failing to or inadequately completing homework), the therapist reflect back concern that the patient may be exhibiting resistance to attempting a different approach to therapy.

4.11 Awareness of therapist reactions

As noted above, the patient with pain-related fear can be particularly challenging and therapists need to take time to reflect and become aware of their own personal reactions to the patient and the effect these reactions may be having on the patient and therapeutic alliance. Being aware of one's own reactions is challenging. It is not easy to stay focused on the patient, while also staying in touch with one's own emotional reactions (Shiang et al. 1997). There is enormous pressure to "do something" when working with patients and feelings of incompetence abound when treatment progresses slowly or fails. More often than not we tend to see patient progress as a reflection of our own ability. As therapists, we can help manage our feelings of incompetence and frustration by setting realistic expectations and recognizing the difficulty of the task that is before us and before our patient (Garfield 1992; Wright and Davis 1994). Exercises that can be helpful for avoiding negative reactions toward patients include taking the role of patient, practicing how to react to hostile and challenging statements, peer review of videotapes, and exploration of one's reactions to patients in the context of supervision (Wright and Davis 1994).

The therapist must recognize that formation of a strong relationship with a patient is not entirely in the hands of the provider. In the context of psychotherapy, there is considerable agreement that patients need to have had some positive experience with forming attachments in order to build a solid working alliance (Kokotovic and Tracey 1990; Mallinckrodt et al. 1995), and that they must have a willingness to collaborate (Horvath et al. 1993). Kokotovic and Tracey (1990) found that patients perceived to be hostile or estimated by their therapists to have had few past or present successful relationships were less likely to form a positive therapeutic alliance during the first session. Corroborating this finding, Muran et al. (1994) found that patients who display a hostile and dominant interpersonal style are likely to have a more difficult time establishing the alliance. Similarly, Mallinckrodt et al. (1995) found that the more one trusts and relies on others, feels comfortable with intimacy, expresses little fear of abandonment, and has experienced strong parental bonds, the easier it is to form a strong therapeutic alliance.

Luborsky *et al.* (1988) have looked beyond interpersonal style and attachment and identified additional patient qualities that contribute to the formation of a positive working relationship, including: Psychological security, good motivation, normal to raised affect, good self-disclosure, and good IQ. Examining patient attributes, Stiles *et al.* (1986) emphasize two characteristics in particular: (1) interest in exploration of self or involvement in therapy, and (2) moderate expectations of a positive outcome. Beyond examination of the therapist and patient as separate entities, it has been suggested that the extent to which both parties possess similar qualities (e.g. age or religious affiliation) may influence relationship formation and quality (Luborsky *et al.* 1983).

4.12 Multidisciplinary involvement

Finally, but certainly not least, collaboration with other professionals is critical to the relationship. Physician endorsement of treatment and safety will help build a better relationship. This recommendation is consistent with evidence that multidisciplinary treatment is more effective for chronic pain compared to single modality treatment (Hilderbrandt *et al.* 1997). Patients are often not initially focused on engaging in pain management, but are looking for a bio-medical explanation and treatment for their difficulties. Through the collaboration of psychologists and physicians, as well as other medically based providers (e.g. physiotherapists), the patient can be presented with a united position regarding treatment. This should help in strengthening the relationship between patient and psychologist as the other team members can quickly address doubts the patient may have regarding the psychologist's knowledge outside their specialty (e.g. knowledge regarding what activities are safe to engage in). For patients with pain-related fear this reassurance may be particularly important for engaging in exposure-based techniques.

Although it is not the psychologist's place to determine what care is provided by other health care professionals, there are some suggestions that the psychologist should make to the patient in this regard. This needs to be done in a highly sensitive manner, and can most easily be accomplished in a multidisciplinary setting, so that the recommendations do not interfere with the relationship between patient and psychologist. For instance, in the treatment of patients with health anxiety it is generally recommended that patients be encouraged to keep regularly timed appointments with physicians rather than ones triggered by a somatic complaint (Skelton *et al.* 1996). It is also important to encourage patients to visit the same health care professional. It is found, for instance, that fewer catastrophizing cognitions are reported when patients see the same physician for repeated consultations (van Dulmen *et al.* 1995). When anxious, there is a tendency to repeatedly seek the same information, even though the patient understands this information. In these cases, it is necessary to prevent the response (Warwick 1992). In other words, once reassurance has been provided effectively, the information is not repeatedly given. If reassurance is repeatedly given, this can serve to increase rather than decrease anxiety (Warwick 1992). If more than one provider is consulted this becomes impossible to monitor.

Also important in the relationship between patient and psychologist is encouraging patients to limit unnecessary medical tests that are primarily designed to reduce anxiety (Warwick 1992; Shen and Soffer 2001). These tests, although initially serving to reduce fear, can in the longer term increase anxiety, typically by providing additional pain-related information for the patient to worry about. The examinations serve to perpetuate the focus on medical treatment and foster the belief that self-management of pain is not needed when, in fact, self-management with *all* medical conditions is required. In general, recommendations regarding how other professionals should provide care are best accomplished within a multidisciplinary context so as to not serve as a barrier to the relationship between patient and therapist.

5 Conclusion

Resolution of pain-related fear is crucial to successful treatment outcome among chronic pain patients (McCracken and Gross 1998). There is significant evidence to suggest that the development of a strong therapeutic relationship is likely to assist with therapeutic change. As described in this chapter, however, development and maintenance of the patient–provider relationship with patients who have pain-related fear represents a significant challenge to psychologists, as well as other providers. Based on research and clinical experience, we have outlined a number of strategies for establishing a relationship with patients who express significant pain-related fear. It is our hope that by writing this chapter we have consolidated and explored themes that are important to the patient with pain-related fear and, as a result, provide useful information for consideration by clinicians and enrich the potential for new and creative research in the field.

Further research in this area is essential and would serve to test many of the above hypotheses regarding the importance of the relationship between provider and patient with pain-related fear and how best to develop and strengthen this relationship to improve therapeutic outcomes. Numerous questions require clarification, such as:

1. How important is the relationship in shielding patients from the development of or exacerbation of pain-related fear?

2. How central is a poor therapeutic relationship in the growth and augmentation of pain-related fear?

3. How critical is the relationship for improving therapeutic outcomes among patients with pain-related fear?

4. If the relationship is critical, what are the most effective strategies for development, maintenance, and enhancement of this bond with patients experiencing pain-related fear?

Currently, our understanding of the impact of the patient–provider relationship on pain-related fear, as well as strategies for improving the affiliation, is based on clinical observations and extrapolation of findings in other areas of research. Direct study of the patient–provider bond among patients with pain-related fear is likely a fruitful area for future research with the potential to improve patient outcomes of countless individuals who suffer from fear of pain.

References

Alexander, L.B. and Luborsky, L. (1986). The Penn helping alliance scales. In L.S. Greenberg and W.M. Pinsoff (eds.), *The Psychotherapeutic Process: A Research Handbook*, pp. 325–66. New York, NY: Guilford Press.

Asmundson, G.J.G. and Norton, G.R. (1995). Anxiety sensitivity in patients with physically unexplained chronic back pain: A preliminary report. *Behaviour Research and Therapy*, **33**, 771–7.

Asmundson, G.J.G., Norton, P.J., and Veloso, F. (1999). Anxiety sensitivity and fear of pain in patients with recurring headaches. *Behaviour Research and Therapy*, **37**, 703–13.

Bandura, A. (1977). Self-efficacy: Toward a unifying theory of behavioral change. *Psychological Review*, **84**, 191–215.

Beck, A.T. and Weishaar, M.E. (1995). Cognitive therapy. In R.J. Corsini and D. Wedding (eds.), *Current Psychotherapies*, 5th ed., pp. 229–61. Itasca, IL: Peacock.

Beck, A.T., Freeman, A.F., and Associates. (1990). *Cognitive Therapy of Personality Disorders*. New York, NY: Guilford Press.

Beutler, L.E. and Harwood, T.M. (2002). What is and can be attributed to the therapeutic relationship? *Journal of Contemporary Psychotherapy*, **32**, 25–33.

Bordin, E.S. (1979). The generalizability of the psychoanalytic concept of the working alliance. *Psychotherapy: Theory, Research, and Practice*, **16**, 252–60.

Brody, D.S., Miller, S.M., Lerman, C.E., Smith, D.G., and Caputo, G.C. (1989). Patient perception of involvement in medical care: Relationship to illness attitudes and outcomes. *Journal of General Internal Medicine*, **4**, 506–11.

Burns, J.W., Higdon, L.J., Mullen, J.T., Lansky, D.L., and Wei, J.M. (1999). Relationships among patient hostility, anger expression, depression, and the working alliance in a work hardening program. *Annals of Behavioral Medicine*, **21**, 77–82.

Butler, S.F. and Strupp, H.H. (1986). Specific and nonspecific factors in psychotherapy: A problematic paradigm for psychotherapy research. *Psychotherapy: Theory, Research, and Practice*, **23**, 30–40.

Carosella, A.M., Lackner, J.M., and Feuerstein, M. (1994). Factors associated with early discharge from a multidisciplinary work rehabilitation program for chronic low back pain. *Pain*, **57**, 69–76.

Chew-Graham, C.A. and May, C. (2000). 'Partners in pain'—the game of painmanship revisited. *Family Practice*, **17**, 285–7.

Deyo, R.A. and Diehl, A.K. (1986). Patient satisfaction with medical care for low back pain. *Spine*, **11**, 28–30.

Eimer, B.N. (1989). Psychotherapy for chronic pain: A cognitive approach. In A. Freeman, K.M. Simon, L.E. Beutler, and H. Arkowitz (eds.), *Comprehensive Handbook of Cognitive Therapy*, pp. 449–65. New York, NY: Plenum Press.

Feuerstein, M. and Zastowny, T.R. (1996). Occupational rehabilitation: Multidisciplinary management of work related musculoskeletal pain and disability. In R.J. Gatchel and D.C. Turk (eds.), *Psychological Approaches to Pain Management: A Practitioner's Handbook*, pp. 458–85. New York, NY: Guilford Press.

Finn, W.F. (1986). Patients' wants and needs: The physicians' responses. *Loss, Grief and Care*, **1**, 1–18.

Galley, P.M. and Foster, A.L. (1987). *Human Movement*. Edinburgh: Churchill Livingstone.

Garfield, S.L. (1992). Major issues in psychotherapy research. In D. Freedheim (ed.), *History of Psychotherapy: A Century of Change*. Washington, DC: American Psychiatric Association.

Gaston, L. (1991). Reliability and criterion-related validity of the California Psychotherapy Alliance Scales—Patient version. *Psychotherapy*, **27**, 143–53.

Gelso, C.J. and Hayes, J.A. (1998). *The Psychotherapy Relationship: Theory, Research, and Practice*. New York, NY: John Wiley & Sons, Inc.

Hadjistavropoulos, H.D. and Williams, A. (2004). Psychological interventions and chronic pain. In T. Hadjistavropoulos and K.D. Craig (eds.), *Pain Psychological Treatment Perspectives*, pp. 271–301. New Jersey, NJ: Lawrence Erlbaum.

Hadjistavropoulos, H.D., Owens, K.M.B., Hadjistavropoulos, T., and Asmundson, G.J.G. (2001). Hypochondriasis and health anxiety among pain patients. In G.J.G. Asmundson, S. Taylor, and B.J. Cox (eds.), *Health Anxiety: Clinical and Research Perspectives on Hypochondriasis and Related Disorders*, pp. 298–321. London: Wiley.

Hadjistavropoulos, H.D., Quine, A., and Asmundson, G.J.G. (submitted). The patient–physician relationship in chronic pain patients: Predicting satisfaction. *European Journal of Pain*.

Hammen, C.L. and Peters, S.D. (1978). Interpersonal consequences of depression: Responses to men and women enacting a depressed role. *Journal of Abnormal Psychology*, **87**, 322–32.

Hanlon, R.B., Turk, D.C., and Rudy, T.E. (1987). A collaborative approach in the treatment of chronic pain. *British Journal of Guidance and Counselling*, **15**, 37–49.

Henry, W.P., Schacht, T.E., and Strupp, H.H. (1986). Structural analysis of social behavior: Application to a study of interpersonal process in differential psychotherapeutic outcome. *Journal of Consulting and Clinical Psychology*, **54**, 27–31.

Hildebrandt, J., Pfingsten, M., Saur, P., and Jansen, J. (1997). Prediction of success from a multidisciplinary treatment program for chronic low back pain. *Spine*, **22**, 990–1001.

Horvath, A.O. and Greenberg, L.S. (1989). Development and validation of the working alliance Inventory. *Journal of Counseling Psychology*, **36**, 223–33.

Horvath, A.O. and Symonds, B.D. (1991). Relation between working alliance and outcome in psychotherapy: A meta-analysis. *Journal of Counseling Psychology*, **38**, 139–49.

Horvath, A.O., Gaston, L., and Luborsky, L. (1993). The therapeutic alliance and its measures. In N.E. Miller, L. Luborsky, J.P. Barber, and J.P. Docherty (eds.), *Psychodynamic Treatment Research: A Handbook for Clinical Practice*, pp. 247–73. New York, NY: Basic Books, Inc.

Houben, R.M.A., Ostelo, R.W.J.G., Vlaeyen, J.W.S., Peters, M.L., Wolters, P.M.J.C, and Stomp-van den Berg, S.G.M. (submitted). Health care providers' orientations towards common low back pain predict harmfulness of physical activities and recommendations regarding return to normal activity. *European Journal of Pain*.

Jensen, M.P. (1996). Enhancing motivation to change in pain treatment. In R.J. Gatchel and D.C. Turk (eds.), *Psychological Approaches to Pain Management: A Practitioner's Handbook*, pp. 78–111. New York, NY: Guilford Press.

Keijsers, G.P.J., Schaap, C.P.D.R., Hoogduin, C.A.L., Hoogsteyns, B., and de Kemp, E.C.M. (1999). Preliminary results of a new instrument to assess patient motivation for treatment in cognitive-behaviour therapy. *Behavioural and Cognitive Psychotherapy*, **27**, 165–79.

Kerns, R.D., Bayer, L.A., and Findley, J.C. (1999). Motivation and adherence in the management of chronic pain. In A.R. Block, E.F. Kremer, and E. Fernandez (eds.), *Handbook of Pain Syndromes: Biopsychosocial Perspectives*, pp. 99–121. Mahwah, NJ: Lawrence Erlbaum Associates, Inc.

Kokotovic, A.M. and Tracey, T.J. (1990). Working alliance in the early phase of counseling. *Journal of Counseling Psychology*, **37**, 16–21.

Kumlin, I.W. and Kroksmark, T. (1992). The first encounter: Physiotherapists' conceptions of establishing therapeutic relationships. *Scandinavian Journal of Caring Sciences*, **6**, 37–44.

Lambert, M.J. and Bergin, A.E. (1994). The effectiveness of psychotherapy. In A.E. Bergin and S.L. Garfield (eds.), *Handbook of Psychotherapy and Behavior Change*, 4th edn., pp. 143–89. Oxford, England: John Wiley & Sons.

Lazarus, A.A. (1989). *The Practice of Multimodal Therapy: Systematic, Comprehensive, and Effective Psychotherapy*. Baltimore, MD: Johns Hopkins University Press.

Luborsky, L., Crits-Christoph, P., Alexander, L., Margolis, M., and Cohen, M. (1983). Two helping alliance methods for predicting outcomes of psychotherapy: A counting signs vs. a global rating method. *Journal of Nervous & Mental Disease*, **171**, 480–91.

Luborsky, L., Crits-Christoph, P., Mintz, J., and Auerbach, A. (1988). *Who will Benefit from Psychotherapy?: Predicting Therapeutic Outcomes*. New York, NY: Basic Books, Inc.

Mallinckrodt, B., Coble, H.M., and Gantt, D.L. (1995). Working alliance, attachment memories, and social competencies of women in brief therapy. *Journal of Counseling Psychology*, **42**, 79–84.

Marquis, M.S., Davies, A.R., and Ware, J.E. Jr. (1983). Patient satisfaction and change in medical care provider: A longitudinal study. *Medical Care*, **21**, 821–9.

McCracken, L.M. (1998). Learning to live with the pain: Acceptance of pain predicts adjustment in persons with chronic pain. *Pain*, **74**, 21–7.

McCracken, L.M. and Gross, R.T. (1998). The role of pain-related anxiety reduction in the outcome of multidisciplinary treatment for chronic low back pain: Preliminary results. *Journal of Occupational Rehabilitation*, **8**, 179–89.

McCracken, L.M., Zayfert, C., and Gross, R.T. (1992). The Pain Anxiety Symptoms Scale: Development and validation of a scale to measure fear of pain. *Pain*, **50**, 67–73.

McCracken, L.M., Gross, R.T., Sorg, P.J., and Edmands, T.A. (1993). Prediction of pain in patients with chronic low back pain: Effects of inaccurate prediction and pain related anxiety. *Behaviour Research and Therapy*, **31**, 647–52.

McCracken, L.M., Klock, P.A., Mingay, D.J., Asbury, J.K., and Sinclair, D.M. (1997). Assessment of satisfaction with treatment for chronic pain. *Journal of Pain and Symptom Management*, **14**, 292–9.

McCracken, L.M., Faber, S.D., and Janeck, A.S. (1998). Pain-related anxiety predicts non-specific physical complaints in persons with chronic pain. *Behaviour Research and Therapy*, **36**, 621–30.

McCullough, L., Winston, A., Farber, B.A., Porter, F., Pollack, J., Laikin, M. *et al.* (1991). The relationship of patient-therapist interaction to outcome in brief psychotherapy. *Psychotherapy: Theory, Research, Practice, Training*, **28**, 525–33.

McNeill, B.W., May, R.J., and Lee, V.E. (1987). Perceptions of counselor source characteristics by premature and successful terminators. *Journal of Counseling Psychology*, **34**, 86–9.

Mead, N. and Bower, P. (2000). Patient-centredness: A conceptual framework and review of the empirical literature. *Social Science and Medicine*, **51**, 1087–110.

Miller, P.C. (1991). The application of cognitive therapy to chronic pain. In T.M. Vallis and J.L. Howes (eds.), *The Challenge of Cognitive Therapy: Applications to Nontraditional Populations*, pp. 159–82. New York, NY: Plenum Press.

Morris, R.J. and Magrath, K.H. (1983). The therapeutic relationship in behavior therapy. In M.J. Lambert (ed.), *Psychotherapy and Patient Relationships*, pp. 154–89. Homewood, IL: Dow Jones-Irwin.

Muran, J.C., Segal, Z.V., Samstag, L.W., and Crawford, C.E. (1994). Patient pretreatment interpersonal problems and therapeutic alliance in short-term cognitive therapy. *Journal of Consulting and Clinical Psychology*, **62**, 185–90.

Orlinski, D., Grawe, K., and Parks, B. (1994). Process and outcome in psychotherapy— noch einmal. In A.E. Bergin and S.L. Garfield (eds.), *Handbook of Psychotherapy and Behavior Change*, 4th edn., pp. 270–376. Oxford, England: John Wiley & Sons.

Pascoe, G.C. (1983). Patient satisfaction in primary health care: A literature review and analysis. *Evaluation & Program Planning*, **6**, 185–210.

Prochaska, J.O. and Di Clemente, C.C. (1982). Transtheoretical therapy: Toward a more integrative model of change. *Psychotherapy: Theory, Research and Practice*, **19**, 276–88.

Rhodes, L.A., McPhillips-Tangum, C.A., Markham, C., Klenk, R. (1999). The power of the visible: The meaning of diagnostic tests in chronic back pain. *Social Science and Medicine*, **48**, 1189–203.

Rothstein, M.M. and Robinson, P.J. (1990). The therapeutic relationship and resistance to change in cognitive therapy. In T.M. Vallis, J.L. Howes, and P.C. Miller, (eds.), *The Challenge of Cognitive Therapy: Applications to Nontraditional Populations*, pp. 43–54. New York, NY: Plenum Press.

Safran, J.D. and Segal, Z.V. (1990). *Interpersonal Process in Cognitive Therapy*. New York, NY: Jason Aronson, Inc.

Safran, J.D., Crocker, P., McMain, S., and Murray, P. (1990). Therapeutic alliance rupture as a therapy event for empirical investigation. *Psychotherapy: Theory, Research, Practice, Training*, **27**, 154–65.

Sanders, S.H. (1996). Operant conditioning with chronic pain: Back to basics. In R.J. Gatchel and D.C. Turk (eds.), *Psychological Approaches to Pain Management: A Practitioner's Handbook*, pp. 112–30. New York, NY: Guilford Press.

Shen, B. and Soffer, E. (2001). The challenge of irritable bowel syndrome: Creating an alliance between patient and physician. *Cleveland Clinic Journal of Medicine*, **68**, 224–37.

Shiang, J., Landry, B., and Bongar, B. (1997). Psychotherapy. In J.R. Matthews and C.E. Walker (eds.), *Basic Skills and Professional Issues in Clinical Psychology*, pp. 83–113. Needham Heights, MA: Allyn & Bacon.

Skelton, A.M., Murphy, E.A., Murphy, R.J., and O'Dowd, T.C. (1996). Patients' views of low back pain and its management in general practice. *British Journal of General Practice*, **46**, 153–6.

Sluijs, E.M., Kok, G.J., van der Zee, J., Turk, D.C., and Riolo, L. (1993). Correlates of exercise compliance in physical therapy. *Physical Therapy*, **73**, 771–82.

Smith, R.C. (1985). A clinical approach to the somatizing patient. *The Journal of Family Practice*, **21**, 294–301.

Stiles, W.B., Shapiro, D.A., and Elliott, R. (1986). "Are all psychotherapies equivalent?" *American Psychologist*, **41**, 165–80.

Thomas, J.W. and Penchansky, R. (1984). Relating satisfaction with access to utilization of services. *Medical Care*, **22**, 553–68.

Thornquist, E. (1992). Examination and communication: A study of first encounters between patients and physiotherapists. *Family Practice*, **9**, 195–202.

Turk, D.C. (1996). Biopsychosocial perspective on chronic pain. In R.J. Gatchel and D.C. Turk (eds.), *Psychological Approaches to Pain Management: A Practitioner's Handbook*, pp. 3–32. New York, NY: Guilford Press.

Turk, D.C. and Rudy, T.E. (1991). Neglected topics in the treatment of chronic pain patients—relapse, noncompliance, and adherence enhancement. *Pain*, **44**, 5–28.

van Dulmen, A.M., Fennis, J.F.M., Mokkink, H.G.A., van der Velden, H.G.M., and Bleijenberg, G. (1995). Doctor-dependent changes in complaint-related cognitions and anxiety during medical consultations in functional abdominal complaints. *Psychological Medicine*, **25**, 1011–18.

Waddell, G., Newton, M., Henderson, I., Somerville, D., and Main, C.J. (1993). A Fear-Avoidance Beliefs Questionnaire (FABQ) and the role of fear-avoidance beliefs in chronic low back pain and disability. *Pain*, **52**, 157–68.

Warwick, H. (1992). Provision of appropriate and effective reassurance. *International Review of Psychiatry*, **4**, 76–80.

Wright, J.H. and Davis, D. (1994). The therapeutic relationship in cognitive–behavioral therapy: Patient perceptions and therapist responses. *Cognitive and Behavioral Practice*, **1**, 25–45.

Appendix: Working with patients with significant pain-related fear

Checklist of barriers to the patient–therapist relationship

Challenges in the therapeutic relationship	Therapist notes
☐ Patient dissatisfaction with care	
☐ Varying perspectives on pain	
☐ Varying goals	
☐ Low readiness for treatment	
☐ Low interest in taking active role in therapy	
☐ Low self-efficacy	
☐ Patient complexity	
☐ Therapist frustration	
☐ Other	

Checklist of approaches to improving the patient–therapist relationship

Approaches for improving alliance	Therapist notes
☐ Attention to relationship	
☐ Empathy	
☐ Comprehensive assessment	
☐ Family involvement	
☐ Education	
☐ Collaborative goal setting	
☐ Expression of affect	
☐ Highlighting self-efficacy	
☐ Technical competence	
☐ Competence in assignment of homework	
☐ Awareness of therapist reactions	
☐ Multidisciplinary involvement	

Part III

Treatment

Chapter 12

The management of pain-related fear in primary care

Benjamin H.K. Balderson, Elizabeth H.B. Lin, and Michael Von Korff

1 Introduction

Fear of pain and activity level are emerging as primary determinants of functional outcomes in patients with chronic or recurrent back pain (e.g. Frost *et al.* 1998; Mannion *et al.* 1999; Moffett *et al.* 1999; Abenhaim *et al.* 2000). In some back pain patients, fears of (re)injury or harmful movements of the spine are common. These fears can result in patients avoiding normal activities; a phenomenon called *fear-avoidance* (Lethem *et al.* 1983; Asmundson *et al.* 1999; Vlaeyen and Linton 2000).

Epidemiologic studies show that most back pain patients seek health care services first in the primary care setting. Two months after seeking care for back pain, a large proportion of primary care back pain patients continue to have significant pain-related worries (Von Korff *et al.* 1998; Moore *et al.* 2000). Optimal back pain management in primary care has the potential to influence subsequent outcomes for these patients. However, barriers to optimal care exist in primary care (Pruitt and Von Korff 2002) and most of the work on improving care for back pain is conducted outside of primary care. This chapter addresses the challenges of managing chronic back pain in primary care. Studies conducted in general health care settings illustrate the potential value of managing fear and disability in the primary care setting. We provide a model visit to guide primary care research and practice. The reorganization of primary care services to achieve optimal management of back pain is discussed.

2 The extent of the problem

In the United States, pain is the fifth leading reason for office visits (Hart *et al.* 1995), and back pain is the most frequently reported site of pain (Cherkin *et al.* 1994; Anderson 1999). Up to 80 percent of adults experience low back problems at some point in their lives (Clinical Standards Advisory Group 1994), and back pain is the most common cause of work-related disability in people under 45 years of age (Agency for Health Care Policy and Research (AHCPR) 1994). When patients decide to pursue medical care for common pain problems they typically turn to their primary care physician for help. Among individuals seeking care for back pain, 91 percent see a physician, predominately primary care physicians (Carey *et al.* 1995). A World Health Organization study found that in an international sample of primary care patients, 22 percent had persistent pain (i.e. pain present on most days in the prior year) and that back pain was the most common site (Gureje *et al.* 1998). Persistent pain was associated with disability, psychological distress, and unfavorable health perceptions.

Historically, back pain was viewed as an acute problem with favorable outcomes. In contrast, studies have demonstrated that a recurrent course of back pain is typical and that chronic back pain problems are more frequent than previously believed (Von Korff *et al.* 1993; Von Korff and Saunders 1996). Approximately 30 percent of patients seen in primary care for back pain have persistent problems 12 months later, and approximately 20 percent continue to experience moderate to severe activity limitations (Von Korff and Saunders 1996).

3 Challenges in the primary care assessment and care of back pain

3.1 Identifying and treating psychosocial factors

Psychosocial factors are often more important determinants of the functional outcome of back pain than physical findings (Waddell 1992; Clinical Standards Advisory Group 1994; Linton 1999). Primary care providers are often ill-prepared to address the psychosocial problems their back pain patients face (Cherkin *et al.* 1988). Evidence suggests that physicians struggle to identify such problems in their patients and experience frustration in trying to change patients' attitudes and behaviors (Alto 1995), rendering back problems among the conditions least liked by primary care physicians (Klein *et al.* 1982; Najman *et al.* 1982). Consequently, providers often view back pain patients as difficult, dependent, and unmotivated (Cherkin *et al.* 1988, 1995). Patients report similar negative emotions, expressing frustration and dissatisfaction with back care (Cherkin and MacCormack 1989).

Unfortunately, skills necessary to assess and modify this situation are not part of traditional medical education and are generally not available in most primary care settings (Von Korff 1999). To expect primary care physicians to provide cognitive–behavioral interventions at the necessary level for the more complex patients is unrealistic (Schorth 1996). Primary care providers may be able to deliver brief educational and behavioral interventions, but practical approaches appropriate to primary care need to be developed and tested for effectiveness.

3.2 Physicians' beliefs and behavior during primary care visits

In a survey of general practitioners and physical therapists, Linton *et al.* (2002) found that some practitioners held beliefs that may encourage fear-avoidance. More than two-thirds reported that they would advise a patient to avoid painful movements, over one-third believed a reduction in pain was necessary for a patient to return-to-work, and more than a quarter believed that sick leave is helpful for back pain patients. These fear-avoidance beliefs of physicians were related to practice behaviors. For instance, practitioners with high levels of fear-avoidance beliefs were more likely to provide low quality information about activities and were more uncertain in identifying patients at risk for poor outcomes (Linton *et al.* 2002).

An audiotape study of primary care back pain visits found that primary care physicians seldom addressed patient's worries and avoidance of normal activities (Turner *et al.* 1998; Von Korff 1999). The study physicians often did not explain their diagnostic actions to their patients, nor what serious conditions they had excluded. Although questions about "red flags" (i.e. signs and symptoms indicating a medically serious condition) were asked in most visits, the clinicians did not systematically explain the "red flags." Among patients who raised worries about disease (e.g. arthritis, spinal nerve problems), these worries were fully addressed only 50 percent of the time. Only 22 percent of the study patients were told to stay active and to avoid bed rest. Even though the primary care physicians often recommended exercise, the physicians did not give clear explanations of why engaging in normal activities and physical exercise is safe, even when back pain continues. These results suggest that there is considerable room for improvement in eliciting and addressing common patient worries in primary care.

Interestingly, in one study physicians who prescribed less bed rest and pain medicines were rated more favorably by their back pain patients and had lower care costs. In a longitudinal study of 1213 back pain patients, 44 primary care physicians were categorized into one of three groups—low, moderate, or high frequency of prescribing bed rest and prescription pain medicines. Patients treated by physicians in the infrequent prescriber group rated their doctors more favorably on quality of education about how to manage back pain and had lower 1-year ambulatory care cost (Von Korff *et al.* 1994).

3.3 Gap between guidelines and routine care for back pain

Despite the availability of clinical practice guidelines (Spitzer *et al.* 1987; AHCPR 1994), physicians' management and diagnostic strategies for back pain continue to vary widely (Freeborn *et al.* 1997; Di Iorio *et al.* 2000). The distribution of evidence-based guidelines was expected to change physicians' clinical practice, presuming that a knowledge deficit was the principle reason for practice variability. Not surprisingly, the dissemination of guidelines alone has not led to their implementation (Lomas *et al.* 1989; Lomas 1991). A variety of explanations for primary care providers' lack of compliance in implementing back pain guidelines have been proposed (Dixon 1990; Mittman *et al.* 1992; Conroy and Shannon 1995; Frost *et al.* 1998; Rainville *et al.* 2000). Greater specificity in the back pain guidelines may be necessary to improve implementation (Shekelle *et al.* 2000). Finally, some propose the key is the lack of organizational support and practical tools to assist physicians in implementing guidelines (Rossignol *et al.* 2000).

3.4 Patient expectations

Patients bring both realistic and unrealistic expectations to the visit. On the one hand, they believe that the most important things physicians offer is reassurance and advice (Klaber-Moffett *et al.* 2000). On the other hand, they believe that back pain is often due to a slipped disc or trapped nerve. Most expect a doctor to order an X-ray and to be able to tell them exactly what is wrong (Klaber-Moffett *et al.* 2000). Patients will often come with underlying fears regarding movement and expect that movement may cause further injury. Further, patients may expect that an intervention such as a prescription or procedure will resolve their back pain. Physicians need to be aware of such underlying expectations and prepared to re-orient patients to more realistic expectations for diagnosis, treatment, and prognosis.

4 Assessing and treating fear-avoidance beliefs and disability

Two months after seeking care for back pain, almost two-thirds of surveyed primary care patients continued to have concerns that a wrong movement might cause a serious problem with their back, and half believed that avoiding certain movements was the safest way to prevent back pain from getting worse (Von Korff *et al.* 1998; Moore *et al.* 2000). Patients who endorse these beliefs tend to have reduced activity levels and increased disability.

Primary care has the potential to influence the subsequent course of back pain and its care by assessing and managing patients' fear of back pain and related activity limitations. However, much of the research on fear-avoidance beliefs and disability is conducted outside of the primary care setting. Such interventions can be difficult to implement given the competing demands in primary care.

Based upon the research literature and our own programmatic research, our team has developed a brief means for addressing fear-avoidance beliefs and activity limitations with primary care patients with back pain. This approach has been used by a psychologist working with primary care back pain patients in combination with trained physical therapists. We recommend that practitioners employ techniques described in a "model back pain visit" that have proven effective in our research. The key elements of this model back pain visit are: (1) assessing fear-avoidance beliefs, (2) addressing identified fear-avoidance beliefs, (3) identifying activity limitations, (4) encouraging activity, (5) identifying and addressing potential "red flags," and (6) providing treatment recommendations and collaborative goal setting.

As part of this model visit we administer a brief questionnaire to be completed by the patient in the waiting room. This questionnaire aids the provider and helps to expedite the visit. The following section highlights data on each of these elements and provides examples of how they might be handled in a primary care back pain visit.

4.1 Assessing fear-avoidance beliefs

As previously mentioned, pain-related fear-avoidance beliefs are rarely assessed during primary care visits. At best, practitioners may ask open-ended questions regarding concerns or painful movement. This type of inquiry is unlikely to uncover patients' underlying fears that may influence their behavior. Further, patients may not view their problem as involving fear at all, but simply a problem involving difficulty performing certain activities or movement. However, further assessment of specific patients' fears and how they influence behaviors is often necessary to guide clinical management.

A number of standardized questionnaires have been developed to assess pain-related fear, avoidance, and anxiety, including the Tampa Scale of Kinesiophobia (TSK; Miller *et al.* 1991), Fear-Avoidance Beliefs Questionnaire (FABQ; Waddell *et al.* 1993), Pain and Impairment Relationship Scale (PAIRS; Riley *et al.* 1988), Pain Catastrophizing Scale (Sullivan *et al.* 1995) and the Pain Anxiety Symptoms Scale (PASS; McCraken *et al.* 1992). However, many of these questionnaires require too much time to administer, have redundant items, provide a score that needs further interpretation, and are generally impractical for primary care use (see Chapter 9 for further review of pain-related fear, avoidance, and anxiety questionnaires).

Our model visit questionnaire is a brief instrument and provides qualitative information to aid the physician in changing patient's worries. The assessment consists of an open-ended question regarding major concerns followed by eight specific questions. These eight questions ask about the most common fears reported by primary care patients (Von Korff *et al.* 1998; Moore *et al.* 2000; Balderson and Von Korff 2002). This is followed by an open-ended question targeting any feared activities or movements (see Appendix).

During the clinical visit the physician should clarify endorsed fear-avoidance beliefs and how they influence behavior. Normalizing concerns and the experience of pain may help patients understand that back pain is experienced by a large number of people and that their pain does not mean that their back is damaged. Because fears have largely been identified via the patient questionnaire, time can now be spent on providing individualized information that addresses specific fears.

4.2 Addressing patient's worries

Recent randomized controlled trials of brief interventions have found significant benefits of addressing fear-avoidance beliefs and encouraging resumption of normal activities. For example, Burton *et al.* (1999) found that an educational booklet addressing fear-avoidance beliefs reduced fears and yielded a short-term reduction in disability. The written material was provided to patients at the end of a physician visit for back pain and emphasized strength of the spine, the lack of serious disease, the association between recovery and activity, and the importance of positive attitudes about getting better. This differs from traditional educational messages and reassurance that a speedy recovery can be expected.

Similarly, Indahl *et al.* (1995) found that provision of reassuring messages about the safety of movement, stressing the importance of normal walking, personal goal setting, and return to normal activity were effective in reducing sick leave time for patients with back pain. It is noted that other studies have shown that providing basic educational material to primary care patients may not result in improvements in worries or functional status (Cherkin *et al.* 1996; Little *et al.* 2001) and, thus, its provision to aid back pain management is not fully understood.

Increasing the intensity of such educational measures has proven beneficial (Turner 1996). Von Korff and colleagues found in two randomized trials that brief group-format interventions addressing worries and concerns and advice to stay active reduced worry about back pain and yielded moderate reductions in activity limitations among primary care back pain patients. These effects were sustained at 1-year follow-up (Von Korff *et al.* 1998; Moore *et al.* 2000; Von Korff and Moore 2001). We further adapted the work conducted in the aforementioned trials and developed standardized messages providers can give in response to the most common back pain-related fears (see Table 12.1 for examples).

Table 12.1 Examples of corrective information scripts to address specific back pain-related worries

Identified fear	Model response to fear
Fears regarding diagnosis or underlying disease	"Many people with back pain are concerned about what is causing their pain or sometimes wonder if there is some undetected disease. The physical exam, in combination with the clinical history of your symptoms, helps us determine if a serious medical problem may be present, such as a tumor, infection, fracture, or pinched nerve and whether further diagnostic tests such as x-rays or CT scans are needed. I will conduct a physical exam today and will explain some of the things I am looking for. For instance during this exam I will be checking for <insert any relevant illnesses the patient expressed concerns about>. The good news is that a majority of people with back pain have what is considered non-threatening back pain. Based on what I know already I suspect your pain is a non-threatening form of back pain. But we will check everything out today to make sure."
Fears regarding movement and activity	"People with back pain are often concerned with particular movements or when is it safe to return to normal activities. I will know more about what may be safe for you after your physical exam, but generally if there are no red flag symptoms present, as a severe flare-up subsides, it is safe and beneficial to resume normal activities. While there is no specific exercise program that is right for all patients, regular aerobic exercise that you enjoy, such as walking, swimming, or cycling, is often helpful in reducing pain and improving a person's quality of life. One of the most important things is to be active and gradually return to normal activity."
Fears regarding prognosis and future disability	"It's normal to worry about the future. Will my pain ever go away or will it get worse? Back pain is often persistent or recurrent. About one in three patients with back pain have persistent back pain, meaning that they have back pain on more than half the days in a year. Flare-ups of pain are more common, over 80% of people seeking care for back pain have recurrences or flare-ups from time to time. Severe flare-ups, when back pain is at its worst, are over for most people within a few days to a week or two. After a flare-up, back pain usually improves gradually, but mild to moderate back pain can continue for months or longer. Thus, totally eliminating pain may not be realistic. The goal of treatment is to improve quality of life. The good news is that as long as people remain active back pain rarely worsens with time."

4.3 Assessing activity limitations

A major goal of addressing back pain-related fear is to reduce activity limitation and disability. In general, many primary care physicians are not aware of the extent back pain interferes with a patient's daily activity. Typically there is inadequate discussion regarding the importance of staying active, avoidance of bed rest, or clear explanations of why engaging in normal activities and physical exercise is safe even when back pain continues. In cases when providers do recommend exercise, there is often a lack of clear instructions regarding what activities are safe and how to regain lost functioning (Turner *et al.* 1998; Von Korff 1999).

As discussed in the assessment of fear-avoidance beliefs, the use of traditional standardized measures of disability may be useful but may require too much time to be used effectively in primary care. Measures used to evaluate back pain disability include the Roland Disability Questionnaire (Roland and Morris 1983; Deyo *et al.* 1998), Oswestry Questionnaire (Fairbank *et al.* 1980; Fairbank 2000), and Quebec Back Pain Disability Scale (Kopec *et al.* 1995, 1996). However, given the time required for administration and scoring, these measures are often not feasible for routine use in primary care.

To overcome some of these difficulties we have employed a brief set of questions about common activity limitations (Appendix). The questionnaire asks patients to rate the level of activity interference based on a 0–10 scale, across three major domains: (1) home and activities of daily living, (2) social and recreational, and (3) work activities. This is followed by an open-ended question regarding activity limitations and a checklist of common activities limited by back pain. Providers should follow-up and clarify these activity limitations. Often patient fears can be linked to activity limitations. This can help the patient understand how fear-avoidance beliefs have led to unnecessary activity limitations and disability. An example dialogue between a primary care physician and a back pain patient is provided below.

Provider: You indicated that back pain is affecting some of your activities.

Patient: Yeah, I can get along at work okay and doing things around the house isn't such a problem, but I avoid exercise.

Provider: What type of exercises do you avoid?

Patient: Just about all of it. I used to be real good . . . jogging, biking, I used to go to a gym. But now all of that sounds like a bad idea.

Provider: A bad idea?

Patient: Yeah, I worry that if I push my back real hard that I will make it worse. Maybe I should just let it rest, not push it too hard.

Provider: It sounds like you are concerned that exercise is unsafe for your back, that exercise will make it worse.

Patient: Yeah. That's it. I wonder what I can do safely now that my back hurts. Like what can or can't I do now, so I just avoid it all. But on the other hand I figure not exercising can't be great for me and I miss going for bike rides.

Provider: So you feel like exercise would be good for your health and even enjoyable but you worry about what is safe so you end up avoiding all exercise. It's true exercise and being active is a good idea, not only for your back but for your overall health. People with back pain are often concerned about particular movements or when is it safe to return to normal activities and exercise. Generally if there are no red flag symptoms present, as a severe flare-up subsides, it is safe and beneficial to resume normal activities. While there is no specific exercise program that is right for all patients, regular aerobic exercise that you enjoy, such as walking, swimming, or cycling, is often helpful in reducing pain and improving a person's quality of life. One of the most important things is to be active and gradually return to normal activity. Were there any specific movements or activities that you were worried about?

4.4 Addressing activity limitations

Activity interventions often overlap with those designed to address patients' worries because misperceptions about back pain are tied to concerns about physical activity. In fact most interventions designed to change fear-avoidance beliefs have components of changing activity limitations as well.

4.4.1 Advice to stay active

Deyo *et al.* (1986) found that recommending 2 days, rather than 7 days, of bed rest reduced days off work among acute back pain patients. This finding contributed to revised thinking regarding the role of prescribed bed rest and activation in back pain care (Quebec Task Force on Spinal Disorders 1987; Abenhaim *et al.* 2000). Burton *et al.* (1999), comparing two educational books, found both books resulted in greater improvement on the Roland Disability Questionnaire when compared to a usual care group. However, there were no significant differences between the two educational groups in Roland scores. Two studies by Von Korff and Moore, utilizing group sessions in primary care to provide educational, activating interventions that addressed fear-avoidance, have shown significant effects on Roland disability scores at follow-up (Von Korff *et al.* 1998; Moore *et al.* 2000; Von Korff and Moore 2001). Rossignol *et al.* (2000) found that adding care coordination efforts to usual care, that encouraged activation, yielded significant between group differences in disability scores at 6-month follow-up. Malmivaara *et al.* (1995) showed that advice to avoid bed rest and to continue routine activity as normally as possible resulted in better functional outcomes than either advice to rest in bed for 2 days or back mobilizing exercises for patients with acute back pain.

In a comparison of primary care patients with acute and subacute back pain, Linton and Andersson (2000) examined a cognitive–behavioral intervention against two written information only groups. The cognitive–behavioral intervention consisted of six group sessions conducted by trained therapists. The groups covered such topics as the causes and prevention of pain, activity scheduling, relaxation skills, cognitive appraisal, and communication skills. The pamphlet group received one pamphlet aimed at preventing fear-avoidance, promoting coping and advice to remain active and think positively. The information package group received information once a week for 6 weeks, to mirror the number of sessions in the CBT group. This material was based on a back school approach and advised how the patient might cope with back pain by such methods as lifting properly, maintaining good posture and maintaining usual activities. All three groups reported benefit, showing improvements in terms of pain, fear-avoidance, and cognitions. However, the cognitive–behavioral group showed comparatively lower long-term sick absence, perceived risk and a significant decrease in use of physician and physical therapy.

4.4.2 Exercise and structured activity programs

There is evidence that exercise is efficacious for the treatment of low back pain (Koes *et al.* 1995; Van Tulder *et al.* 1997, 2002). Fitness programs with aerobics, stretching, and strengthening components have been evaluated and found effective for patients with chronic back pain problems (Frost *et al.* 1998; Mannion *et al.* 1999; Moffett *et al.* 1999). Systematic reviews conclude that exercise improves functional outcomes of back pain patients, but evidence does not favor one form of exercise over another (Mior 2001; Van Tulder *et al.* 2002). A recent comparison of activating interventions (i.e. active physical therapy, muscle reconditioning using training equipment, aerobics) suggested that clinical improvements were not due to change in physical status as a result of specific treatment but, rather, to a change in patients' beliefs or perceptions of pain and disability (Mannion *et al.* 1999).

In addition, graded activity programs have been evaluated and appear to be more effective than information alone (Frost *et al.* 1998). Graded activity programs gradually increase activity levels, setting initial exercise levels according to the patient's baseline capacity. The effect size in these intervention studies has typically ranged from small to moderate, suggesting the difficulties in increasing activity levels in a patient population impaired by back pain.

In vivo exposure to feared activities might offer an approach to increase the effect size of activating interventions. Crombez *et al.* (1996) found that repetition of exercises at maximal force lowered future predictions of back pain. Single-case crossover studies have found that *in vivo* exposure to feared activities is more effective than graded activity (Vleayen *et al.* 2001, 2002). Results indicate that fear reduction only happened during exposure and not during graded activity. In addition, reductions in pain-related fear were accompanied by reductions in pain vigilance and disability and by increases in physical activity (Vleayen *et al.* 2001). Furthermore, treatment gains produced during exposure generalized to the home setting (Vleayen *et al.* 2002). *In vivo* exposure is discussed in detail in Chapter 14 of this volume.

The crucial point seems to be that patients alter the way they think about pain and their perceptions of their physical abilities when they become physically active. These findings are encouraging as exercise programs are relatively inexpensive, easily administered, and the type of exercise may not be so critical. However, adherence to activity recommendations becomes a concern in primary care because patients with pain problems may find it difficult to incorporate an exercise regimen into their daily routine (Deyo and Weinstein 2001), and primary care providers are not able to offer extensive support for adopting an exercise regimen. Adherence to any medical recommendation is increasingly more difficult as patients are asked to learn new behaviors, alter their daily patterns, and maintain changes over time (Marlatt and Gordon 1985; Meichenbaum and Turk 1987). Future investigations of exercise for long-term back pain management will need to address maintenance issues, especially in primary care settings.

Whether advised to remain active or to participate in a structured exercise program, a *key feature* of the activation concept is to avoid giving patients the message that they need bed rest to promote recovery from back pain. Although there is evidence of increased awareness in clinical practice about the importance of exercise and the avoidance of bed rest, a recent survey of family physicians identified continued problems with physician's advice. Physicians often recommended that patients with ongoing back problems restrict work and activities (Rainville *et al.* 2000) rather than encouraging return to normal activities and exercise. Some have suggested that a straightforward but fundamental change in physicians' advice could significantly improve outcomes and reduce costs associated with back pain (Waddell *et al.* 1997). A critical question is how to care for patients who require more guidance than simple advice. Organizing graded activity or *in vivo* exposure programs in physical therapy or other ancillary care settings may provide a means of reaching these patients.

4.5 **Clinical assessment and review of red flags**

As part of the clinical assessment physicians should not only check for "red flags" (i.e. indication of potential serious medical pathology) (AHCPR 1994; Atlas and Deyo 2001) but also explain them to patients. As previously mentioned, physicians do not appear to systematically explain red flags and only fully address disease-related fears about half the time. Physicians can use the clinical exam as an opportunity to explain what diagnoses are being ruled out and to further address illness-related fears. Explaining positive and negative findings of the physical examination may help to build patient confidence that a thorough examination has been conducted and particular problems ruled out. Explaining the importance of "red flags" can broaden patients understanding of medically important reasons for consulting a physician, and help them understand when self-care is appropriate.

The clinical exam should end with a clear explanation of the diagnosis and its likely prognosis. Allowing patients to clarify their understanding may help curb unnecessary confusion or concerns. Providing an understanding of the expected prognosis and potential difficulties may prepare patients for these difficulties and lay the ground work for discussion of how to manage them. If possible, reassurance that activity is beneficial, even if pain continues, is critical.

Provider: Your neurological exam shows that you have good muscle strength and no evidence of damage to the nerve. For example when I raised your leg up you did not show signs of significant pinching of the spinal nerve to your lower extremities. Overall you are not showing any signs of the alarming symptoms or red flags we were talking about. This is good news.

Patient: That's good to hear. So if its not one of these red flag symptoms what is it?

Provider: The type of back pain you are experiencing is pretty common, typically called mechanical or non-specific back pain.

Patient: Mechanical back pain. How come I got it, what caused it?

Provider: The cause of recurrent back pain is usually difficult to pinpoint. In most cases, physicians don't find any specific injury or condition in the muscles, joints, ligaments or nerves of the back that fully explains the pain. One idea is that after an injury, back pain causes people to tense their back muscles and limit their movement. These in turn may cause the muscle and ligaments to shorten, which can cause more pain. Have you ever tried tensing a muscle as long as you can? It quickly becomes tired and then painful. This may be happening in the back, if normal movement is restricted and muscles are tense.

This can happen without even being aware of how tense the back muscles are. Since your examination was normal, and you do not have any of red flag symptoms, your back problem is unlikely to be medically dangerous. However, it is common for people to have continued difficulties with pain.

Patient: Continued difficulties? Will my pain ever go away?

Provider: It's normal to wonder: Will my pain ever go away or will it get worse? Typically, severe pain gets better over a few days to a week, but mild to moderate back pain can be present in varying degrees for months or longer. Back pain is usually recurrent and sometimes persistent. Over 80 percent of people seeking care for back pain will have future episodes. Pain that continues or recurs does not mean that the body is injured. Nerve fibers can continue to send pain signals to our brain without significant tissue damage. So, becoming totally pain-free is often not possible. Rather, the goal of treatment is to improve quality of life. The good news is that you can do things to reduce the severity of pain, improve your activities and that for people who stay active, back pain rarely gets progressively worse with time.

Patient: You've mentioned keeping active earlier, that seems to be one of the key things I need to do to help make this better.

4.6 Treatment recommendations and collaborative goal setting

Following a clear explanation of the diagnosis and prognosis, any recommended diagnostic tests should be explained. If no diagnostic tests are needed, then this should be made explicit. Medications should be prescribed on a time-limited basis as a palliative measure and explained as such to patients. Any referrals to other providers, such as a physical therapist, should be considered and the potential benefits explained to the patient.

Time should be spent on recommending self-care behaviors that can help manage back pain, explaining that research has shown that self-care strategies including gradual return to normal activities and physical exercise are beneficial, improve quality of life, and can reduce awareness of back pain. Patients should be encouraged to set clearly defined behavioral goals or "action plans" aimed at encouraging the resumption of activities or exercise that the patient enjoys (Lorig 1993; Bodenheimer *et al.* 2002). Recommendations may be given but it is important that the patient, not the provider, set the "action plan". The physician should refrain from being prescriptive, providing only guidance as necessary. For instance the patient may need guidance in determining if selected goals are safe and manageable. Confidence in carrying out such plans should be checked to make sure the patient feels ready.

Provider: The [medicines/other palliative treatments] will help reduce your pain over the next few days, but research has consistently shown that self-care strategies including gradual return to normal activities and physical exercise are beneficial. Being physically active can improve the quality of your daily life and even help reduce awareness of back pain. Gradually returning to normal activities and physical exercise will be important for long term care for your back. If you were to think of how back pain has affected your life, what do you think you would like to get back to most?

Patient: A lot of things. Biking, gardening, going for walks with my wife. All the things I used to enjoy doing. But I know I can't just jump right back doing all of them, it's been awhile.

Provider: If you were to select one activity that you would like to do more of, something that is important to you and would really improve your day, what would that be?

Patient: I guess walking more, my wife and I used to walk the dog together every night.

Provider: When was the last time you went walking?

Patient: I haven't gone much, I went once last month. But I think I pushed it too hard. I really wanted to walk around the lake and afterwards my back really hurt.

Provider: It sounds like you would really like to go walking, how far do you think you can go with no problems?

Patient: I wish I could go for three miles like I used to, I used to do that a few times a week. But now I think I could only walk for about 15 minutes before I needed to take a break. But 15 minutes is that even worth it?

Provider: Sure, I think it would be great if you could get some walking in and every bit helps. It's important for you to realize what you can do now and where you would like to be. It sounds like you feel you can only walk for about 15 minutes but would like to get back to walking three miles a few times a week.

Patient: I guess that's true. I guess walking a little bit is better than none at all. I guess I could try walking for 15 minutes a few times and see how that feels.

Provider: That sounds like a great idea, when do you think you might go for a walk?

5 Reorganizing primary care

Primary care services are currently organized in a fashion that makes adequate management of chronic pain difficult. Some have proposed that pain problems are exacerbated by current pain management practices (Waddell 1996;

Crombez *et al.* 1999). Despite these difficulties, primary care is still the most appropriate setting for the management of non-specific back pain (Waddel 1996; Freeborn *et al.* 1997). With pragmatic restructuring, primary care has the potential to provide effective management of back pain and not only improve quality of life, but also potentially prevent chronic disability, thereby reducing back pain's societal costs (Malmivaara *et al.* 1995).

As the view of back pain shifts from an acute, rapidly resolving problem to a chronic, recurrent problem, primary care services need to change accordingly. Patients need accurate prognostic information regarding the expected course of their problem. For many patients, explicit reassurance, information, and education during an initial visit may be adequate. In fact, most patients may not desire or need additional primary care services if adequately educated during the early phase of back pain care. Unfortunately, effective reassurance and education are not routinely provided in primary care settings (Turner *et al.* 1998).

Back pain is the most common chronic pain problem, yet primary care services are not structured to address back pain as a chronic condition. To do so would involve changes in approach, such as those called for in the management of other chronic conditions such as asthma, diabetes, and arthritis (Davis *et al.* 2000). However, reorganization of care may not be as overwhelming as it initially appears. There is increasing recognition that management strategies for chronic conditions share common themes that make differences among specific chronic conditions less critical. Self-care tasks, shared by all chronic conditions including back pain, include engaging in health-promoting activities, minimizing impact on daily activities, monitoring and adapting to changes, collaborating with health care providers, and adhering to the management plan (Lorig 1993; Von Korff *et al.* 1997; Bodenheimer *et al.* 2002).

5.1 Collaborative care

In managing a chronic-recurrent illness, a collaborative approach between patients and providers can improve outcomes. Collaborative management has been defined as care that strengthens and supports self-care while assuring that effective medical, preventive, and health maintaining interventions take place (Von Korff *et al.* 1997). Preparing patients for care is an effective approach to enhancing patient–provider collaboration. Interventions that prepare patients for care typically orient patients about what to expect in the visit, educate patients about their condition, and coach patients in using this information to improve decisions and communication with their provider. Patient preparation has been shown to improve a range of outcomes including self-reported physical and psychological health, functioning, physiological outcomes, and satisfaction with care (Greenfield *et al.* 1985, 1988; Kaplan *et al.*

1989; Maly *et al.* 1999; Oliver *et al.* 2001). Better prepared patients may initiate care with more realistic expectations, better aligned with the expectations of the provider. Preparation may also enable back pain patients to assume a more active role in their care.

5.2 Stepped care

A stepped care approach may help by targeting intervention efforts. Stepped care provides a framework for distributing limited resources to the greatest effect on a population basis, while individualizing care. A stepped care approach initiates care with the least expensive, intensive, and restrictive treatment deemed sufficient to meet the patient's needs, increasing treatment intensity until a favorable outcome has been achieved (Donovan and Marlatt 1993). Thus, stepped care seeks to optimize care at both the individual and population level by providing each patient the level and kind of care needed to achieve a favorable outcome, no more and no less. Stepped care approaches have been advocated for the treatment of a wide range of chronic conditions (Von Korff and Tiemens 2000) including chronic back pain (Von Korff 1999; Von Korff and Moore 2001; Balderson and Von Korff 2002).

Drawing on data from studies conducted by our research group (Von Korff *et al.* 1998; Moore *et al.* 2000) patients needs were identified and used to help guide a stepped care approach. The lowest-intensity intervention (Step One) consists of addressing patients' fear-avoidance beliefs through education and information, and through advice about the importance of returning to usual activities as quickly as possible. This level of intervention is brief and can occur during a primary care office visit. Moreover, it may be all that is necessary for a majority of patients with nonspecific low back pain.

In Step Two, more intense interventions are employed, reserved for patients who continue to report activity limitations 6–8 weeks after seeking care. An intervention at Step Two could include a structured exercise program or other educational and activating strategies to address fears and help patients resume their usual work and leisure activities. Interventions at this level require more than can be offered in a single, 15-min office visit. Providers from other disciplines (e.g. physical therapists, nurses, psychologists) will be important for providing these kinds of interventions. One-third to one-half of primary care back pain patients may benefit from activating interventions that address common activity limitations that continue weeks and months after the primary care visit, although a smaller percentage of more severely impaired patients could be targeted.

Step Three is reserved for a smaller percentage of back pain patients (10–20 percent) who are experiencing significant work disability and are at risk of becoming permanently work disabled. This step consists of case management that addresses patient and work environment factors that contribute to work disability. Step Three may also include identification and treatment of psychiatric comorbidities (e.g. major depression). Step Three interventions may be provided in primary care if personnel, time, and space are available. For instance the treatment of depression can often be very effectively handled in primary care. The provision of more intensive supervised activity training, such as *in vivo* exposure or work hardening, also calls for the inclusion of other care providers (e.g. multidisciplinary pain team, occupational therapy, physical therapy).

6 Conclusion

Primary care is and will most likely continue to be the major entry point for care for patients with back pain. As the modal provider of back pain care, primary care is responsible for providing effective treatments to the widest group of back pain patients. Primary care providers are expected to not only provide effective and cost-considerate treatments to a diverse population of back pain patients but also help patients access appropriate diagnostic and therapeutic services.

The growing body of evidence on addressing back pain-related fear and activity limitation is promising. Research on the development of fear and chronic pain may help identify ways to target patients at risk of developing chronic problems (Sieben *et al.* 2002). Research on the optimal management of pain-related fears, such as *in vivo* exposure, has the potential to improve patient outcomes.

There continues to be many difficulties in the effective management of back pain in primary care. Although we have provided findings regarding the assessment and treatment of fears and activity limitations in primary care, more research is needed. How to best deliver patient education and self-management interventions in the primary care setting is an unanswered question. How to optimize the provision of quality back pain care in a time efficient manner given the time constraints of primary care? The content and timing of self-management interventions also need further study. Answering these questions will help primary care providers respond more effectively to the significant demands of back pain care in the primary care setting.

References

Abenhaim, L., Rossignol M., Valat, J.P. *et al.* (2000). The role of activity in the therapeutic management of back pain. Report of the International Paris Task Force on Back Pain. *Spine*, **25**(Suppl. 4), 1S–33S.

Agency for Health Care Policy and Research (1994). *Acute Low Back Problems in Adults. Clinical Practice Guidelines*, No. 14. U.S. Department of Health and Human Services: Rockville, MD.

Alto, W.A. (1995). Prevention in practice. *Primary Care*, **22**, 543–4.

Andersson, G.B.J. (1999). Epidemiologic features of chronic low-back pain. *Lancet*, **354**, 581–5.

Asmundson, G.J., Norton P.J., and Norton, G.R., (1999). Beyond pain: the role of fear and avoidance in chronicity. *Clinical Psychology Review*, **19**, 97–119.

Atlas, S.J. and Deyo, R.A. (2001). Evaluating and managing acute low back pain in the primary care setting. *Journal General Internal Medicine*, **16**, 120–31.

Balderson, B.H.K., and Von Korff, M. (2002). The stepped care approach to chronic back pain. In S.J. Linton (ed.), *New Avenues for the Prevention of Chronic Musculoskeletal Pain and Disability: Pain Research and Clinical Management*, Volume 12. pp. 238–43. Amsterdam: Elevsier.

Bodenheimer, T., Lorig, K., Holman, H., and Grumbach, K. (2002). Patient self-management of chronic disease in primary care. *Journal of the American Medical Association*, **288**, 2469–75.

Burton, A.K., Waddell, G., Tillotson, K.M., and Summerton, N. (1999). Information and advice to patients with back pain can have a positive effect. A randomized controlled trial of a novel educational booklet in primary care. *Spine*, **24**, 2484–91.

Carey, T.S., Evans, A., Hadler, N., Kalsbeek, W., McLaughlin, C., and Fryer, J. (1995). Care-seeking among individuals with chronic low back pain. *Spine*, **20**, 312–17.

Cherkin, D.C. and MacCornack, F.A. (1989). Patient evaluations of low back pain care from family physicians and from chiropractors. *Western Journal of Medicine*, **150**, 351–5.

Cherkin, D.C., MacCornack, F.A., and Berg, A.O. (1988). The management of low back pain: A comparison of the beliefs and behaviors of family physicians and chiropractors. *Western Journal of Medicine*, **149**, 475–80.

Cherkin, D.C., Deyo, R.A., Wheeler,K., and Ciol, M.A. (1994). Physician variation in diagnostic testing for low back pain: Who you see is what you get. *Arthritis and Rheumatism*, **37**, 15–22.

Cherkin, D.C., Deyo, R.A., Wheeler, K., and Ciol, M.A. (1995). Physician views about treating low back pain. The results of a national survey. *Spine*, **20**, 1–9.

Cherkin, D.C., Deyo, R.A., Street, J.H., Hunt, M., and Barlow, W. (1996). Pitfalls of patient education. Limited success of a program for back pain in primary care. *Spine*, **21**, 345–55.

Clinical Standards Advisory Group. (1994). *Report of a CSAG Committee on Back Pain*. London: HMSO.

Conroy, M. and Shannon, W. (1995). Clinical guide-lines: Their implementation in general practice. *British Journal of General Practice*, **45**, 317–75.

Crombez, G., Vervaet, L., Baeyens, F., Lysens, R., and Eelen, P. (1996). Do pain expectancies cause pain in chronic low back patients? A clinical investigation. *Behavior Research and Therapy* , **34**, 919–25.

Crombez, G., Vlaeyen, J.W., Heuts, P.H., and Lysens, R. (1999). Pain-related fear is more disabling than pain itself: Evidence on the role of pain-related fear in chronic back pain disability. *Pain*, **80**, 329–39.

Davis, R.M., Wagner, E.G., and Groves, T. (2000). Advances in managing chronic disease. *British Medical Journal*, **320**, 525–6.

Deyo, R.A. and Weinstein, J.N. (2001). Low back pain. *New England Journal of Medicine*, **344**, 363–70.

Deyo, R.A., Diehl, A.K., and Rosenthal, M. (1986). How many days of bed rest for acute low back pain? A randomized clinical trial. *New England Journal of Medicine*, **315**, 1064–70.

Deyo, R.A., Battie, M., Beurskens, A.J.H.M. *et al.* (1998). Outcomes measures for low back pain research: A proposal for standardized use. *Spine*, **23**, 2003–13.

Di Iorio, D., Henley, E., and Doughty, A. (2000). A survey of primary care physician practice patterns and adherence to acute low back problem guidelines. *Archives of Family Medicine*, **9**, 1015–21.

Dixon, A.S. (1990). The evolution of clinical policies. *Medical Care*, **28**, 201–20.

Donovan, D.M. and Marlatt, G.A. (1993). Recent developments in alcoholism behavioral treatment. *Recent Developments in Alcoholism*, **11**, 397–411.

Fairbank, J. (2000). Revised Oswestry Disability questionnaire. *Spine*, **25**, 218–23.

Fairbank, J.C., Coupler, J., Davies, J.B., and O'Brien, J.P. (1980). The Oswestry low back pain disability questionnaire. *Physiotherapy*, **66**, 271–3.

Freeborn, D.K., Shye, D., Mullooly, J.P., Eraker, S., and Romero, J. (1997). Primary car physicians use of lumbar spine imaging tests. Effects of guidelines and practice pattern feedback. *Journal of General Internal Medicine*, **12**, 619–25.

Frost, H., Lamb, S.E., Moffett, J.A., Fairbank, J.C.T., and Moser, J.S. (1998). A fitness programme for patients with chronic low back pain: 2-year follow-up of a randomized controlled trial. *Pain*, **75**, 273–9.

Greenfield, S., Kaplan, S.H., and Ware, J.E. Jr. (1985). Expanding patient involvement in care. Effects of patient outcomes. *Annals of Internal Medicine*, **102**, 520–8.

Greenfield, S., Kaplan, S.H., Ware, J.E. Jr., Yano, E.M., and Frank, H.J. (1988). Patients' participation in medical care: Effects of blood sugar control and quality of life in diabetes. *Journal of General Internal Medicine*, **3**, 448–57.

Gureje, O., Von Korff, M., Simon, G.E., and Gater, R. (1998). Persistent pain and well being: A World Health Organization study in primary care. *Journal of the American Medical Association*, **280**, 147–51.

Hart, L.G., Deyo, R.A., and Cherkin, D.C. (1995). Physician office visits for low back pain frequency, clinical evaluation, and treatment patterns from a U.S. national survey. *Spine*, **20**, 11–19.

Indahl, A., Velund, L., and Reikeraas, O. (1995). Good prognosis for low back pain when left untampered. A randomized clinical trial. *Spine*, **20**, 473–7.

Kaplan, S.H., Greenfield, S., and Ware, J.E. Jr. (1989). Assessing the effects of physician–patient interactions on the outcomes of chronic disease. *Medical Care*, **27**, S110–S127.

Klaber-Moffett, J.A., Newbronner, E., Waddell, G., Croucher, K., and Spear, S. (2000). Public perceptions about low back pain and its management: A gap between expectations and reality? *Health Expectations*, **3**, 161–8.

Klein, D., Najman, J., Kohrman, A.F., and Munro, C. (1982). Patient characteristics that elicit negative responses from family physicians. *Journal of Family Practice*, **5**, 881–8.

Koes, B.W., Bouter, L.M., and van der Heijden, G.J.M.G. (1995). Methodological quality of randomised clinical trials on treatment efficacy in low back pain. *Spine*, **20**, 228–35.

Kopec, J., Esdaile, J., Abrahamowics, M. *et al.* (1995). The Quebec Back Pain Disability Scale: Measurement properties. *Spine*, **20**, 341–52.

Kopec, J.A., Esdaile, J.M., Abrahamowicz, M. *et al.* (1996). The Quebec back pain disability scale: Conceptualization and development. *Journal of Clinical Epidemiology*, **48**, 151–61.

Lethem, J., Slade, P.D., Troup, J.D., and Bentley, G. (1983). Outline of a fear-avoidance model of exaggerated pain perception. *Behavioral Research and Therapy*, **21**, 401–8.

Linton, S.J. (1999). Prevention with special reference to chronic musculoskeletal disorders. In R.J. Gatchel and D.C. Turk (eds.), *Psychosocial Factors in Pain: Critical perspectives*, pp. 374–89. New York: Guilford Press.

Linton, S.J. and Andersson, T. (2000). Can chronic disability be prevented? A randomized trial of a cognitive-behavior intervention and two forms of information for patients with spinal pain. *Spine*, **25**, 2825–31.

Linton, S.J., Vlaeyen, J., and Ostelo, R. (2002). The back pain beliefs of health care providers: Are we fear-avoidant? *Journal of Occupational Rehabilitation*, **12**, 223–32.

Little, P., Roberts, L., Blowers, H. *et al.* (2001). Should we give detailed advice and information booklets to patients with back pain? A randomized controlled factorial trial of self-management booklet and doctor advice to take exercise for back pain. *Spine*, **26**, 2065–72.

Lomas, J. (1991). Words without action? The production, dissemination, and impact of consensus recommendations. *Annual Review of Public Health*, **12**, 41–65.

Lomas, J., Anderson, G.M., Domnick-Pierre, K., Vayda, E., Enkin, M.W., and Hannah, W.J. (1989). Do practice guidelines guide practice? The effect of a consensus statement on the practice of physicians. *New England Journal of Medicine*, **321**, 1306–11.

Lorig, K. (1993). Self-management of chronic illness: A model for the future. *Generations*, 11–14.

Malmivaara, A., Hakkinen, U., Aro, T. *et al.* (1995). The treatment of acute low back pain—bed rest, exercises, or ordinary activity? *New England Journal of Medicine*, **332**, 351–5.

Maly, R.C., Bourque, L.B., and Engelhardt, R.F. (1999). A randomized controlled trial of facilitating information giving to patients with chronic medical conditions: Effects on outcome of care. *Journal of Family Practice*, **48**, 356–63.

Mannion, A.F., Muntener, M., Taimela, S., and Dvorak, J. (1999). A randomized clinical trial of three active therapies of chronic back pain. *Spine*, **24**, 2435–48.

Marlatt, G.A. and Gordon, W.H. (1985). Relapse prevention: Introduction and overview of the model. *British Journal of Addiction*, **79**, 261–73.

McCraken, L.M., Zayfert, C., and Gross, R.T. (1992). The Pain Anxiety Symptoms scale: Development and validation of a scale to measure fear of pain. *Pain*, **50**, 67–73.

Meichenbaum, D. and Turk, D.C. (1987). *Facilitating Treatment Adherence: A Practitioner's Guidebook*. New York: Plenum Press.

Miller, R.P., Kori, S.H., and Todd, D.D. (1991). The Tampa Scale of Kinesiophobia. Unpublished Report. Tampa, FL.

Mior, S. (2001). Exercise in the treatment of chronic pain. *Clinical Journal of Pain*, **17**: S77–S85.

Mittan, B.S., Tonesk, X., and Jacobson, P.D. (1992). Implementing clinical guidelines: Social influence strategies and practitioner behavior change. *Quality Review Bulletin*, **18**, 413–22.

Moffett, J.K., Torgerson, D., Bell-Syer, S. *et al.* (1999). Randomized controlled trial of exercise for low back pain: Clinical outcome, costs, and preferences. *British Medical Journal*, **319**, 279–83.

Moore, J.E., Von Korff, M., Cherkin, D., Saunders, K., and Lorig, K. (2000). A randomized trial of a cognitive-behavioral program for enhancing back pain self-care in primary care setting. *Pain*, **88**, 145–53.

Najman, J.M., Klein, D., and Munro, C. (1982). Patient characteristics negatively stereotyped by doctors. *Social Science in Medicine*, **16**, 1781–9.

Oliver, J.W., Kravitz, R.L., Kaplan, S.H., and Meyers, F.L. (2001). Individualized patient education and coaching to improve pain control among cancer outpatients. *Journal of Clinical Oncology*, **19**, 2206–12.

Pruitt, S.D. and Von Korff, M. (2002). Improving the management of low back pain: A paradigm shift for primary care. In D.C. Turk and R.J. Gatchel (eds.), *Psychological Approaches to Pain Management: A Practitioner's Handbook*, 2nd edn., pp. 301–16. New York: Guilford Press.

Quebec Task Force on Spinal Disorders (1987). Scientific approach to the assessment and management of activity-related spinal disorders. A monograph for clinicians. Report of the Quebec Task Force for Spinal Disorders. *Spine*, **12**(Suppl. 7): S1–S59.

Rainville, J., Carlson, N., Polatin, P., Gatchel, R.J., and Indahl, A. (2000). Exploration of physicians' recommendations for activities in chronic low back pain. *Spine*, **25**, 2210–20.

Riley, J.F., Ahern, D.K., and Follick, M.J. (1988). Chronic pain and functional impairment: Assessing beliefs about their relationship. *Archives of Physical Medicine and Rehabilitation*, **69**, 579–82.

Roland, M. and Morris, R.A. (1983). A study of the natural history of back pain. Part I: Development of a reliable and sensitive measure of disability in low-back pain. *Spine*, **8**, 141–4.

Rossignol, M., Abenhaim, L., Suguin, P. *et al.* (2000). Coordination of primary health car for back pain. A randomized controlled trial. *Spine*, **25**, 251–9.

Schroth, W.S. (1996). Educational and behavioral interventions for back pain in primary care. Point of view. *Spine*, **21**, 2858.

Shekelle, P.G., Kravits, R.L., Beart, J., Marger, M., Wang, M., and Lee, M. (2000). Are nonspecific practice guidelines potentially harmful? A randomized comparison of the effect of nonspecific versus specific guidelines on physician decision making. *Health Services Research*, **34**, 1429–48.

Sieben, J.M., Vlaeyen, J.W.S., Tuerlinckx, S., and Portegijs, P.J.M. (2002). Pain-related fear in acute low back pain: The first two weeks of a new episode. *European Journal of Pain*, **6**, 229–37.

Spitzer, W.O., Leblanc, F.E., Dupuis, M. *et al.* (1987). Scientific approach to the assessment and management of activity-related spinal disorders: A monograph for clinicians. Report of the Task Force on Spinal Disorders. *Spine*, **12**(Suppl.), 1–59.

Sullivan, M.J.L., Bishop, S.R., and Pivik, J. (1995). The Pain Catastrophizing Scale: Development and validation. *Psychological Assessment*, 7, 524–32.

Turner, J.A. (1996). Educactional and behavioral interventions for back pain in primary care. *Spine*, 21, 2851–9.

Turner, J., Le Resche, L., Von Korff, M., Saunders, K., and Ehrlich, K. (1988). Back pain in primary care: Patient characteristics, content of initial visit, and short-term outcomes. *Spine*, 23, 463–9.

Turner, J.A., LeReche, L., Von Korff, M., and Ehrlich, K. (1998). Primary care back pain patient characteristics, visit content and short-term outcomes. *Spine*, 23, 463–9.

Van Tudler, M.W., Malmivaara, A., Esmail, R., and Koes, B.W. (2002). Exercise Therapy for Low Back Pain. The Cochran Library Issue 3. Oxford: Update Software.

Van Tulder, M.W., Koes, B.W., and Bouter, L.M. (1997). Conservative treatment of acute and chronic nonspecific low back pain: A systematic review of randomized controlled trials of the most common interventions. *Spine*, 22, 2128–56.

Vlaeyen, J.W. and Linton, S.J. (2000). Fear-avoidance and its consequences in chronic musculoskeletal pain: A state of the art. *Pain*, 85, 317–32.

Vlaeyen, J.W., de Jong, J., Geilen, M., Heuts, P.H., and van Breukelen, G. (2001). Graded exposure *in vivo* in the treatment of pain-related fear: A replicated single-case experimental design in four patients with chronic low back pain. *Behavariol Research and Therapy*, 39, 151–66.

Vlaeyen, J.W., de Jong, J., Geilen, M., Heuts, P.H., and van Breukelen, G. (2002). The treatment of fear of movement/(re)injury in chronic low back pain: Further evidence on the effectiveness of exposure *in vivo*. *Clinical Journal of Pain*, 18, 251–61.

Von Korff, M. (1999). Pain management in primary care: An individualized stepped-care approach. In R.J. Gatchel and D.C. Turk (eds.), *Psychosocial Factors In Pain*, pp. 360–73. New York: Guilford Press.

Von Korff, M. and Moore, J. (2001). Stepped care for back pain: Activating approaches for primary care. *Annals of Internal Medicine*, 134 (Suppl. 9, Pt. 2), 911–17.

Von Korff, M. and Saunders, K. (1996). The course of back pain in primary care. *Spine*, 21, 2833–7.

Von Korff, M. and Tiemens, B. (2000). Individualized stepped care of chronic illness. *Western Journal of Medicine*, 172, 133–7.

Von Korff, M., Deyo, R.A., Cherkin, D., and Barlow, W. (1993). Back pain in primary care: Outcomes at one year. *Spine*, 18, 855–62.

Von Korff, M., Barlow, W., Cherkin, D., and Deyo, R.A. (1994). Effects of practice style in managing back pain. *Annals of Internal Medicine*, 121, 187–95.

Von Korff, M., Gruman, J., Schaefer, J., Curry, S.J., and Wagner, E.H. (1997). Collaborative management of chronic illness. *Annals of Internal Medicine*, 127, 1097–2002.

Von Korff, M., Moore, J., Lorig, K. *et al.* (1998). A randomized trial of a lay person-led self-management group intervention for back pain patients in primary care. *Spine*, 23, 2608–15.

Waddell, G. (1992). Biopsychosocial analysis of low back pain. *Baillieres Clinical Rheumatology*, 6, 523–57.

Waddell, G. (1996). Keynote address for primary care forum. Low back pain: A twentieth century health care enigma. *Spine*, 21, 2820–5.

Waddell, G., Fader, G., and Lewis, M. (1997). Systematic reviews of bed rest and advice to stay active for acute low back pain. *The British Journal of General Practice*, **47**, 647–52.

Waddell, G., Newton, M., Henderson, I., Sommerville, D., and Main, C.J. (1993). A fear-avoidance beliefs questionnaire (FABQ) and the role of fear-avoidance beliefs in chronic low back pain and disability. *Pain*, **52**, 157–68.

Appendix: Instrument for assessing back pain patient's worries, concerns, and activity limitations in the primary care setting

Please list any worries or concerns you may have regarding your back.

_____

_____

_____

Below is a list of common worries and concerns that many patients have about back pain. Please mark any that apply to you?

☐ Your back pain may worsen or become chronic

☐ You will not be able to participate in activities that you enjoy

☐ You may become permanently disabled

☐ Physical activity or exercise may worsen your condition

☐ Severe back pain means that there is something dangerously wrong with your back

☐ Back pain during physical activity means that you are harming your back

☐ You may not be able to keep your current job due to back pain

☐ Your back pain may be due to a serious condition that has been missed or overlooked

Many people with back pain are fearful that certain movements or activities will cause further injury or pain. Please list any activities that you fear or avoid doing because of back pain.

_____

_____

Are you currently working: YES   NO

What do you do for work: _____

Over the past month (30 days) how many days of work do you feel you missed due to back pain? _____

Rating on a scale from 0–10, how much do you think back pain have interfered with the following activities where zero is no interference and 10 is unable to carry on any activities.

1. In the past <u>month</u>, how much have your back pain interfered with your ability to take care of yourself and home.

0	1	2	3	4	5	6	7	8	9	10

No
Interference

Moderate
Interference

Unable to carry
on any activities

2. In the past <u>month</u>, how much have your back pain interfered with your ability to take part in recreational, social and family activities.

0	1	2	3	4	5	6	7	8	9	10

No
Interference

Moderate
Interference

Unable to carry
on any activities

3. In the past <u>month</u>, how much have your back pain interfered with your ability to work.

0	1	2	3	4	5	6	7	8	9	10

No
Interference

Moderate
Interference

Unable to carry
on any activities

Please list activities that you are unable to do, or have difficulties doing, due to back pain?

_____

_____

How much have back pain affected each of these.

	Not at all	A little	A lot
Work activities			
Sitting for long periods of time, for example, in meetings			
Working at tasks that require bending or stooping			
Lifting objects			
Standing			
Driving			
Concentrating on your work			
Being able to go to work			
Household, family and self-care activities			
Doing jobs around the house			
Getting up stairs			
Getting out of bed			
Grocery shopping, carrying groceries			
Walking short or long distances			
Bathing			
Getting dressed or undressed			
Social and recreational activities			
Getting out of the house to do things			
Gardening, working in the yard			
Going to movies or plays			
Doing things for fun with others			
Going on a plane trip			
Exercising			
Participating in sports or activities that you enjoy			
Having sex or enjoying it as much as you would like			

Please list any activities that you fear or avoid doing because of back pain:

Chapter 13

Cognitive–behavioral therapy for chronic pain: An overview with specific reference to fear and avoidance

Amanda C. de C. Williams and
Lance M. McCracken

1 Introduction

Behavioral methods were introduced into the treatment of pain (Fordyce *et al.* 1968; Fordyce 1976; Sanders 1979) with a mixture of concern for patients for whom the rapidly developing techniques and pharmacopeia for pain relief were disappointing, and of therapeutic optimism about the scope of application of behavioral principles. Within the behavioral framework, pain was not the problem as it was unknowable by any direct means, but pain behavior was a problem both to the patient and to those around him or her. Such behavior as limping, guarding, moaning, grimacing, and withdrawal from normal activities caused secondary disability by deconditioning and created social distance and practical and material problems for the patient and his or her family. Repeated recourse to medical consultations and the armoury of possible treatments, particularly strong analgesics and those with intrinsic rewarding properties—the opioids—frustrated and defeated medical and paramedical professionals and third party funders of treatment attempts.

A fundamental tenet of behavioral methods, and of other treatment components built on or incorporating behavioral methods, is that everything the patient says and does is behavior. This includes the central focus of many treatments for pain, the patient's report of pain severity, influenced by past experience and current situation (Fordyce 1976). This was not to deny the influence of various anatomical and physiological conditions, but represented a major change in focus from these alone as the explanation for patients' behaviors. However, as will become clear, investigation of the various social, cultural, and emotional factors influencing pain behaviors is rather uneven.

Nevertheless, the focus on behavior sharpened the definition of treatment out-come, not only in terms of pain relief and a description of pain at the lower end of pain scales, but whatever the pain level, in terms of a more productive and satisfying range and extent of daily activity, reduced emotional suffering, and judicious use of medical services. Regardless of other interventions to reduce pain, behavioral and cognitive methods deserve consideration for their effects on these outcomes.

Some of the treatment literature represents a version of operant, relaxation, and behavioral technology significantly short of the standards and formula-tions of their pioneers. First, although the main impact of Fordyce's behav-ioral model was to shift the emphasis from pain, as a cue for and consequence of other behaviors, toward other, particularly social, cues, the model was rooted in the contemporary gate control model of pain. However, some pain researchers and clinicians seem to have overlooked the subsequent explosion of understanding of pain, particularly of the functional changes in the CNS that generate or amplify pain signals (see Wall 1994; Loeser and Melzack 1999). Second, behavioral concepts were, by definition, value-free, yet psychopatho-logical models of chronic pain were grafted on (see Turk and Salovey 1984; Sharpe and Williams 2002). Third, pain behaviors, originally established by observation of behavior, cues, and contingencies, came to be defined descrip-tively without reference to context or consequences. This obscured any sense of function, so that *avoidance*—as an undesirable behavior—was often addressed without reference to its object or to short and long-term effects (rarely identical, not infrequently completely different). This may have con-tributed to the slowness with which models of fear and avoidance, flourishing in mainstream psychology and the treatment of anxiety disorders, were recog-nized as relevant for many chronic pain patients: After fear and avoidance were originally mooted in relation to chronic pain by Lethem *et al.* (1983), it was only in the 1990s that this was revisited by Vlaeyen, McCracken, and others (McCracken *et al.* 1992; Vlaeyen *et al.* 1995; see Asmundson *et al.* 1999; Vlaeyen and Linton 2000 for reviews). Their work is extensively described and reviewed in other chapters in this book.

Although research has increasingly focused on models of fear and avoidance as a way to understand chronic pain and disability, treatment methods in gen-eral do not yet specifically address fear and avoidance. Recent treatment trials using exposure-based methods, as described in Chapter 14, give strong grounds for doing so. Behavioral and cognitive–behavioral treatments (BT or CBT) can vary in many ways in practice. The literature may obscure different practices, as short descriptions cannot specify important details. Nevertheless, all the inter-ventions described in Table 13.1 may be applied alone or in combination,

Table 13.1 Common components of BT or CBT of chronic pain

- ◆ Reorientation and promotion of a self-management approach
- ◆ Education about pain; distinction between pain and damage; treatment issues
- ◆ Behavioral activation and management including goal-setting and pacing strategies
- ◆ Development of an exercise and fitness regimen to underpin increased activity
- ◆ Relaxation training and application to areas of difficulty such as sleep and pain cues
- ◆ Cognitive therapy; also know as cognitive restructuring, or self-statement analysis
- ◆ Training in problem-solving
- ◆ Self-application of operant-based, contingency management strategies
- ◆ Other interventions to change perception or emotional response to pain such as guided imagery, desensitization, hypnosis, or attention control exercises
- ◆ Communication skills training or family interventions
- ◆ Stress inoculation training and relapse prevention
- ◆ Reduction of analgesic and/or psychotropic drugs, particularly any with sedating properties

briefly or at length, superficially or intensively. The most minimal may fall below the level of therapeutic efficacy. One of the purposes of this chapter will be to consider the potential utility of these interventions to address pain-related fear and avoidance.

2 **Review of treatment trials**

A meta-analysis, of BT and CBT combined or not with physical and occupational rehabilitation strategies and conservative medical treatments (multicomponent programs), was conducted by Flor *et al.* (1992) on 65 randomized and non-randomized studies of multidisciplinary treatment published between 1960 and 1990, involving 3089 patients. The mean between-group effect size across outcome variables was 0.62 at short-term follow-up and 0.81 at follow-up beyond 6 months (selective attrition from follow-up should be borne in mind in interpreting these results). Pain was reduced by 37 percent in treated patients compared to 4 percent in control patients; treated patients achieved a 63 percent reduction in drug use and 53 percent improvement in activity compared to 21 and 13 percent, respectively, for control patients. Flor *et al.* (1992) reported the likelihood of returning to work at 68 percent for treated patients compared to 32 percent for control patients. A slightly later meta-analysis of 37 trials of multicomponent treatments for chronic pain, with return to work as the main outcome (Cutler *et al.* 1994), reported a more modest 41 percent return for patients not working at the beginning of treatment, over a mean follow-up interval of 14 months.

The first meta-analytic review restricted to randomized trials (Turner 1996) reported significant improvement in pain reports, self-reported pain behavior, and disability but not observed pain behavior or mood. However, only four trials met inclusion criteria, so conclusions were limited. A larger meta-analysis by Morley *et al.* (1999), based on a systematic review conducted to explicit protocols, found 30 randomized controlled trials (RCTs) for chronic pain, of which 25 provided analyzable data on 1672 patients randomized to BT–CBT or two control conditions (no treatment or treatment as usual). In outcome domains categorized as pain experience, mood/affect, positive cognitive coping and appraisal, negative cognitive coping and appraisal, behavior/expression, behavior/activity, and social role performance, effect sizes for treatment compared to waiting list were about 0.50 in each domain, but were lower (and nonsignificant for mood/affect, negative coping and appraisal, and social role functioning, with no data for behavior/activity) for BT–CBT compared to treatment as usual.

Two further systematic reviews with meta-analyses reported qualified effectiveness. Van Tulder *et al.* (2000) found effect sizes for BT–CBT of 0.62 for pain and 0.36 and 0.40 for function and behavioral outcomes, respectively, but from only six trials for low back pain. Guzmán *et al.* (2001) combined 10 trials of low back pain and concluded that only intensive (longer, rather than brief) multicomponent treatment with a CBT approach reduced pain and improved function when all were compared with treatment as usual. Both studies were weakened by unnecessary restriction on trial inclusion, through (1) the use of quality scoring methods appropriate to medical trials some of which are inapplicable to psychological trials, and (2) limiting their scope to low back pain, neither a psychologically nor probably medically meaningful category. Further, the Guzmán *et al.* primary outcome of return to work was inapplicable to some of the populations in the trials entered, guaranteeing a poor result, where a more general disability or function effect size would have served better. Also, the authors unaccountably attributed all variability in outcomes only to treatment length, ignoring patient variables, treatment content, and their interaction.

Overall, there are numerous methodological shortcomings with the treatment trials reviewed, as discussed by Morley *et al.* (1999), but their improvement relies on the application of appropriate psychological concepts and methods. Work status, medication use, or health care use were not addressed frequently enough in treatment trials to be evaluated. However, significantly reduced health care use from CBT for chronic pain has been demonstrated (Caudill *et al.* 1991; Williams *et al.* 1996, 1999), as have substantially reduced costs compared to other treatment approaches (Goossens and Evers 1997; Okifuji *et al.* 1999*b*).

While the use of the meta-analytic methods allows pooling of data, obtaining Ns greater than is likely ever to be achieved in single or multicenter trials, effect sizes and confidence intervals around them are used to determine statistical significance, but few authors address the issue of clinical significance which might be marked by smaller or larger changes than those which attain statistical significance. It is an issue rarely discussed in public: What is an excellent outcome? What is a good enough outcome? And what is apparently ineffective, such that the program should be urgently reviewed and revised?

3 Refining treatment: Selection of patients

Much research has sought to identify patient variables that may predict treatment effectiveness. This is of concern to treatment providers, to patients on long waiting lists (which may contain patients for whom treatment is unsuitable), and not least to treatment funders. Unfortunately, studies of predictors of treatment are limited in a number of ways. These issues are reviewed in detail elsewhere (Kleinke and Spangler 1988; Turk 1990; Fishbain *et al.* 1993; McCracken and Turk 2002; Morley and Williams 2002). Briefly, these limits include a lack of theory driving selection of measures, a diversity of outcome domains that demonstrate no unique relations with potential predictors, differences in treatment methods and samples across studies, and differences in follow-up interval. The current status, therefore, is that what positive findings there are lack replication and demonstration of generalizability.

We did not identify any studies of treatment outcome prediction that utilized measures of pain-related fear responses. Although findings about predictors are not yet ready to offer firm guidance on treatment-related decisions, they may nonetheless shed light on the potential roles of pain-related fear in the selection of patients for appropriate treatment, and suggest avenues for further research that may improve our understanding of treatment mechanisms.

The search for predictors has often been pragmatic rather than theory-driven. Findings concerning patient demographic and medical data are inconsistent. This is not surprising given how little these factors represent psychological constructs of significance that might interact with treatments to affect outcome. By contrast, depression and depressed mood, an important problem for chronic pain sufferers (Banks and Kerns 1996), has emerged in some studies as a predictor of poorer treatment outcome (e.g. Dworkin *et al.* 1986; Polatin *et al.* 1989). However, this is not a consistent finding across studies, and problems with assessment of depression in the presence of chronic pain (Williams 1998; Pincus and Williams 1999) suggest that findings should be interpreted with caution. Nevertheless, depression and fear response classes share many features including avoidance, socially recognizable signs of distress, ineffective thinking, physiological disturbance, and unhelpful and distressing habits such as catastrophic thinking (Sullivan *et al.* 2001). Measures of depression and pain-related fear are often highly correlated (McCracken *et al.* 1992; Vlaeyen *et al.* 1995), thus some of what we learn about depression in relation to treatment outcome may also apply to pain-related fear. Despite these concerns about interpretation of findings on depression and depressed mood, the findings that depressed chronic pain sufferers demonstrate less return to work (Barnes *et al.* 1989), involvement in work (Dolce *et al.* 1986), treatment program completion (Kerns and Haythornthwaite 1988), and exercise participation (Harkapaa *et al.* 1991) are worth consideration. Consistent with BT of depression (Williams 1992), Dworkin *et al.* (1986) suggested that participation in the activity component of treatment might be particularly important for pain patients with depression.

Researchers have developed patient typologies with the aim of identifying patient suitability for particular treatments. For example, Turk and Rudy (1988) used a measure (West Haven Yale Multidimensional Pain Inventory (MPI), Kerns *et al.* 1985) to classify patients as dysfunctional, interpersonally distressed (in addition to dysfunction), and adaptive copers. This categorization strategy appears reasonably, although not universally, robust across populations (Okifuji *et al.* 1999*a*). Further study showed that patients classified as dysfunctional reported significantly more pain-related fear and avoidance than patients classified as interpersonally distressed or adaptive copers (Asmundson *et al.* 1997; McCracken *et al.* 1999). However, the psychological meaning of the profiles derived from cluster analysis of MPI scores remains unclear, and tests of their validity in relation to prediction of treatment needs is at an early stage (Rudy *et al.* 1995; Turk *et al.* 1996, 1998).

4 Behavior change processes during treatment

What about relationships between changes in psychological variables during treatment and outcomes? There are fewer studies of these, covering a narrower range of areas, particularly pain coping strategies, pain beliefs, depression, and fear of pain. Certain cognitive changes during the course of treatment, including reduced helplessness, reduced catastrophizing, and increased perceived control (Spinhoven and Linssen 1991; Tota-Faucette *et al.* 1993), predict treatment gains in depression and other symptoms of psychological distress. Another study (Jensen *et al.* 1994) reported that favorable treatment outcome in physical disability, depression, and health care use was a product of decreased beliefs in pain as harmful and disabling, decreased catastrophizing, and increased beliefs in control over pain, but not a product of the practice of physical exercise, relaxation, and strategies to increase activity. In general, findings on the relationship between change in physical capacity or performance and functional gain are mixed (Fredrickson *et al.* 1988; Hildebrandt *et al.* 1997; Burns *et al.* 1998; Vendrig 1999).

It has been suggested that the benefits of psychological approaches to pain may lie in reducing fear and depression associated with pain, rather than reducing the pain itself (Malone and Strube 1988). This was investigated in a study of injured workers with low back pain (McCracken and Gross 1998). All patients participated in a 3-week multidisciplinary program including physical rehabilitation and BT. Results showed that decreased pain-related anxiety significantly predicted improvement in pain, depression, disability, general emotional distress, and daily activity. Additional analyses showed that change in pain-related anxiety was a significant predictor of each outcome independent of change in depression. Decreased depression did not predict improvement in disability or daily activity, independent of change in pain-related anxiety. In a follow-up study, it was shown that the role of reduced pain-related anxiety in treatment outcome was independent of change in physical capacity and, in general, changes in pain-related anxiety during treatment accounted for more variance than improvement in physical capacity in the prediction of outcome (McCracken *et al.* 2002).

5 How does cognitive–behavioral treatment for pain reduce specific fear and avoidance?

There are a few trials of CBT for chronic pain that show anxiety reduction as one of their outcomes (e.g. Nicholas *et al.* 1991). Likewise, to the extent that other trials demonstrate increased daily activity from treatment (e.g. Deardorff *et al.* 1991), these results at least imply that cognitive–behavioral approaches reduce avoidance associated with chronic pain. However, the outcome measures used in these studies have been generic and do not specify that the anxiety and avoidance are directly related to pain. While we are not aware of any controlled treatment trials specifically showing reduced pain-related fear and avoidance, there are uncontrolled studies showing reduction on a composite measure of pain-related fear and avoidance during combined physical rehabilitation and CBT (McCracken and Gross 1998; McCracken *et al.* 2002). Recent unpublished data ($N = 70$) from one of our centers in the United Kingdom demonstrate a reduction during treatment in each of the four subscales from the Pain Anxiety Symptoms Scale (McCracken *et al.* 1992). Changes in avoidance, cognitive anxiety responses, and fearful thinking each amounted to greater than a one half a standard deviation in magnitude. The change in physiological anxiety responses was somewhat smaller but still statistically significant. Treatment included general physical reconditioning exercises, and self-management training, based on behavioral and cognitive behavioral principles. All scores remained significantly below baseline at 3-month follow-up with the exception of the score for physiological anxiety responses. Again, no control group was used for comparison so effects cannot be unambiguously attributed to the treatment package.

Cognitive–behavioral treatment for chronic pain is effective for many patients. Pain-related fear and avoidance responses appear to decrease during treatment, presumably as a function of active treatment components, and reduction of pain-related fear and anxiety responses may be a key process in treatment outcome overall. However, it is not yet clear which components of treatment are most effective for reducing fear and anxiety and how they operate. Since fear and avoidance are responses to threat, presumably the treatment features that reduce the threats associated with pain and promote engagement in avoided activity should be critical.

Other chapters in this volume review models of pain-related fear and anxiety and, thus, they will not be reviewed again here. However, we must consider the influences that maintain fear and anxiety responses before considering the interventions to alter them. Clearly, individual patients vary in terms of the frequency and type of fear and avoidance responses they demonstrate. They also vary in terms of their experiences and the learning that gave rise to these responses, and in terms of the situations that maintain them over time. Among the influences to consider are contingencies of behavioral avoidance, emotional avoidance, verbally mediated associations between pain situations and threat, social influences, coupled with weak environmental support for alternative, fear-incompatible behaviour (see Chapter 3 of this volume).

The literature on treatment of anxiety disorders clearly supports the utility of exposure therapies for fear and avoidance in conditions such as panic disorder (Craske *et al.* 1991; Margraff *et al.* 1993), posttraumatic stress disorder (Foa *et al.* 1999), and obsessive compulsive disorder (Foa *et al.* 1980; Abramowitz 1997; McClean *et al.* 2001). There may be advantages to graded *in vivo* trials, spaced over time (Tsao and Craske 2000), including self-directed exposure (Barlow 1988). In order to be effective, exposure must include (1) a convincing rationale, (2) contact with specific feared situations, (3) methods that prevent treatment dropout, (4) continuation of treatment until fear and avoidance are reduced, (5) generalization of behavior changes to relevant situations, and (6) some maintenance enhancement strategy. To the extent that the reorientation, education, physical exercise, and behavioral activation

strategies of general CBT packages for chronic pain include these components, they are likely to be effective at reducing fear and avoidance. As they are
standardly applied, however, it is likely that these strategies are not as useful as
they could be, or may even inadvertently worsen the situation, because they
normally do not include the exposure rationale, they may not specifically
target feared situations, they may allow avoidance to continue, and they may be
discontinued before fear and avoidance are effectively reduced. It is likely that
patients with significant pain-related fears require more structured and specific treatment before they can start to increase activities by steady increments,
as in the exercise and activity components of CBT for chronic pain. There is a
high risk of premature confrontation of a feared activity, such as walking
without support, or lifting a heavy weight, provoking a rapid rise in fear. The
circumstances under which escape during the course of exposure treatment
might enhance fear are not precisely certain. Escape before fear reduction may
not strengthen avoidance in all cases (DaSilva and Rachman 1984); it may
depend on what the patient learns from the experience. However, punishing
experiences from confronting activity may discourage further rehabilitation
efforts and may strengthen patients' convictions that pain-producing activities
are dangerous. At this point, if the activity is abandoned, the fear is strengthened and avoidance will be even more pronounced. While both of us have
seen this occur in clinical settings, the extent to which it may be responsible
for treatment failure or attrition is unknown.

Education and instruction about pain can reduce perceived threats related
to pain and strengthen renewed approaches to normal activity. Patients may
respond to exacerbation of pain from activity as if all hurt equals harm; they
may feel they have an undiagnosed and threatening condition. Some patients
have received frightening information in the past or have been given instructions that lead them to avoid activities, and they may interpret ambiguous
information—sensations such as stiffness, or comments on nonpathological
investigation findings—as threatening. Education and instruction can resolve
uncertainties and mitigate the threatening information contained in inappropriate and inaccurate descriptions of the problem. The more specifically the
patient's fears are addressed, the better. Clearly, generic information that does
not identify and address specific fearful notions of pain is not likely to have
much impact on the behavior of pain sufferers with high levels of fear of pain
and interconnected and strongly held beliefs.

In general, although there is evidence supporting the use of relaxation-
based techniques with patients, it appears not to be a matter of reducing general muscle tension in the painful area by voluntary control (Knost et al. 1999)
but more of reducing the muscle tension response in the painful area

to specific emotional stressors (Flor *et al.* 1992), and retraining patterns of muscle overactivity and slow return to baseline on simple movement (Watson *et al.* 1997). Interestingly, although relaxation has long been recommended for treatment of anxiety, to increase a patient's sense of control and to facilitate participation with exposure methods (Barlow 1988), it may not be necessary to the effectiveness of exposure (Margraff *et al.* 1993) and may be only half as effective as exposure methods when used alone (Margraff *et al.* 1993; Abramowitz 1997).

One of the real strengths of BT in its original form was its focus on the individual and his or her history and current circumstances. Assessment included identification of behavior for change and manipulation of the most remediable circumstances. For many cases of pain-related fear and avoidance, education, instruction, and graded activation may produce successful change. But, a minority of patients show pain-related fear and avoidance that are more like an anxiety disorder, which are likely to be intractable to standard CBT methods as currently delivered in pain-management group programs. For instance, strong fear may prompt partial or complete avoidance of particular activities in exercise sessions; safety behaviors, including thoughts, may immunize patients from cognitive and emotional change as a result of behavioral exposure; and, outside influences may maintain fear and avoidance in a way that may not manifest during a brief pain-management program. In all of these cases, individual treatment will be required to be much closer to BT for anxiety disorders. The challenge is to discover how best to identify patients needing intensive treatment before they fail to make behavioral changes toward their goals in a CBT program, or if not, as soon as possible after that failure.

Our experiences of trying to integrate such individual treatment into intensive (inpatient) group CBT programs have taught us much. First, patients do not identify themselves as fearful, and their avoidance as far as they are concerned is primarily because of pain: This needs to be explored further and sensitively, to uncover fears about damage and the effects of increased pain. The beliefs uncovered are unlike many in people with phobias in that patients who fear damage from increased activity, or unmanageable pain, are often drawing on advice and information they have received from authorities such as doctors, and on critical pain events in their past. They do not in any way identify the fears as unfounded, nor do any but a small minority experience physiological arousal in relation to confrontation of the activity. In these ways fear of pain and damage do not resemble the classic phobia.

Despite high scores (>40) on the Tampa Scale for Kinesiophobia (Kori *et al.* 1990), and identification of fear-related avoidance of some activities using photo assessment (see Chapter 14), some patients rapidly lose these fears during interactive group education on pain from an authoritative source. However, other patients identify such avoidance during goal setting, exercise sessions, or physical assessment, so it is important to share the framework with physiotherapist and occupational therapist colleagues. Within a patient-centered way of working, it can be hard to strike a balance between patients setting their own goals (and abandoning or discounting some) and encouraging them to envisage attempting some goals which they have avoided and discounted because of their fears. A recent study that allowed patients to select the treatment components of CBT found that a majority did not opt to work on improving physical function but preferred to gain skills in goal-setting, activity scheduling, problem-solving and cognitive restructuring for fatigue and negative mood (Evers *et al.* 2002). When working with patients on avoided activities, it is important to distinguish those that are treated by exposure, with increments decided by level of anxiety, and those that progress by graded activity, using increments of time or performance; these can be hard to integrate in complex goals, which involve both. In addition, therapists need to be alert to possible safety behaviors (Sharp 2001), including their own presence, "ergonomically correct" movements, elaborate relaxation procedures, and others. At worst, an overemphasis on ergonomics, posture, and pain-management techniques can exacerbate fears, or make them more specific to particular conditions, and so sabotage the overall aims of pain management.

Cognitive therapy procedures, such as cognitive restructuring or self-statement analysis, are commonly applied to treat anxiety disorders today. Cognitive therapy can successfully reduce symptoms of anxiety disorders (see Chambless and Gillis 1993; Margraff *et al.* 1993 for reviews) and, therefore, may helpfully reduce pain-related fear and avoidance when used as a part of treatment packages for chronic pain sufferers. A relatively recent systematic review demonstrated that anxiety-related cognitive variables change during the course of CBT for anxiety disorders and change in these variables is correlated with outcome (Chambless and Gillis 1993). One explanation for this is a causal connection, but other findings from structural equation modeling do not support a *causal* relationship to outcome in treatment of anxiety (Burns and Spangler 2001). And, when cognitive change occurs in treatment, it can be produced by a number of treatment methods, including exposure alone or pharmacological therapy (Chambless and Gillis 1993; Newman *et al.* 1994; Abramowitz 1997). In fact, cognitive therapy may be no more effective than other treatment modalities for producing change in cognitive variables (Barlow 1988; Chambless and Gillis 1993; Abramowitz 1997; McClean *et al.* 2001). Admittedly, these issues of the relative importance of exposure versus cognitive therapy are controversial. There is, additionally, a risk of overemphasis on thoughts and beliefs and an associated overemphasis on "cognitive restructuring" treatments.

Changing thoughts and feelings is not the only route to behavior change. Talking about distressing emotions is standardly included in CBT for chronic pain. Obviously, negative emotional experiences produce a tendency to avoid possible recurrence in most people. Some have argued that emotional avoidance is at the core of many common human behavioral problems such as anxiety disorders (Hayes *et al.* 1996). Naturally, emotional avoidance will contribute to fear and avoidance if it interferes with the chronic pain sufferer examining problem situations, planning alternative responses, and confronting difficulties. Discussing personally relevant anxiety-provoking circumstances is likely to help patients with significant fear and avoidance, if structured within an appropriate format. Sharing with others may make their distress more acceptable. The exposure to memories, descriptions, and images may have a desensitizing or exposure-oriented effect (e.g. Linehan 1993; Hayes *et al.* 1999), and being brought in contact with the distressing material may show practical ways to move forward toward goals.

Many of the components of CBT as it is currently practiced for chronic pain (see Table 13.1) are potentially appropriate treatments for pain-related fear and avoidance. We presume that they are not yet optimal for this purpose but a base for development exists. What is less clear is the role of the broader treatment context in fear and avoidance reduction. CBT is rarely practised in isolation from other health care experiences and treatments; physiotherapists, occupational therapists, nurses, and physicians often participate in treatment with varying degrees of integration with those who directly provide CBT. We know very little of the effect on fears and avoidance of medication use, interventional pain management, further examination or diagnostic investigations, or any other palliative or analgesia-oriented strategies. We have presumed for some time that medicalizing the problem or promising a simple fix may discourage self-management efforts and behavior change and may perpetuate a sense of threat by conveying the impression of a situation in need of medical treatment. Any interventions that promise comfort may deliver, or they may simply provide a sense of security; that is, a "treated" problem may feel less threatening than an untreated problem. In this sense, medications or other comfort measures may undermine the effects of exposure-based treatments to some degree. Patients may learn, "I can do that activity but only if . . ." a particular condition is met, such as the use of an analgesic, the recent use of massage or other palliative strategy, the presence of a therapist, or the safety of a hospital setting. Adoption of these conditions as necessary to confront fear and attempt activity presents real challenges to exposure-based treatments, constituting other forms of avoidance and undermining generalization of gains from exposure.

6 Refining treatment: New directions

In addition to the increasing body of work directly related to pain-related fear and avoidance, researchers have also focused on the related areas of attention to pain and pain-related attitudes. These separate areas appear likely to converge, increasing our understanding of negative emotional responses to pain and pain-related disability.

The role of attention to pain has received a new impetus from research approaches with a more secure theoretical basis than those that led to simply training patients to ignore or distract themselves from pain. These latter techniques are largely ineffective for patients with chronic pain (Cioffi 1991; Jensen et al. 1992). It has been argued that the problem of pain is that its presence sets the occasion for distressed and pain-related behavior on the part of the pain sufferer and inhibits the influence of other life circumstances that would occasion more healthy behavior, directed toward important life goals (McCracken 1997). Pain presents interruptions in ongoing functioning (Eccleston and Crombez 1999) and while there is evidence to suggest that greater and selective attention to bodily cues is a feature of anxiety disorders (Barlow 1988; Asmundson et al. 1992; Ehlers and Breuer 1992), and also that pain-related attention is associated with pain-related fear (Crombez et al. 1999) and with catastrophic interpretation of physical sensations (Hadjistavropoulos et al. 2000), treatment to decrease attention to pain would decrease the behavior-influencing effects of pain and increase the behavior-influencing effects of non-pain-related circumstances. This reduced *preoccupation* with pain would no doubt decrease other pain-related fear and avoidance responses as well; indeed, panic disorder patients show decreased vigilance to body sensations associated with reduction in anxiety symptoms during CBT (Schmidt et al. 1997).

Behavioral intervention for pain-related fear and avoidance may also bear on changes in the patient's relationship with the pain. It has been suggested that positive treatment results for patients with chronic pain come from acceptance of the concept of "functioning regardless of pain" (Deardorff et al. 1991). Studies of persons with chronic pain seeking treatment in comparison to those not seeking treatment suggest that those not seeking treatment have accepted their chronic problem (Reitsma and Meijler 1997). Acceptance of pain has been defined as a willingness to have pain without trying to avoid or reduce it (McCracken 1999), basically not construing it as a threat or impediment to functioning. Schmitz et al. (1996) found less distress among those pain patients who modified existing goals or substituted new ones (accommodation) compared to those who pursued unmodified goals, counting on eventual relief of pain for their realization. Acceptance would appear to have clear implications for pain-related fear and avoidance in that these imply incompatible response classes. In fact, studies have now shown that acceptance of pain is associated with good/better adjustment (McCracken 1998; McCracken *et al.* 1999) and with lower pain-related anxiety and avoidance (McCracken 1998). Treatment approaches intended to foster acceptance in relation to other behavior problems may be useful for pain-related fear and avoidance in chronic pain (Hayes *et al.* 1999).

7 Conclusion

Research into pain-related fear and avoidance has provided a valuable opportunity to refine BTs for chronic pain, making them much more potent for some patients. There is good evidence that CBT is generally effective when conducted in group formats for diverse patients with chronic pain. However, group treatment does not imply identical treatment, although for reasons of economy and of insufficient staff skill, many BT and CBT packages are applied with relatively little appreciation for specific patient behavior problems and the continuing influences that maintain them. The function of behaviors that represent obstacles to patients' achievement of important goals needs to be examined in a broad psychological framework, not with *a priori* assumptions of operant influences, fears, or other important but not universal factors in chronic pain.

Many current CBT treatment components resemble standard treatments for anxiety disorders. However, as in the treatment of anxiety, their full effectiveness is likely compromised where clinicians miss opportunities to use clear case conceptualization and rationales, to design implicit exposure trials graded by anxiety level, and of an intensity and duration of exposure adequate to produce lasting change. In turn, generalization and maintenance may not be fully addressed. The problem here is with treatment conceptualization: Both patient and clinician are treating the problem as pain when in fact it is fear. Chapter 14 describes a promising approach to treating fear in chronic pain, that of graded exposure *in vivo*.

Clearly not all patients with chronic pain have a history of fear and avoidance responses that contribute significantly to their disability, but for those who respond to chronic pain as a threat, who experience extreme feelings of anxious distress, and show life-disrupting avoidance, functional improvement will come from treatments that reduce these responses. Even when this level of treatment specificity has been achieved more work may be needed. When significant pain-related fear and avoidance exist, they may be a function of any combination of a range of influences, social, emotional, or physical. We are at last moving on from universal assumptions of operant reinforcement of all avoidance; treatments in the future are likely to achieve better results as they increasingly come to address patients' unique combinations of behavioral and emotional problems.

References

Abramowitz, J.S. (1997). Effectiveness of psychological and pharmacological treatments for obsessive-compulsive disorder: A quantitative review. *Journal of Consulting and Clinical Psychology*, **65**, 44–52.

Asmundson, G.J.G., Sandler, L.S., Wilson, K.G., and Walker, J.R. (1992). Selective attention toward physical threat in patients with panic disorder. *Journal of Anxiety Disorders*, **6**, 295–303.

Asmundson, G.J.G., Norton, G.R., and Allderdings, M.D. (1997). Fear and avoidance in dysfunctional chronic back pain patients. *Pain*, **69**, 231–6.

Asmundson, G.J.G., Norton, P.J., and Norton, G.R. (1999). Beyond pain: The role of fear and avoidance in chronicity. *Clinical Psychology Review*, **19**, 97–119.

Banks, S.M. and Kerns, R.D. (1996). Explaining high rates of depression in chronic pain: A diathesis–stress framework. *Psychological Bulletin*, **199**, 95–110.

Barlow, D.H. (1988). *Anxiety and its Disorders*. New York: The Guilford Press.

Barnes, D., Smith, D., Gatchel, R., and Mayer, T.G. (1989). Psychosocioeconomic predictors of treatment success/failure in chronic low back pain patients. *Spine*, **14**, 427–30.

Burns, D.D. and Spangler, D.L. (2001). Do changes in dysfunctional attitudes mediate changes in depression and anxiety in cognitive behavioral therapy? *Behavior Therapy*, **32**, 337–69.

Burns, J.W., Johnson, B.J., Mahoney, N., Devine, J., and Pawl, R. (1998). Cognitive and physical capacity process variables predict long-term outcome after treatment of chronic pain. *Journal of Consulting and Clinical Psychology*, **66**, 434–9.

Caudill, M., Schnable, R., Zuttermeister, P., Benson, H., and Friedman, R. (1991). Decreased clinic use by chronic pain patients: Response ot behavioral medicine intervention. *Clinical Journal of Pain*, **7**, 305–10.

Chambless, D.L. and Gillis, M.M. (1993). Cognitive therapy of anxiety disorder. *Journal of Consulting and Clinical Psychology*, **61**, 248–60.

Cioffi, D. (1991). Beyond attentional strategies: A cognitive-perceptual model of somatic interpretation. *Psychological Bulletin*, **109**, 25–41.

Craske, M.G., Brown, T.A., and Barlow, D.H. (1991). Behavioral treatment of panic disorder: A two-year follow-up. *Behavior Therapy*, **22**, 289–304.

Crombez, C., Eccleston, C., Baeyens, F., Van Houdenhove, B., and Van Den Broeck, A. (1999). Attention to chronic pain is dependent upon pain-related fear. *Journal of Psychosomatic Research*, **47**, 403–10.

Cutler, R.B., Fishbain, D.A., Rosomoff, H.L., Abdel-Moty, E., Khalil, T.M., and Rosomoff, R.S. (1994). Does nonsurgical pain center treatment of chronic pain return patients to work? A review and meta-analysis of the literature. *Spine*, **19**, 643–52.

DaSilva, P. and Rachman, S. (1984). Does escape strengthen agoraphobic avoidance? A preliminary study. *Behaviour Research and Therapy*, **22**, 87–91.

Deardorff, W.W., Rubin, H.S., and Scott, D.W. (1991). Comprehensive multidisciplinary treatment of chronic pain: A follow-up study of treated and untreated groups. *Pain*, **45**, 35–43.

Dolce, J.J., Crocker, M.F., and Doleys, D.M. (1986). Prediction of outcome among chronic pain patients. *Behaviour Research and Therapy*, **24**, 313–19.

Dworkin, R.H., Richlin, D.M., Handlin, D.S., and Brand, L. (1986). Predicting treatment response in depressed and non-depressed chronic pain patients. *Pain*, **24**, 343–53.

Eccleston, C. and Crombez, G. (1999). Pain demands attention: A cognitive-affective model of the interruptive function of pain. *Psychological Bulletin*, **125**, 356–66.

Ehlers, A. and Breuer, P. (1992). Increased cardiac awareness in panic disorder. *Journal of Abnormal Psychology*, **101**, 371–82.

Evers, A.W.M., Kraaimaat, F.W., van Riel, P.L.C.M., and de Jong, A.J.L. (2002). Tailored cognitive-behavioral therapy in early rheumatoid arthritis for patients at risk: A randomized controlled trial. *Pain*, **100**, 141–53.

Fishbain, D.A., Rosomoff, H.L., Goldberg, M., Cutler, R., Abdel Moty, E., Khalil, T.M., and Rosomoff, R.S. (1993). The prediction of return to the workplace after multidisciplinary pain center treatment. *Clinical Journal of Pain*, **9**, 3–15.

Flor, H., Fydrich, T., and Turk, D.C. (1992). Efficacy of multidisciplinary pain treatment centers: A meta-analytic review. *Pain*, **49**, 221–30.

Foa, E.B., Steketee, G., and Milby, J.B. (1980). Differential effects of exposure and response prevention in obsessive compulsive washers. *Journal of Consulting and Clinical Psychology*, **48**, 71–9.

Foa, E.B., Dancu, C.V., Hembree, E.A., Jaycox, L.H., Meadows, E.A., and Street, G.P. (1999). A comparison of exposure therapy, stress inoculation training, and their combination for reducing posttraumatic stress disorder in female assault victims. *Journal of Consulting and Clinical Psychology*, **67**, 194–200.

Fordyce, W.E. (1976). Behavioral *Methods for Chronic Pain and Illness*. St Louis: The C. V. Mosby Company.

Fordyce, W.E., Fowler, R.S., Lehman, J.F., and DeLateur, B.J. (1968). Some implications of learning in problems of chronic pain. *Journal of Chronic Disease*, **21**, 179–90.

Fredrickson, B.E., Trief, P.M., VanBeveren, P., Yuan, H.A., and Baum, G. (1988). Rehabilitation of the patient with chronic pain: A search for outcome predictors. *Spine*, **13**, 351–3.

Goossens, M.E.J.B. and Evers, S.M.A.A. (1997). Economic evaluation of back pan interventions. *Journal of Occupational Rehabilitation*, **7**, 15–32.

Guzmán, J., Esmail, R., Karjalainen, K., Irvin, E., and Bombadier, C. (2001). Multidisciplinary rehabilitation for chronic low back pain: Systematic review. *British Medical Journal*, **322**, 511–16.

Hadjistavropoulos, H.D., Hadjistavropoulos, T., and Quine, A. (2000). Health anxiety moderates the effects of distraction versus attention to pain. *Behaviour Research and Therapy*, **38**, 425–38.

Harkapaa, K., Jarvikoski, A., Mellin, G., Hurri, H., and Luoma, J. (1991). Health locus of control beliefs and psychological distress as predictors for treatment outcome in low-back pain patients: Results of a 3-month follow-up of a controlled intervention study. *Pain*, **46**, 35–41.

Hayes, S.C., Strosahl, K.D., and Wilson, K.G. (1999). *Acceptance and Commitment Therapy: An Experiential Approach to Behavior Change.* New York, NY: The Guilford Press.

Hayes, S.C., Wilson, K.G., Gifford, E.V., Follette, V.M., and Strosahl, K. (1996). Experiential avoidance and behavioral disorders: a functional dimensional approach to diagnosis and treatment. *Journal of Consulting Clinical Psychology*, **64**, 1152–68.

Hildebrandt, J., Pfingsten, M., Saur, P., and Jansen, J. (1997). Prediction of success from a multidisciplinary treatment programme for chronic back pain. *Spine*, **9**, 990–1001.

Jensen, M.P., Turner, J.A., and Romano, J.M. (1992). Chronic pain coping measures: Individual vs. composite scores. *Pain*, **51**, 273–80.

Jensen, M.P., Turner, J.A., and Romano, J.M. (1994). Correlates of improvement in multidisciplinary treatment of chronic pain. *Journal of Consulting and Clinical Psychology*, **62**, 172–9.

Kerns, R.D. and Haythornthwaite, J.A. (1988). Depression among chronic pain patients: Cognitive-behavioral analysis and effect on rehabilitation outcome. *Journal of Consulting and Clinical Psychology*, **56**, 870–6.

Kerns, R.D., Turk, D.C., and Rudy, T.E. (1985). The West Haven-Yale Multidimensional Pain Inventory (WHYMPI). *Pain*, **23**, 345–56.

Kleinke, C.L. and Spangler, A.S. (1988). Predicting treatment outcome of chronic back pain patients in a multidisciplinary pain clinic: Methodological issues and treatment implications. *Pain*, **33**, 41–8.

Knost, B., Flor, H., Birbaumer, N., and Schugens, M.M. (1999). Learned maintenance of pain: Muscle tension reduces central nervous system processing of painful stimulation in chronic and subchronic pain patients. *Psychophysiology*, **36**, 755–64.

Kori, S.H., Miller, R.P., and Todd, D.D. (1990). Kinisophobia: A new view of chronic pain behavior. *Pain Management*, Jan/Feb, 35–43.

Lethem, J., Slade, P.D., Troup, J.D., and Bentley, G. (1983). Outline of a fear-avoidance model of exaggerated pain perception—1. *Behaviour Research and Therapy*, **21**, 401–8.

Linehan, M.M. (1993). *Cognitive-behavioral Treatment of Borderline Personality Disorder.* New York, NY: Guilford Press.

Loeser, J.D. and Melzack, R. (1999). Pain: An overview. *Lancet*, **353**, 1607–9.

Malone, M.D. and Strube, M.J. (1988). Meta-analysis of non-medical treatments for chronic pain. *Pain*, **34**, 231–44.

Margraff, J., Barlow, D.H., Clarke, D.M., and Telch, M.J. (1993). Psychological treatment of panic: Work in progress on outcome, active ingredients, and follow-up. *Behavior Research and Therapy*, **31**, 1–8.

McClean, P.D., Whittal, M.L., Sochting, I. *et al.* (2001). Cognitive versus behavior therapy in group treatment of obsessive-compulsive disorder. *Journal of Consulting and Clinical Psychology*, **69**, 205–14.

McCracken, L.M. (1997). "Attention" to pain in persons with chronic pain: A behavioral approach. *Behavior Therapy*, **28**, 271–84.

McCracken, L.M. (1998). Learning to live with the pain: Acceptance of pain predicts adjustment in persons with chronic pain. *Pain*, **74**, 21–7.

McCracken, L.M. (1999). Behavioral constituents of chronic pain acceptance: Results from factor analysis of the Chronic Pain Acceptance Questionnaire. *Journal of Back and Musculoskeletal Rehabilitation*, **13**, 93–100.

McCracken, L.M. and Gross, R.T. (1998). The role of anxiety reduction in the outcome of multidisciplinary treatment for chronic low back pain. *Journal of Occupational Rehabilitation*, **8**, 179–89.

McCracken, L.M. and Turk, D.C. (2002). Behavioral and cognitive behavioral treatment for chronic pain: Outcome, predictors of outcome, and treatment process. *Spine*, **27**, 2564–73.

McCracken, L.M., Gross, R.T., and Eccleston, C. (2002). Multimethod assessment of treatment process in chronic low back pain: Comparison of reported pain-related anxiety with directly measured physical capacity. *Behaviour Research and Therapy*, **40**, 585–94.

McCracken, L.M., Zayfert, C., and Gross, R.T. (1992). The Pain Anxiety Symptoms Scale: Development and validation of a scale to measure fear of pain. *Pain*, **50**, 67–73.

McCracken, L.M., Spertus, I.L., Janeck, A.S., Sincliar, D., and Wetzel, F.T. (1999). Behavioral dimensions of adjustment in persons with chronic pain: Pain-related anxiety and acceptance. *Pain*, **80**, 283–9.

Morley, S. and Williams, A.C. de C. (2002). Conducting and Evaluating Treatment Outcome Studies. In D.C. Turk and R. Gatchel (eds.) *Psychological Approaches to Pain Management: A Practitioners Handbook*, 2nd edn., pp. 52–68. New York, NY: Guilford Press.

Morley, S., Eccleston, C., and Williams, A.C. de C. (1999). Systematic review and meta-analysis of randomized controlled trials of cognitive behaviour therapy and behaviour therapy for chronic pain in adults, excluding headache. *Pain*, **80**, 1–13.

Newman, M.G., Hoffman, S.G., Trabert, W., Roth, W.T., and Taylor, C.B. (1994). Does treatment of social phobia lead to cognitive changes? *Behavior Therapy*, **25**, 503–17.

Nicholas, M.K., Wilson, P.H., and Goyen, J. (1991). Operant-behavioural and cognitive-behavioural treatment for chronic low back pain. *Behaviour Research and Therapy*, **29**, 225–38.

Okifuji, A., Turk, D.C., and Eveleigh, D.J. (1999*a*). Improving the rate of classification of patients with the multidimensional pain inventory (MPI): Clarifying the meaning of "significant other". *Clinical Journal of Pain*, **15**, 290–96.

Okifuji, A., Turk, D.C., and Kalauokalani, D. (1999*b*). Clinical outcome and economic evaluation of multidisciplinary pain centers. In A.R. Block, E.F. Kremer, and E. Fernandez (eds.), *Handbook of Pain Syndromes*, pp. 77–97. Mahwah, NJ: Lawrence Erlbaum Associates.

Pincus, T. and Williams, A. (1999) Models and measurements of depression in chronic pain. *Journal of Psychosomatic Research*, **47**, 211–19.

Polatin, P.B., Gatchel, R.J., Barnes, D., Mayer, H., Arens, C., and Mayer, T.G. (1989). A psychosociomedical prediction model of responses to treatment by chronically disabled workers with low-back pain. *Spine*, **14**, 956–61.

Reitsma, B. and Meijler, W.J. (1997). Pain and patienthood. *Clinical Journal of Pain*, **13**, 9–21.

Rudy, T.E., Turk, D.C., Kubinski, J.A., and Zaki, H.S. (1995). Differential treatment responses of TMD patients as a function of psychological characteristics. *Pain*, **61**, 103–12.

Sanders, S.H. (1979). *Behavioral Assessment and Treatment of Clinical Pain: Appraisal of Current Status*. In M. Hersen, R.M. Eisler, and P.M. Miller (eds.), *Progress in Behavior Modification*, Vol. 8, pp. 249–91. New York, NY: Academic Press.

Schmidt, N.B., Lerew, D.R., and Trakowski, J.H. (1997). Body vigilance in panic disorder: Evaluating attention to bodily perturbations. *Journal of Consulting and Clinical Psychology*, **65**, 214–20.

Schmitz, U., Saile, H., and Nilges, P. (1996). Coping with chronic pain: Flexible goal adjustment as an interactive buffer against pain-related distress. *Pain*, **67**, 41–51.

Sharpe, M. and Williams, A.C. de C. (2002). Treating patients with somatoform pain disorder and hypochondriasis. In D.C. Turk and R. Gatchel (eds.) *Psychological Approaches to Pain Management: A Practitioners Handbook* 2nd edn., pp. 515–33. New York, NY: Guilford Press.

Spinhoven, P. and Linssen, A.C.G. (1991). Behavioral treatment of chronic low back pain: I. Relation of coping strategy use to outcome. *Pain*, **45**, 29–34.

Sullivan, M.J.L., Thorn, B., Haythornthwaite, J.A., Keefe, F., Martin, M., Bradley, L.A., and Lefevre, J.C. (2001). Theoretical perspectives on the relation between catastrophising and pain. *Clinical Journal of Pain*, **17**, 53–61.

Tota-Faucette, M.E., Gil, K.M., Williams, D.A., Keefe, F.J., and Goli, V. (1993). Predictors of response to pain management treatment: The role of family environment and changes in cognitive processes. *Clinical Journal of Pain*, **9**, 115–23.

Tsao, J.C.I. and Craske, M.G. (2000). Timing of treatment and return of fear: Effects of massed, uniform-, and expanding-spaced exposure schedules. *Behavior Therapy*, **31**, 479–7.

Turk, D.C. (1990). Customizing treatment for chronic pain patients: Who, what, and why. *Clinical Journal of Pain*, **6**, 255–70.

Turk, D.C. and Rudy, T.E. (1988). Toward an empirically derived taxonomy of chronic pain patients: Integration of psychological assessment data. *Journal of Consulting & Clinical Psychology*, **56**, 233–8.

Turk, D.C. and Salovey, P. (1984). "Chronic pain as a variant of depressive disease": A critical reappraisal. *Journal of Nervous and Mental Disease*, **172**, 398–404.

Turk, D.C., Rudy, T.E., Kubinski, J.A., Zaki, H.S., and Greco, C.M. (1996). Dysfunctional patients with temporomandibular disorders: Evaluating the efficacy of a tailored treatment protocol. *Journal of Consulting & Clinical Psychology*, **64**, 139–46.

Turk, D.C., Okifuji, A., Sinclair, J.D., and Starz, T.W. (1998). Differential responses by psychosocial subgroups of fibromyalgia syndrome patients to an interdisciplinary treatment. *Arthritis Care & Research*, **11**, 397–404.

Turner, J.A. (1996). Educational and behavioral interventions for back pain in primary care. *Spine*, **21**, 2851–57.

Van Tulder, M.W., Ostelo, R., Vlaeyen, J.W.S., Linton, S.J., Morley, S.J., and Assendelft, W.J. (2000). Behavioral treatment of for chronic low back pain: A systematic review within the framework of the Cochrane Back Review Group. *Spine*, **25**, 2688–99.

Vendrig, A.A. (1999). Prognostic factors and treatment-related changes associated with return to work in the multimodal treatment of chronic back pain. *Journal of Behavioral Medicine*, **22**, 217–32.

Vlaeyen, J.W.S. and Linton, S.J. (2000). Fear-avoidance and its consequences in chronic musculoskeletal pain: A state of the art. *Pain*, **85**, 317–32.

Vlaeyen, J.W.S., Kole-Snijders, A.M.K., Boeren, R.G.B., and Van Eek, H. (1995). Fear of movement/(re)injury in chronic low back pain and its relation to behavioral performance. *Pain*, **62**, 363–72.

Wall, P.D. (1994). Introduction. In P.D. Wall and R. Melzack (eds.), *Textbook of Pain* 3rd edn. Edinburgh: Churchill Livingstone.

Watson, P.J., Booker, C.K., Main, C.J., and Chen, A.C. (1997). Surface electromyography in the identification of chronic low back pain patients: The development of the flexion relaxation ratio. *Clinical Biomechanics*, 11, 165–71.

Williams, J.M.G. (1992). *The Psychological Treatment of Depression: A Guide to the Theory and Practice of Cognitive Behavioural Therapy*. London: Routledge.

Williams, A.C. de C. (1998). Depression in chronic pain: Mistaken models, missed opportunities. *Scandinavian Journal of Behavior Therapy*, 27, 61–80.

Williams, A.C. de C., Richardson, P.H., Nicholas, M.K. *et al.* (1996). Inpatient vs. outpatient pain management: Results of a randomised controlled trial. *Pain*, 66, 13–22.

Williams, A.C. de C., Nicholas, M.K., Richardson, P.H., Pither, C.E., and Fernandes, J. (1999). Generalizing from a controlled trial: The effects of patient preference versus randomization on the outcome of inpatient versus outpatient chronic pain management. *Pain*, 83, 57–65.

Chapter 14

Fear reduction in chronic pain: Graded exposure *in vivo* with behavioral experiments

Johan W.S. Vlaeyen, Jeroen de Jong,
Maaike Leeuw, and Geert Crombez

1 Introduction

In acute injury, the escape from the harmful situation and the associated withdrawal behavior promotes the healing process. In majority of the cases, healing occurs within a couple weeks and the pain resolves quickly. However, in certain people with pain, the immediate withdrawal behaviors do not lead to the anticipated reduction of pain, which then is interpreted as a signal of a continuous threat to the integrity of the body. In fact, a mismatch occurs between what the patient expects (quick decrease of pain) and what actually happens (increasing or lasting pain). Negative interpretation may not always reflect a real threat and, in such cases, catastrophic misinterpretations of benign physical sensations may occur. Sometimes, these misinterpretations may be fuelled by external information, such as unfavorable pain histories of relatives or acquaintances, verbal and visual information provided by health care providers suggesting the probability of a serious illness causing the pain complaints. Catastrophic misinterpretations consequently lead to an increase of the individual distress level, and fear reactions in particular.

In pain patients, errors in interpretation inevitably result in pain-related fear—fear of pain, fear of injury, fear of physical activity, and so forth—depending on the anticipated source of threat. These negative emotions are currently conceptualized by most theorists as *fundamental action tendencies* whose purpose is to motivate behavior related to successful survival. Some of these behaviors include preparing for, avoiding, or escaping potentially dangerous life-threatening events, which are at the heart of the emotions of fear and anxiety (Barlow 2002). One of the most prominent theories of emotion is the bio-informational theory (Lang 1979; Lang *et al.* 1998). This theory conceptualizes emotions as networks of action tendencies stored in memory along three levels: A perceptual level, a response level, and a semantic level. The theory predicts that events that match elements of the network can activate the whole network. The better the match, the stronger the emotion. In other words, fear and anxiety are behavior programs (much like computer programs) comprising stimulus, response, and meaning structures (i.e. data files). Data at the stimulus level will prompt action and define the function and direction of the act.

Consider the following situation of a fearful patient with back pain:

> I am cleaning the house. When picking up a book from the table, I hear a crack in my back and feel a shooting pain. The slightest movement is painful. I keep thinking how bad the pain is. There might be something wrong. I better stay still, otherwise I might be in danger of (re)injuring myself.

In this situation, stimulus information is the recognition of the frightening object (bodily sensations, such as the shooting pain). Response propositions are relevant responses, such as avoiding movement and staying still. The meaning propositions tie these two together. For example, they may include the following statement: "In this situation, these pain sensations are unpredictable and dangerous, and my responding indicates that I am afraid." Following this line of thought, and in an attempt to explain how and why some people develop a chronic pain syndrome, biopsychosocial models have been developed (for recent review see Asmundson and Wright 2004). These include the "fear-avoidance model of exaggerated pain perception" (Lethem *et al.* 1983), and more recently, a cognitive–behavioral model of fear of movement/(re)injury (Vlaeyen *et al.* 1995*a,b*). The central concept of these models is fear of pain, or the more specific *fear that physical activity will cause (re)injury.* Two opposing behavioral responses to pain are postulated. These include confrontation and avoidance (see Fig. 14.1). In the absence of a serious somatic pathology, confrontation is conceptualized as an adaptive response that eventually may lead to the reduction of fear and the promotion of recovery of function. In contrast, avoidance leads to the maintenance or exacerbation of fear, possibly resulting in a condition comparable to a phobia. The avoidance results in the reduction of both social and physical activities, which in turn leads to a number of physical and psychological consequences that augment disability (Philips 1987). Prospective studies in acute low back pain patients (Klenerman *et al.* 1995) and healthy people (Linton *et al.* 2000; Picavet *et al.* 2002) have provided support for the idea that pain-related fear may be an important precursor of pain disability.

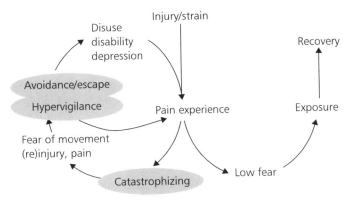

Fig. 14.1 Cognitive-behavioral model of pain-related fear. If pain, possibly caused by an injury or strain, is interpreted as threatening (pain catastrophizing), pain-related fear evolves. This leads to avoidance/escape, followed by disability, disuse, and depression. The latter will maintain the pain experiences thereby fuelling the vicious circle of increasing fear and avoidance. A more direct causal link between pain-related fear and pain is assumed to be mediated by hypervigilance. In non-catastrophizing patients, no pain-related fear and rapid confrontation with daily activities is likely to occur, leading to fast recovery. Based on Vlaeyen *et al.* (1995) with permission of IASP Press, Seattle.

2 Characteristics of pain-related fear

In 1990, Kori *et al.* introduced the term *kinesiophobia* (kinesis = movement) to describe the condition in which a patient has "an excessive, irrational, and debilitating fear of physical movement and activity resulting from a feeling of vulnerability to painful injury or reinjury" (p. 37). Recent evidence indicates that during confrontation with feared movements, chronic low back pain patients who are fearful of movement/(re)injury typically show cognitive (worry), psychophysiological (muscle reactivity), and behavioral (escape and avoidance) responses, rendering support for the idea that chronic pain and chronic fear share important characteristics (Philips 1987; Asmundson *et al.* 1999; Vlaeyen and Linton 2000). Indeed, when comparing the major features of specific phobia according to *Diagnostic and Statistical Manual of Mental Disorders-IV* (*DSM-IV*) (APA 1994) and pain-related fear in chronic pain patients, there is much similarity between the two conditions (Kori *et al.* 1990). One point on which they differ is that people with a phobia are aware that the fear is excessive and irrational, while most pain patients reporting pain-related fear are convinced that their avoidance has a protective function and is in no way excessive. Other researchers have proposed that fear of pain can better be understood as a manifestation of anxiety sensitivity rather than a specific phobia (Greenberg and Burns 2003). Pain-related fear is most likely phenomenologically distinct from circumscribed phobias.

There is evidence that pain-related fear is associated with specific worries, often referred to as pain catastrophizing. Pain catastrophizing is considered an exaggerated negative orientation toward noxious stimuli, and has been shown to mediate distress reactions to painful stimulation (Sullivan *et al.* 1995). Crombez *et al.* (1998*a*) found that pain-free volunteers with a high frequency of catastrophic thinking about pain became more fearful when threatened with the possibility of occurrence of intense pain than did students with a low frequency of catastrophic thinking. Chronic pain patients who catastrophize report more pain intensity, feel more disabled by their pain problem, and experience more psychological distress (Severeijns *et al.* 2001). A strong association has been found between pain catastrophizing and pain-related fear, and it has been suggested that pain catastrophizing is likely to be a precursor of pain-related fear (McCracken and Gross 1993; Vlaeyen *et al.* 1995*a*). In addition, there is evidence that people who catastrophize about pain or are fearful of it do not respond well to pain coping strategies training, such as attention diversion and applied relaxation (Heyneman *et al.* 1990; Vlaeyen *et al.* 1997).

In line with the cognitive theory of anxiety, a number of studies have also shown that pain-related fear is associated with increased body awareness and attentional focus toward pain and innoxious body stimuli. Indirect evidence on the association between pain-related fear and body hypervigilance is found using a primary task paradigm in which chronic pain patients are requested to direct their attentional focus toward an attentionally demanding task. Degradation in task performance on the task can be taken as an index of attentional interference due to hypervigilance (see Chapter 4).

It has repeatedly been shown that pain-related fear is associated with escape/avoidance behaviors. In a study where chronic pain sufferers volunteered to undergo cold pressor pain, Cipher and Fernandez (1997) showed that expected danger significantly predicted avoidance of another cold pressor immersion. Chronic pain patients who associate pain with damage tend to avoid activities that produce pain. Other studies that used physical performance tests reported that poor behavioral performance appeared to be more strongly associated with pain-related fear than with pain severity (Crombez *et al.* 1999*a*) or biomedical findings (Vlaeyen *et al.* 1995*b*). The effects of pain-related fear on behavioral performance also appear to generalize towards restrictions in daily life situations. Waddell *et al.* (1993) demonstrated that fear-avoidance beliefs about work are strongly related to disability of daily living and work lost in the past year, and more so than pain variables such as anatomical pattern of pain, time pattern, and pain severity. This led these investigators to conclude that "Fear of pain and what we do about it may be more disabling than pain itself" (Waddell *et al.* 1993: 164).

3 Disconfirmations of harm beliefs

What are the clinical implications of above-mentioned findings? Philips (1987) was one of the first to argue for the systematic application of graded exposure to produce disconfirmations between expectations of pain and harm, the actual pain, and the other consequences of the activity. She suggested that:

> These disconfirmations can be made more obvious to the sufferer by helping to clarify the expectations he or she is working with, and by delineating the conditions or stimuli which he feels are likely to fulfill his expectations. Repeated, graded, and controlled exposures to such situations under optimal conditions are likely to produce the largest and most powerful disconfirmations (Philips 1987: 279).

Experimental support for this idea is provided by the match–mismatch model of pain (Rachman 1994). This model states that people initially tend to over-predict how much pain they will experience but, after some exposures, tend to correctly match their predictions with actual experience.

A similar pattern of results was reported by Crombez *et al.* (1996) in a sample of chronic low back pain patients who were requested to perform four exercises (two with each leg) at maximal force. During each exercise the baseline pain, the expected pain, and experienced pain were recorded. As predicted, the chronic low back pain patients initially overpredicted pain, but after repetition of the exercise the overprediction was readily corrected. Recently, these findings were replicated with two other physical activities, including bending forward and straight leg raising (Goubert *et al.* 2002). In sum, it is quite plausible that, as with the treatment of phobias, graded exposure to back-stressing movements may indeed be a successful treatment approach for back pain patients reporting substantial fear of movement/(re)injury, although special attention should be drawn to generalization issues.

4 Graded exposure *in vivo* versus graded activity

At first sight, graded exposure *in vivo* may appear quite similar to the usual graded activity programs (Fordyce *et al.* 1986; Lindstrom *et al.* 1992), in that it gradually increases activity levels despite pain. However, both conceptually and practically, exposure *in vivo* is different from graded activity.

1. Graded activity is based on instrumental learning principles. Selected health behaviors are shaped through positively reinforcing a pre-defined quota of activities. Exposure *in vivo*, originally based on extinction of

Pavlovian conditioning (Bouton 1988), is currently viewed as a cognitive process in which fear is activated, catastrophic expectations are challenged and disconfirmed (resulting in reductions of the threat value of the originally fearful stimuli).

2. During graded activity attention is given to the identification of positive reinforcers that can be provided when the individual quotas are met, whereas in graded exposure, attention is given to establishing an individual hierarchy of the pain-related fear stimuli.

3. Usual graded activity programs include individual exercises according to functional capacity and observed individual physical work demands, while graded exposure includes activities that are selected based on a fear hierarchy and the idiosyncratic aspects of the fear stimuli. For example, if the patient fears the repetitive spinal compression produced by riding a bicycle on a bumpy road, then the graded exposure should include an activity that mimics that specific activity, and not just riding on a stationary bicycle.

5 Cognitive–behavioral assessment

In this section, we will address specific questionnaires, the interview, methods to establish graded hierarchies, and behavioral tests that can be used to gain sufficient information about the idiosyncratic aspects of pain-related fear responses in patients with chronic musculoskeletal pain.

5.1 Specific questionnaires

A basic question that may be asked is what the patient is afraid of or, in other words, what is the nature of the perceived threat? An answer to this question is not as simple as it seems. Patients may not view their problem as involving fear and may simply see difficulty or harm in performing certain movements or activities. In addition, the specific nature of pain-related fear varies considerably, making an idiosyncratic approach almost indispensable. Most patients fear pain itself. Other patients may not fear current pain, but pain that will be experienced at a later time (e.g. the day after an increase in physical exercise). Finally, patients may not fear pain itself, but the impending (re)injury that it is supposed to indicate, such as fear of becoming permanently handicapped. For these patients, pain is considered a warning signal for a seriously threatening situation. The literature reflects this variety of fear stimuli by including measures for the assessment of fear of pain, fear of work and physical activity, and fear of (re)injury as a result of movement. Questionnaires include the Pain and Impairment Relationship Scale (PAIRS), developed to study chronic pain patient's attitudes concerning activity and pain (Riley *et al.* 1988), the

Fear-Avoidance Beliefs Questionnaire (FABQ), focusing on patients' beliefs about how work and physical activity affect their low back pain (Waddell *et al.* 1993), the Pain Anxiety Symptoms Scale (PASS) developed to measure cognitive anxiety symptoms, escape and avoidance responses, fearful appraisals of pain and physiologic anxiety symptoms related to pain (McCracken and Dhimaga 2002), the Survey of Pain Attitudes (SOPA) (Jensen and Karoly 1992) measuring patients attitudes towards five dimensions of the chronic pain experience, and the Tampa Scale of Kinesiophobia (TSK) (Miller *et al.* 1991) aimed at the assessment of fear of (re)injury due to movement. For clinical purposes, these questionnaires seem appropriate as screening instruments to identify patients who suffer excessive pain-related fear (see Chapter 9). However, the questionnaires do not conclusively tell us what the individual is fearful of. In case of elevated scores, the above mentioned fear questionnaires are only indicative of the presence of pain-related fear. The assessment should be continued to further validate the hypothesis that the patient's disability is determined mainly by these fears.

5.2 Interview

The semi-structured interview is an additional and important tool that can be used to obtain information about the cognitive, behavioral, and psychophysiological aspects of the patient's symptoms and to better estimate the role of pain-related fear in the maintenance of their pain problem. It also includes information about the antecedents (situational or internal) of the pain-related fear, and about the direct and indirect consequences. Other areas of life stresses may also be addressed, as these might increase arousal levels and indirectly fuel pain-related fear. Phobogenic beliefs of fearful patients with chronic pain often take the form of conditional assumptions of the type "if P, then Q" whereby P is the predictor of a catastrophic consequence (Q). For example, "If I do this particular movement, pain will increase" and "If I feel pain, it means that my injury is getting worse." Often these forms of reasoning follow a confirmation bias in the sense that the rule "if P, then Q" is seldom falsified. Falsification would be to test if there are instances in which P is followed by non-Q. In the case of dysfunctional assumptions, the selective search of confirming evidence and the lack of falsifying evidence reinforces the credibility of the false assumptions (Smeets *et al.* 2000).

During the interview, it is essential to gather as much information as possible about the patient's logical assumptions regarding the relationships between physical activities, pain, and (re)injury. One possibility is to make use of the catastrophizing interview described by Vasey and Borkovec (1992). They argue that many of the cognitive products that are associated with the internal dialogue of anxious individuals take the form of "What if?" questions. In practice, clinicians can inquire during the interview about the nature of the worry by asking, "What is it about _____ that worries you?" (where the blank is filled with the response of the previous prompt). This procedure is repeated until the individual is unable to generate additional responses. Such a procedure is known to produce thoughts with deeper levels of meaning than typically accessed during a naturally occurring worrying process. Because in the assessment phase no attempts are made to subject the responses to logical analysis, such an interview is not likely to have a decatastrophizing effect (Vasey and Borkovec 1992).

It has to be kept in mind that chronic pain patients do not always conceive their problem as a phobia and, thus, they may not talk about fear. We suggest the interview be geared to the patient's perception of his or her pain problem. Based on our clinical experience with these patients, we recommend paraphrasing their personal story in terms of harmfulness (e.g. "You feel that it might be better not to do these activities," "I understand that you think that these activities might further harm your back") rather than using the words *fear* or *anxiety*. As often is the case, patients spontaneously start reconceptualizing their pain problem as a fear problem later on during treatment.

Factors that are often associated with the development of pain-related fear are (1) the characteristics of pain onset, and (2) the ambiguity around presence or absence of positive findings on medico-diagnostics. For example, a person involved in a traffic accident may develop a fear of driving as a result of the traumatic experience. Likewise, a back pain patient may develop a fear of lifting after experiencing pain while lifting or after receiving information from a medical doctor that lifting can damage nerves in the spinal cord. Most chronic back pain patients who report increased pain-related fear appear to have found their conviction about vulnerability to (re)injury following the results of diagnostics tests such as X-rays and MRI. The combination of (threatening) information conveyed by the medical specialist and the experience of pain and discomfort seem to strengthen that conviction. The visual confrontation with the X-rays and simply hearing the diagnosis can be upsetting to some patients and can be interpreted as being more threatening than intended by the specialist.

Although reports about misconceptions and misinterpretations of information can be clarified during the educational part of the intervention, it is more useful to identify the current level of severity and the maintaining factors of the pain problem and associated pain-related fear. The severity can often be estimated by inquiring about the extent to which the pain problem interferes with daily life, including the ability to carry on paid work, leisure activities, and normal relationships. Maintaining factors usually include negative thoughts about the consequences of the physical activities, the avoidance of these activities, and hypervigilance to signals of threat. Negative thoughts can be elicited by inquiring about the patient's personal theory about his or her pain and associated functional incapacity. Expectations about the future are also worth assessing: "What do you think will happen if the pain is left untreated?" For example, the back and pelvic pain complaints of one of our female patient's started during her first pregnancy and increased after the delivery. She started worrying about the future because a relative who received the same diagnosis ended up in a wheelchair. Her main belief was that during certain movements the tissue and nerves around the ridged symphysis pubis could be damaged or ruptured, possibly resulting in paralysis of the lower limbs. In most cases these thoughts make people cognisant of bodily sensations that may signal impending danger. Situations that provoke these sensations are then fearfully avoided. To gain insight into avoidance behaviors, the therapist may ask questions such as, "What does the pain prevent you from doing?" and "If you no longer had this pain problem, what differences would it make to your daily life?" One can also ask directly about the situations that may worsen the pain problem. Finally, from the assessment, it should become clear whether other problems, such as major depression, marital conflicts, or disability claims, warrant specific attention before or after treatment. When more complicated problems are expected to arise following the reduction of pain, it may be advisable to leave the pain disability problem untreated. A summary of the topics covered during the interview is provided in Table 14.1.

5.3 Determining treatment goals

There are several reasons why it is important to spend some time on the specification of treatment goals (Kirk 1989).

1. Cognitive–behavioral treatments (CBTs) for pain, including exposure *in vivo*, never primarily aim at reducing pain but at the restoration of functional abilities despite pain (Turk and Okifuji 2002). It helps to make this general goal explicit, and both the patient and therapist should agree on one or more realistic and specific goals that are formulated in positive terms. Typical examples include

   (a) being able to go shopping to the supermarket,

   (b) swimming twice a week for half an hour, and

   (c) return to work.

   In cases in which the goal is to return to work, it is appropriate to consult with the occupational physician or vocational counsellor. Often the exposure treatment can be conducted in synchrony with a graded resumption of work activities.

2. Goal-setting helps to structure the treatment and to design the hierarchy of stimuli that will be introduced during the actual *in vivo* exposure. For example, if a patient wishes to resume their sports activities, the therapist will make sure that aspects of these will be included in the graded exposure exercises.

3. Setting functional goals redirects the focus of attention from pain and physical symptoms toward daily life activities, emphasizing the possibility of change away from the disability status. Finally, as the patient is invited to formulate his or her own goals, goal setting inadvertently reinforces the notion that active participation is an essential part of the treatment.

5.4 Graded hierarchies

Once it has become clear that pain-related fear is pivotal in the maintenance of a patient's pain disability, it is useful to inquire about the essential stimuli—what is the patient actually afraid of? To date, there are no standardized questionnaires for identifying these stimuli. In our experience, it is difficult for pain patients to verbally estimate the threat value of different situations.

Table 14.1 Summary of topics covered during the interview

◆ Description of the current pain problem

◆ Detailed description when the pain problem first occurred:
  ● Situation: Where and when did it occur? What were you doing?
  ● Behavior: How did you respond to the pain? What did other people do?
  ● Cognitions: What did you think was going on?
  ● Information provided by others: What did other people say about the pain?
  ● Bodily reactions: How did you feel?

◆ Current situations: List of situations the pain is most likely to occur or to be most severe

◆ Avoidance: What are you not doing anymore because of the pain?

◆ Modulators: What are the things that make it better or worse?

◆ Current cognitions: What do you think is the cause of the pain problem?

◆ Attitudes and behaviors of others: What do other people (spouse/doctor/therapists) think is the cause of the pain problem?

◆ Previous treatments

◆ Personal strengths and assets

◆ Social and financial circumstances

◆ Medication use

One of the problems is that their avoidance behaviors are not really acknowledged as consequences of fear, but as a direct consequence of the pain and the experienced vulnerability for (re)injury. In addition to checklists of daily activities, the presentation of visual materials, such as pictures of back-stressing activities and movements, is worthwhile. These can be quite helpful in the development of graded hierarchies, reflecting the full range of situations avoided by the patient, beginning with those that provoke only mild discomfort, and ending with activities or situations that are beyond the patient's present abilities.

The Photograph Series of Daily Activities (PHODA) is a standardized method that is appropriate to design graded hierarchies (Kugler *et al.* 1999). PHODA uses 98 photographs representing various physical daily life activities, (e.g. lifting, bending, walking, bicycling), which are presented to the patients. The patient is requested to place each photograph along a fear thermometer. This consists of a vertical line with 11 anchor points (ranging from 0 to 100) printed on a 60 cm × 40 cm hardboard. The fear-thermometer is placed on a table in front of the patient with the following instruction: "*Please watch each photograph carefully, and try to imagine you performing the same movement. Place the photograph on the thermometer according to the extent in which you feel that this movement is harmful to your back.*" In our experience, abrupt changes in movements (e.g. suddenly being hit) or activities consisting of repetitive spinal compressions (e.g. riding a bicycle on a bumpy road) are frequently mentioned stimuli in chronic back pain patients who score high on the pain-related fear measures. These situations are feared because of beliefs about the causes of pain, such as ruptured or severely damaged nerves (e.g. "If I lift heavy weights, the nerves in my back might be damaged"). Also of interest is that the same activity can be rated differently depending on the context in which the activity is performed. For example, the activity "running" receives an 80 when performed in a wood, and 50 when performed on an even terrain. It is, therefore, essential to expose patients to physical activities in a variety of contexts.

5.5 Behavioral tests

Sometimes, patients find it hard to accurately estimate the harmfulness of an activity when it has been avoided extensively. In such cases, behavioral tests can be introduced. These consist of performing an activity that has been previously avoided, while performance indices (such as time, distance, or number of repetitions) are measured. Target behaviors can be derived from PHODA items, and in most cases the behavioral tests can be considered as a variant of the exercise tolerance test described by Fordyce (1976). To assess the extent to which avoidance occurs, patients are asked to perform the activity ". . . until pain, weakness, fatigue or any other reason causes you to wish to stop" (Fordyce 1976: 170). Behavioral tests are advantageous because anticipatory fear and the overall fear during exposure can be measured separately (Butler 1989). In addition, they provide a more objective measure of avoidance behavior.

6 **Fear reduction in chronic pain**

Lang's (1979; Lang *et al.* 1998) bio-informational theory of fear predicts that there are two main conditions required to reduce fear: (1) The fear network needs to be activated and (2) new information needs to be available to disconfirm the fear expectations that are inherent to the fear memory. In clinical practice, several techniques can be applied to reduce fear in patients with chronic pain. These include verbal reassurance, education, physical exercise and/or graded activity, and exposure *in vivo* with behavioral experiments. As will become apparent below, the success of these techniques in reducing fear is not equivalent.

6.1 **Verbal reassurance**

Verbal reassurance generally consists of two classes of verbal cues: Verbal statements intended to emotionally reassure patients directly (e.g. "I wouldn't worry if I were you"), and verbal statements that indicate the absence of a medically relevant diseases (e.g. "There is nothing wrong with your back," Coia and Morley 1998). Medical doctors can tell their patients that they do not have the particular disease they fear, often supported by showing them negative test results, and sometimes by providing an alternative non-disease explanation such as stress, muscle pain, or physical overuse. The major problem with verbal reassurance is its inherent ambiguity "How can it be that there is nothing wrong with my back and yet I still feel pain?" A surprisingly small number of studies have examined the effects of verbal reassurance. Notwithstanding, the available evidence indicates that verbal reassurance does not reduce fears, and can even have paradoxical effects. In the long run, reassurance can increase fear in a number of patients (McDonald *et al.* 1996; Donovan and Blake 2000). These results are not surprising, as verbal reassurance does not activate the fear network (but rather attenuates it), nor does it provide new information that disqualifies previous beliefs. What moderately fearful patients may need is a credible explanation of their pain and disability that provides a better account for the current situation than the disease model. To achieve this in the area of chronic musculoskeletal pain, a number of researchers have developed educational material aimed at modifying beliefs about hurting and harming.

6.2 **Education**

Another way of reducing fear is to provide new information about the irrationality of the feared consequences. Educating patients in a way that leads them to view their pain as a common condition that can be self-managed, rather than as a serious disease or a condition that needs careful protection, is a useful *first* step. One of the major goals of the educational component is to increase the willingness of the patient to eventually engage in activities that they have been avoiding for a long time. That is, the aim is to correct the misinterpretations and misconceptions that have occurred early on during the development of the pain-related fear. To date, empirical evidence suggests that education is an effective means of reducing pain-related fear and disability. One study evaluated a booklet (the "back book") especially designed for lay people in a group of patients consulting their family physician with a new pain episode (Burton *et al.* 1999). Although there were no differences in pain, patients receiving the experimental booklet showed a significantly greater early improvement in beliefs that were maintained at 1 year. A greater proportion of patients with an initially high pain-related fear who received the experimental booklet had clinically significant reductions in pain-related fear at 2 weeks, followed by a significant improvement in their disability levels. Moore *et al.* (2000) examined the effects of a two-session group intervention for back pain patients in primary care settings that were based on education. Besides the group meeting, there was also one individual meeting and a telephone conversation with the group leader, and with a psychologist experienced in chronic pain management. The intervention was supplemented by educational materials (book and videos) supporting active management of back pain. A control group received usual care supplemented by a book on back pain care. Participants assigned to the self care intervention showed significantly greater reductions in back-related worry and fear-avoidance beliefs than the control group (Moore *et al.* 2000). There is also evidence that sub-chronic low back pain may be managed successfully with an approach that includes clinical examination combined with information for patients about the nature of the problem, provided in a manner designed to reduce fear and give them reason to resume light activity (Indahl *et al.* 1998).

Education is a helpful prerequisite for an exposure *in vivo* treatment. The patient is given a careful explanation of the fear-avoidance model, using the patient's individual symptoms, beliefs, and behaviors to illustrate how vicious circles (pain → catastrophic thought → fear → avoidance → disability → pain) maintain the pain problem. For example, consider a 40-year old married woman who works in a cleaning service. Her pain started 5 years earlier, while lifting a trash bag to throw it into a big container. During this movement, she heard a "crack" in her lower back, immediately followed by a "shooting" pain.

She was very frightened that she might have injured herself seriously, because she had never felt anything like this before and did not understand what was going on. From then on, she experienced about 4–6 of these "cracks" per day, which she interpreted as signs of tissue or nerve damage. She can now almost predict which movements provoke these frightening cracks, and tries to avoid them as much as possible. As a result of this "protective" behavior, she stopped cleaning, both at work as at home. She also needed to stop her favored leisure activity (gardening), and spends most of her time reclining and watching TV. As a result of her concerns and the absence of usual distractors, she focuses on her body, thereby amplifying her pain.

In cases where the pain-related fear appears to be fueled by the visual confrontation with (presumably "positive") diagnostic tests, it may be useful to review these tests together with a physician. It can be explained to the patient that he or she has probably overestimated the value of these tests, and that similar abnormalities can also be found in symptom free people (Jensen *et al.* 1994). Additionally, the therapist can suggest one of the existing patient books and leaflets such as the British Back Book (Burton *et al.* 1996), the New Zealand acute back pain patient brochure (Kendall *et al.* 1997), and the recently developed Dutch brochure (Goossens *et al.* 2000). One of the essential messages conveyed during the educational session is that pain and disability are likely to be a signal of too much protection, rather than a signal of harm.

6.3 Exercise/operant graded activity

Although most exercise and operant graded activity programs are not intended to reduce pain-related fear, but rather to directly increase activity levels despite pain, they may have fear-reducing effects. For example, one study compared three active treatments: (1) modern active physiotherapy, (2) muscle reconditioning on training devices, and (3) low-impact aerobics. After therapy, significant reductions were observed in pain intensity, frequency, pain disability, pain catastrophizing, and pain-related fear across all treatment modalities (Mannion *et al.* 1999). These effects were maintained over the subsequent 6 months, with the exception of the patients receiving physiotherapy. For those patients, levels of pain-related fear and disability increased. A subsequent study suggested that the improvements were likely to be a result of the positive experience of completing the prescribed exercises without undue harm (Mannion *et al.* 2001). Similar findings have been reported after an operant graded activity program (Van den Hout 2002).

7 Exposure *in vivo* with behavioral experiments

7.1 Exposure *in vivo*

Current treatments of excessive fears and anxiety are based on the experimental work of Wolpe (1958) on systematic desensitization. In this keystone treatment method, individuals progress through an incremental series of anxiety provoking encounters with phobic stimuli, while utilizing relaxation as a reciprocal inhibitor of increasing anxiety. Because relaxation was intended to compete with the anxiety response, a graded format was chosen to keep anxiety levels as weak as possible. Later studies revealed that the exposure to the feared stimuli appeared to be a most essential component of the systematic desensitization, and produced comparable effects applied without relaxation (Craske and Rowe 1997). For fearful patients, first-hand evidence of behaving differently is far more convincing than rational argument. The most essential step consists of graded exposure to the situations the patient has identified as "dangerous" or "threatening." Further, the general principles for exposure are followed.

1. Establish a fear hierarchy, for example, using the PHODA (Kugler *et al.* 1999).

2. Obtain patients agreement to perform certain activities or movements that she or he typically avoids.

3. Encourage patients to engage in these fearful activities as much as possible until disconfirmation has occurred and anxiety levels have decreased.

4. Demonstrate that the activity is harmless and not extraordinary by modeling it first.

5. Monitor expectations by asking patients to predict the occurrence of harm, and repeat the same question after the first exposure to that activity: *"How would you rate the probability that you may experience a severe pain attack after doing this activity?"*

6. If these ratings significantly decrease, consider moving on to the next item of the hierarchy. Alternatively, the therapist can ask the patient to report their subjective units of distress on a scale from 0 to 10 and repeat the exposure task until the level of distress has substantially decreased.

7. In order to facilitate independence and to promote more exposures, gradually withdraw your presence (as it may serve as an initial safety signal).

8. In order to generalize extinction of pain-related fear, create contexts that mimic those of the home situation.

7.2 **Behavioral experiments**

Following from cognitive theory that assumes that cognitive "errors" can be corrected through conscious reasoning, behavioral experiments have been developed in which a collaborative empiricism is the bottom line. The essence of a behavioral experiment is that the patient performs an activity to challenge the validity of his catastrophic assumptions and misinterpretations. As noted above, these assumptions take the form of "if P, then Q" statements, and are empirically tested with so-called behavioral experiments. Usually, these consist of nine steps (ten Broeke *et al.* 2003):

1. The patient formulates the dysfunctional belief or proposition, and rates its credibility. For example, a back pain patient may expect that jumping down from a stair will inevitably cause nerve damage in the spine and excruciating pain (credibility = 75 percent).

2. A realistic alternative belief is formulated. For example, this patient may formulate that, alternatively, he will be able to continue walking without excruciating pain after jumping down from a chair (credibility = 25 percent).

3. An appropriate behavioral experiment is designed and described as specifically as possible. For example, if the patient is convinced that jumping down is harmful, the therapist can further inquire about the minimal height that is needed to cause nerve injury.

4. Next, the following question is presented to the patient: Suppose the original belief is true, what do you expect will happen during the experiment?

5. The same question is repeated, but then for the alternative belief.

6. The experiment is carried out.

7. The patient describes what happened.

8. Both therapist and patient discuss what conclusions can be drawn from this experiment.

9. Finally, the patient is requested to reflect on what he did learn from this experience, and whether there is more information needed to increase the credibility of the (more adaptive) alternative belief. In this example, the therapist would invite the patient to jump down from the stair and the consequences of doing so would be evaluated.

In practice, behavioral experiments are difficult to separate from exposure, and they can best be used simultaneously. We will describe two cases, in which fear has originated from direct trauma and informational transmission, respectively.

7.3 Case illustrations

7.3.1 Mrs A

Mrs A is a 40-year old married shopkeeper with chronic neck and shoulder pain. Eight years ago she was hit by a ball while swimming in a swimming pool. She reportedly heard a crack in her neck when the ball hit the left side of her head. Initially, she did not feel any pain, but when her husband moved her head to inspect whether she was injured, she felt another crack accompanied by a severe shooting pain that increased over the day. The next day, the general practitioner told her that pain was probably caused by a muscle sprain in the neck region, and his advice consisted of rest and warm packs. She stopped working at the shop and never returned. Several treatments, including massage, electrotherapy, exercise, and wearing a corset, were unsuccessful. A neurologist performed nerve blocks that relieved the pain for a couple of months. When playing with her children, she experienced another crack that reportedly set on the pain again. Repeated nerve blocks did not produce any effect this time. Finally, she was referred for a comprehensive rehabilitation program. Mrs A is convinced that structures in her neck were damaged when she was hit by the ball. She is afraid that she will have to continually wear the corset, and feels that she has to move very carefully not to worsen her condition. Using the PHODA, a fear hierarchy was made (Table 14.2). A single case AB design was set up consisting of a 1-week baseline period, followed by an exposure *in vivo* treatment of 15 sessions, 60 min. each, spread over 5 weeks. During these 6 weeks, measures of pain, pain-related fear, and difficulties encountered with three daily life activities were kept in a diary. During the first educational session, Mrs A was provided with a rationale explaining that painful body sensations can occur without signaling muscle or nerve damage. She was also provided information on how protective behaviors (such as resting, guarding, and vigilance) in the long run can maintain the pain problem. This session was followed by the first exposure session, starting with activities with a PHODA rating of about 40. It was decided to start the exposure with simple tasks such as picking up light objects from the floor, followed by lifting, and reaching tasks. Using behavioral experiments, the belief that sudden movements are harmful was systematically challenged. During subsequent sessions, the activities became physically more intense as the patient ascended the fear hierarchy. At the end, Mrs A was able to do somersaults and learned to kick a ball with her head. After 15 sessions of exposure therapy, the TSK score decreased from 48 to 17, and the PHODA from 690 to 110. Of interest also was that pain ratings decreased significantly (Fig. 14.2). Daily activities that were chosen as important goals, but avoided because of the fear, were gradually resumed (Fig. 14.3).

Table 14.2 Fear hierarchy of Mrs A

Fear hierarchy	PHODA item
100	Sudden, unexpected movements Running Jumping down Falling Bicycling Walking down stairs Trampolining Sneeze
80	Reaching forward Cleaning windows Lifting heavy objects (baby, crate, garbage bin) Gardening
50	Climbing stairs Bending forward Vacuuming Lifting light objects
40	Driving a car Dressing a child Washing dishes Ironing

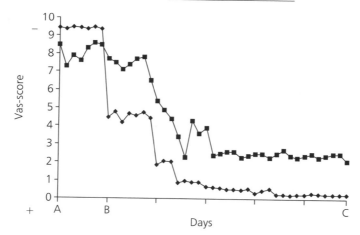

Fig. 14.2 Daily measures of pain-related fear (diamonds) and pain (squares) of Mrs A during baseline (A–B) and exposure treatment (B–C).

7.3.2 Mrs B

Mrs B is a 30-year old student with knee pain that has gradually developed over the last 4 years. The pain is reportedly associated with some kind of "twitch" in the knee. The orthopedic surgeon diagnosed strained muscles

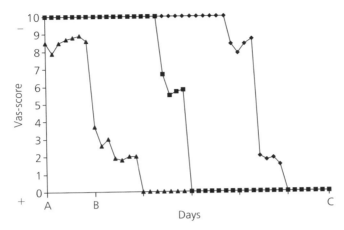

Fig. 14.3 Daily disability ratings of Mrs A during baseline (A–B) and exposure treatment (B–C). Activity 1: Horse around with the children (diamonds), Activity 2: Bicycling (squares), Activity 3: Go out shopping (triangles).

around the knee and suggested that the pain would decrease with rest. Mrs B consulted a second orthopedic surgeon who performed an exploratory operation, which worsened the pain problem. Mrs B, who used to be physically active and enjoyed running, decided to quit sports activities altogether. Moreover, she gradually began avoiding an increasing number of daily activities, terminated her studies, and seldom left the house. She was eventually referred for a comprehensive rehabilitation program. Mrs B is convinced that some part of the knee has been severely damaged, and that physical activity will cause further damage. She is afraid that she will ultimately end up in a wheelchair. She also expresses resentment to others, including the health care providers who did not solve her problem but, instead, made it worse. She has decided not to listen to anyone but herself, as she feels that she is the only one who knows what is good for her at this moment. Like Mrs A, a single case AB design was set up consisting of a 1-week baseline period, followed by an exposure *in vivo* treatment of 15 sessions, 60 min. each, spread over 5 weeks. Table 14.3 provides a brief summary of her fear hierarchy. The exposure treatment proceeded slowly, as she was very reluctant to engage in exposure sessions. Mrs B wondered whether her pain problem was taken seriously enough. The therapist reassured her that there was no doubt that her pain problem was real, but explained to her that the behavioral experiments were set up to challenge the validity of her catastrophic interpretations. During subsequent sessions, the activities became physically more intense as she ascended the fear hierarchy. The final exposure sessions consisted of jumping down from a desk. At the end, Mrs B was convinced to start running again.

Table 14.3 Fear hierarchy of Mrs B

Fear hierarchy	PHODA item
100	Running
	Jumping down
	Falling
	Bicycling
	Walking stairs
	Walking with the dog
	Swimming
90	Bending through the knees
80	Reaching
	Bending forward
	Vacuuming
	Loading washing machine
70	Driving a car for more than 1 h
	Carrying a trash bag
40	Washing dishes
	Ironing

After 15 sessions of exposure therapy, the TSK score decreased from 52 to 24, and the harm scores from the PHODA from 810 to 140. Although pain ratings initially increased somewhat, a steady decrease was observed over the treatment period (Fig. 14.4). Daily activities that were chosen as important goals, but avoided because of the fear, were gradually resumed (Fig. 14.5).

7.4 Treatment barriers

7.4.1 Pain increase

Although patients have agreed that the treatment is not aimed at reducing pain levels, it is often frightening to experience a sudden pain increase during exposure. In most cases, increases in pain are *temporary* and wane after a few hours. In such cases, the following steps can be taken:

1. The therapist can check whether there are medical reasons for the pain increase. If not, the patient can be provided with an acceptable rationale in which it is reiterated that although pain is bothersome, it is not a signal of danger. For example, pain can be explained as the possible result of disuse of the muscles, or as the reaction of the muscles to increased exertion during therapy.

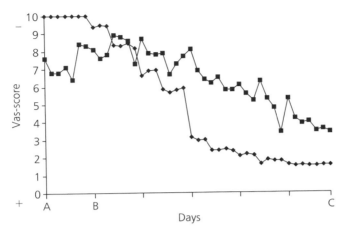

Fig. 14.4 Daily measures of pain-related fear (diamonds) and pain (squares) of Mrs B during baseline (A–B) and exposure treatment (B–C).

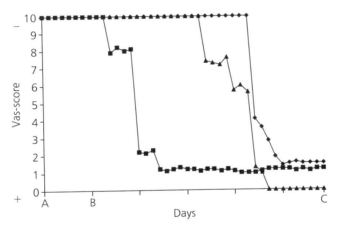

Fig. 14.5 Daily disability ratings of Mrs B during baseline (A–B) and exposure treatment (B–C). Activity 1: Running (diamonds), Activity 2: Walking with the dog (square), Activity 3: Buying clothes (triangle).

2. Preferably, directly following the first step, exposure to physical activity can be continued. If patients are excessively reluctant, the therapist may decide to repeat some of the previous activities at a lower level on the fear hierarchy.

3. Again a behavioral experiment can be set up to challenge the belief that something serious might have happened to cause the pain increase. Our experience is that fear levels quickly go down and, when encountering a similar pain increase in the future, patients are less worried and pain increases

tend to interfere less with their current activities. Actually, the occurrence of an increase in pain during the treatment can be beneficial, as it provides the possibility for both the patient and the therapist to discuss post-treatment planning for times when pain increases re-occur.

7.4.2 Safety behaviors

There are a number of behavioral reactions, more volitional in nature, that have to be considered important in the maintenance of pain-related fear, especially during the exposure procedure. For example, a chronic back pain patient who is exposed to a lifting task with his dominant arm may do so while holding their other arm on their back as to protect it. Or they may focus more attention to the precise lifting motion, or try to relax before starting the lifting task. These subtle and sometimes covert responses constitute safety behaviors (Salkovskis *et al.* 1999) that are intended to avert feared events. Safety behaviors are known to play a significant role in the maintenance of avoidance (see Chapter 2). While the behavior may relieve anxiety in the short-term, it unintentionally maintains the belief in the catastrophic consequences by preventing exposure to disconfirmations of irrational beliefs. In other words, combining exposure *in vivo* treatment with coping strategies such as relaxation or attention diversion techniques may actually weaken the impact of the exposure. Indeed, patients may attribute the non-occurrence of the feared catastrophe to the use of safety behaviors rather than correctly attributing it to the fact that catastrophe will not occur. For example, coming down on one foot at once, instead of both feet simultaneously, during a jump was a typical safety behavior emitted by Mrs A. Other frequent safety behaviors include bracing, guarded walking, seeking physical support, and other behaviors often described as pain behaviors. The therapist should be aware of these often subtle behaviors and closely observe patients during exposure sessions. When safety behaviors are identified, we suggest the therapist repeat the exposure session with the instruction to leave out the safety behavior. That is, response prevention strategies can be combined with exposure.

Firm ergonomic advice about lifting, carrying, and sitting, often provided in the so-called "back schools," conveying the message that activities are only safe when performed in an ergonomically "justified" way, can best be omitted in fearful patients undergoing an exposure *in vivo* procedure. Indeed, they may be interpreted as evidence that if not followed as suggested, the feared catastrophe may occur. Of course, this does not mean that patients can be exposed to any kind of stimulus. All stimuli used in the exposure procedure should be reasonable and safe for anyone, and always be modeled by the therapist and negotiated with the patient.

7.5 **Generalizations and maintenance of change**

What is actually learned during exposure? Although some researchers assume that exposure leads to a disconfirmation of overpredictions of the aversive characteristics of fear stimuli, there is growing evidence that exposure cannot simply be equated with unlearning (see Chapter 2). It appears that during successful exposure, exceptions to the rule rather than a fundamental change of that rule are learned (Bouton 1988). Recent studies have shown that in chronic low back pain patients, exposure to one movement (e.g. bending forward) does not generalize to another, dissimilar movement (e.g. straight leg raising (Crombez *et al.* 2002; Goubert *et al.* 2002). These authors conclude that, during exposure, patients appear to learn exceptions to the rule (if P, then Q). This is in line with animal studies on learning (Bouton 2000). In other words, exposure to physical activities is not likely to result immediately in a fundamental change in the belief that certain movements are harmful or painful but, rather, that the movements involved in the exposure treatment are less harmful or painful than anticipated.

Research findings on exposure in patients with anxiety disorders suggest that generalization and maintenance can be enhanced by a number of measures:

1. The therapist should provide exposure to the full variety of contexts and natural settings in which fear has been experienced. (e.g. Mineka *et al.* 1999). The PHODA might be a useful tool in eliciting information about these contexts in chronic pain patients. It is preferable to carry out an exposure session in the context in which the fear has been acquired. For example, in one patient (reported in Vlaeyen *et al.* 2001) the fear started at work when she heard a "crack" in her lower back while lifting a trash bag and throwing it into a big container. A shooting pain immediately followed the crack, and the patient interpreted subsequent cracking sounds in the back as signs of tissue or nerve damage. In this patient, one of the final exposure sessions consisted of going back to that same place at the work site and repeating the behavior.

2. The therapist should vary the stimuli during exposure (Rowe and Craske 1998*b*). Activities to be included in the exposure procedure can best be extended from those derived from PHODA to other activities as well. For example, bicycling can be done in very different ways, including using a sports bike rather than a regular bike, biking uphill as well as downhill, and biking on rough as well as even terrain.

3. The therapist might enhance generalization and maintenance by using an expanded and spaced exposure schedule rather than one that is presented en masse (Rowe and Craske 1998*a*). That is, it may be preferable to spread

the treatment over a longer period of time instead of concentrating it within a very limited number of weeks.

As exposure *in vivo* with behavioral experiments is a cognitive–behavioral intervention, training in cognitive–behavioral principles is a necessary prerequisite, and supervision by a psychologist experienced in working in the field of behavioral medicine and the area of chronic pain, in particular, is a sine qua non. In addition, the treatment will work best when delivered by therapists who feel comfortable exposing patients to movements, and who are not fearful themselves that too much physical activity will be harmful to the patient. Rainville *et al.* (1995) conjectured that "patients' attitudes and beliefs (and thereby patients disability levels) may be derived from the projected attitudes and beliefs of health care providers" (p. 288). In line with this, a recent study on health care providers attitudes reported that therapists who hold a more biomedical or biomechanical view of chronic pain evaluate daily physical activities as more harmful for patients with common back pain than their colleagues whose attitudes toward pain are more behaviorally oriented (Houben *et al.* 2004).

8 **Effectiveness**

A number of recent studies have examined the effectiveness of a graded exposure *in vivo* treatment with behavioral experiments in reducing pain-related fears, catastrophizing, and pain disability in chronic low back pain patients reporting substantial fear of movement/(re)injury. In two studies, a replicated single case crossover design was applied with four and six consecutive chronic low back pain patients each. Only patients who reported substantial fear of movement/(re)injury (TSK score > 40), and who were referred for outpatient behavioral rehabilitation were included (Vlaeyen *et al.* 2001, 2002*a*). After a no-treatment baseline measurement period, the patients were randomly assigned to one of two interventions. In intervention A, patients received the exposure first, followed by graded activity. In intervention B, the sequence of treatment modules was reversed. Daily measures of pain-related cognitions and fears were recorded with visual analog scales. Before and after the treatment, pain-related fear, pain catastrophizing, pain control, and pain disability were measured.

Although the supplemental value of the graded activity program cannot be ruled out in these studies, the remarkable improvements observed whenever the graded exposure was initiated suggests that its therapeutic power is much stronger. Not only were improvements found on the self-report measures of pain-related fear, pain catastrophizing, and pain disability, but these also generalized to increases in physical activity in the home situation as measured with ambulatory activity monitors (Vlaeyen *et al.* 2002*a*). The crossover design gave the opportunity to examine the differential effects of graded exposure and graded activity, and the additional treatment effect of the second treatment module. As the order of treatment modules did not make any difference on the final outcome of the exposure treatment, it can be concluded that exposure *in vivo* is not enhanced when preceded by graded activity training. On the other hand, carry-over effects were clearly observed when graded exposure was followed by graded activity. A third study revealed similar effects in two low back pain patients (Vlaeyen *et al.* 2002*b*). In this study, exposure *in vivo* was delivered as the only treatment, and without the background rehabilitation program. This suggests that it is the exposure treatment that is responsible for the results. One drawback of these studies is that they were performed by the same treatment staff in similar settings. However, the external validity of the exposure treatment has recently been supported by two Swedish studies in which patients were given the treatment in a different hospital setting (Linton *et al.* 2002; Boersma *et al.* in press). Although the effects seem somewhat weaker than in the Dutch studies described above, the results demonstrate clear decreases in pain-related fear and substantial increases in function. As in the previous studies (Vlaeyen *et al.* 2002*a,b*), marked decreases in pain report are observed despite the resumption of daily activities. Thus, the results replicate and extend the findings of previous studies to a new setting, with other therapists, and a new research design. Together with the initial studies, these results provide a basis for pursuing and further developing the exposure technique—testing it with larger samples and extending it to group designs.

What can be said about the possible mediators of treatment effects? Treatment durations examined were much too short to produce significant increases in muscle strength. The abrupt change in the daily measures is suggestive of cognitive changes. Although the exposure was provided during a period of 3 weeks, the reduction of catastrophizing and fear was achieved within 7 days, or three exposure sessions. Rachman and Whittal (1989) have proposed that such abrupt changes are more characteristic of insight learning, rather than the usual gradual progression of trial and error learning. In our studies, the presentation of the rationale at the start of the exposure might have contributed to this insight. Many patients reported that, for the first time, they received a credible rationale for their current level of disability. To tease apart the differential effects of the educational and exposure components, we have randomized four low back pain patients over two conditions (de Jong *et al.* 2002). Both conditions started with a 3-week baseline wait list period.

Thereafter, patients were randomized over a condition in which (1) one session of education and 3 weeks waiting-list period was followed by exposure *in vivo* or (2) one session of education was followed by graded activity. The results were striking. During the education and waiting-list period, subjective ratings of pain-related fear and catastrophizing decreased substantially in all patients. However, the self-reported difficulties in performance of daily activities at home remained unchanged during that period, and only decreased in the patients who received the exposure *in vivo*. This suggests that education may change patients' perceptions about the harmfulness of physical activity and threat value of pain, but, alone or in combination with graded activity, is not powerful enough to change actual escape and avoidance behaviors.

Although these results are promising, there are a number of caveats to be considered. First, the preliminary evidence reported here is limited in that it is based on a relatively small number of patients. On the other hand, a single-case experimental design was chosen with appropriate time series statistical analyses. Because in crossover designs all patients receive both interventions, long-term differential effects cannot be established. Replication studies in the form of randomized, controlled trials using larger samples and long-term follow-up measurements are warranted.

9 **Conclusion**

"Fear of pain and what we do about it may be more disabling than pain itself" (Waddell *et al.* 1993: 164). With this statement, the intuitively appealing idea that the lowered ability to accomplish tasks of daily living in chronic pain patients is merely the consequence of pain severity is refuted. The recent literature supports the early conjecture that chronic pain and phobia share important characteristics. Indeed, studies have shown that during the confrontation with feared movements, chronic low back pain patients who are fearful of movement/(re)injury typically show psychophysiological (muscle reactivity), behavioral (escape and avoidance), and cognitive (worry) responses. It was not until recently that this line of thought was extended to the behavioral assessment and management of chronic pain. Specific pain-related fear measures, for pain patients whose level of disability is likely to be controlled by pain-related fears, have been developed. For its use in primary care, a screening questionnaire aiming at the identification of acute back pain patients at risk has been developed that include several items on fear and avoidance (Kendall *et al.* 1997; Linton and Hallden 1998). In addition, cognitive–behavioral assessment also includes the semistructured interview, the development of graded hierarchies, and the application of behavioral tests. In this chapter we described an exposure *in vivo* treatment for the reduction of pain-related fear in chronic pain patients. Preliminary outcome data show that an exposure *in vivo* with behavioral experiments consist of individually tailored practice tasks based on a graded hierarchy of fear-eliciting situations, and not just a physical training program or usual graded activity that does not take into account these essential and idiosyncratic fear stimuli. These data also show that such an exposure procedure may help the patient to confront rather than avoid physical movement, and that a reduction in disability levels is likely to follow. Although CBTs for chronic pain are quite favorable (Morley *et al.* 1999), there is an urgent need for further refinement of our treatments, including a better match between treatment modalities and patient characteristics. We hope that our chapter will contribute to the process of customization of CBTs in the care of chronic pain patients.

Acknowledgments

The authors wish to thank Peter Heuts, Mario Geilen, Maria Kerckhoffs-Hanssen, Herman Mulder, Noel Dortu, the staff of the Department of Pain Rehabilitation of the Hoensbroeck Rehabilitation Centre and the staff of the Department of Rehabilitation of the University Hospital Maastricht for their contribution in making the application of the exposure treatment possible. This contribution is supported by Grant no. 904-65-090 of the Council for Medical and Health Research of the Netherlands (NWO-MW) to the first author.

References

APA (1994). *Diagnostic and Statistical Manual of Mental Disorders.* Washington DC: American Psychiatric Association.

Asmundson, G.J.G., Norton, P.J., and Norton, G.R. (1999). Beyond pain: The role of fear and avoidance in chronicity. *Clinical Psychology Review*, **19**, 97–119.

Asmundson, G.J.G. and Wright, K.D. (2004). The biopsychosocial model of pain. In T. Hadjistavropoules and K.D. Craig (eds.), *Pain: Psychological perspectives*, pp. 35–7. New Jersey, NJ: Elbaum.

Barlow, D.H. (2002). *Anxiety and its Disorders. The Nature and Treatment of Anxiety and Panic.* New York: The Guilford Press.

Bouton, M.E. (1988). Context and ambiguity in the extinction of emotional learning: Implications for exposure therapy. *Behaviour Research and Therapy*, **26**, 137–49.

Bouton, M.E. (2000). A learning theory perspective on lapse, relapse, and the maintenance of behavior change. *Health Psychology*, **19**, 57–63.

Burton, A.K., Waddell, G., Burtt, R., and Blair, S. (1996). Patient educational material in the management of low back pain in primary care. *Bulletin (Hospital for Joint Diseases)*, **55**, 138–41.

Burton, A.K., Waddell, G., Tillotson, K.M., and Summerton, N. (1999). Information and advice to patients with back pain can have a positive effect. A randomized controlled trial of a novel educational booklet in primary care. *Spine*, **24**, 2484–91.

Butler, G. (1989). Phobic disorders. In: K. Hawton, P.M. Salkovskis, J. Kirk, and D.M. Clark (eds.), *Cognitive Behaviour Therapy for Psychiatric Problems. A Practical Guide*, pp. 97–128. Oxford: Oxford University Press.

Coia, P. and Morley, S. (1998). Medical reassurance and patients' responses. *Journal of Psychosomatic Research*, **45**, 377–86.

Craske, M.G. and Rowe, M.K. (1997). A comparison of behavioral and cognitive treatments of phobias. In: G.C.L. Davey (ed.), Phobias. *A Handbook of Theory, Research and Treatment*, pp. 247–80. Chichester: Wiley & Sons.

Crombez, G., Vervaet, L., Baeyens, F., Lysens, R., and Eelen, P. (1996). Do pain expectancies cause pain in chronic low back patients? A clinical investigation. *Behaviour and Research Therapy*, **34**, 919–25.

Crombez, G., Vlaeyen, J.W., Heuts, P.H., and Lysens, R. (1999a). Pain-related fear is more disabling than pain itself: Evidence on the role of pain-related fear in chronic back pain disability. *Pain*, **80**, 329–39.

Crombez, G., Eccleston, C., Vlaeyen, J.W., Vansteenwegen, D., Lysens, R., and Eelen, P. (2002). Exposure to physical movements in low back pain patients: Restricted effects of generalization. *Health Psychology*, **21**, 573–8.

de Jong, J.R., Vlaeyen, J.W.S., Geilen, M., Onghena, P., and Goossens, M.E.J.B. (2002). Fear of Movement/(Re)injury in Chronic Low Back Pain: Education or Exposure *in vivo* as a Mediator to Fear Reduction? Paper presented at the10th World Conference on Pain, San Diego.

Donovan, J.L. and Blake, D.R. (2002). Qualitative study of interpretation of reassurance among patients attending rheumatology clinics: "just a touch of arthritis, doctor?". *British Medical Journal*, **320**, 541–4.

Fordyce, W.E., Brockway, J.A., Bergman, J.A., and Spengler, D. (1986). Acute back pain: A control-group comparison of behavioral vs traditional management methods. *Journal of Behavioral Medicine*, **9**, 127–40.

Goossens, M.E.J.B., Vlaeyen, J.W.S., Portegeijs, P., de Vet, H.C.W., and Weber, W. (2000). Het rugboekje: patiëntenbrochure 'omgaan met lage rugpijn' [The little back book: brochure *How to Deal with Low Back Pain*]. Maastricht.

Goubert, L., Francken, G., Crombez, G., Vansteenwegen, D., and Lysens, R. (2002). Exposure to physical movement in chronic back pain patients: No evidence for generalization across different movements. *Behaviour and Research Therapy*, **40**, 415–29.

Goubert, L., Crombez, G., Van Damme, S., Vlaeyen, J.W.S., Bijttebier, P., and Roelofs, J. (in press). Confirmatory factor analysis of the Tampa Scale for Kinesiophobia: Invariant two-factor model across low back pain patients and fibromyalgia patients. *Clinical Journal of Pain*.

Greenberg, J. and Burns, J.W. (2003). Pain anxiety among chronic pain patients: Specific phobia or manifestation of anxiety sensitivity? *Behaviour and Research Therapy*, **41**, 223–40.

Heyneman, N.E., Fremouw, W.J., and Gano, D. (1990). Individual differences and the leffectiveness of different coping strategies for pain. *Cognitive Therapy and Research*, **14**, 63–77.

Houben, R.M.A., Vlaeyen, J.W.S., Peters, M.L., Ostelo, R., Wolters, P.M.J.C., and Stomp-van den Berg, S.G.M. (in press). Health care providers' attitudes and beliefs towards common low back pain. Factor structure and psychometric properties of the HC-PAIRS. *The Clinical Journal of Pain*, **20**, 37–44.

Indahl, A., Haldorsen, E.H., Holm, S., Reikeras, O., and Ursin, H. (1998). Five-year follow-up study of a controlled clinical trial using light mobilization and an informative approach to low back pain. *Spine*, **23**, 2625–30.

Jensen, M.P. and Karoly, P. (1992). Pain-specific beliefs, perceived symptom severity, and adjustment to chronic pain. *Clinical Journal of Pain*, **8**, 123–30.

Jensen, M.C., Brant-Zawadzki, M.N., Obuchowski, N., Modic, M.T., Malkasian, D., and Ross, J.S. (1994). Magnetic resonance imaging of the lumbar spine in people without back pain [see comments]. *New England Journal of Medicine*, **331**, 69–73.

Kendall, N.A.S., Linton, S.J., and Main, C.J. (1997). *Guide to Assessing Psychosocial Yellow Flags in Acute Low Back Pain: Risk Factors for Long-term Disability and Work Loss.* Accident Compensation Corporation, New Zealand: Wellington.

Kirk, J. (1989). Cognitive–behavioral assessment. In: K. Hawton, P.M. Salkovskis, J. Kirk, and D.M. Clark (eds.), *Cognitive Behaviour Therapy for Psychiatric Problems. A Practical Guide*, pp. 13–51. Oxford: Oxford University Press.

Klenerman, L., Slade, P.D., Stanley, I.M., Pennie, B., Reilly, J.P., Atchison, L.E., Troup, J.D., and Rose, M.J. (1995). The prediction of chronicity in patients with an acute attack of low back pain in a general practice setting. *Spine*, **20**, 478–84.

Kori, S.H., Miller, R.P., and Todd, D.D. (1990). Kinesiophobia: A new view of chronic pain behavior, *Pain Management*, **Jan/Feb**, 35–43.

Kugler, K., Wijn, J., Geilen, M., de Jong, J., and Vlaeyen, J.W.S. (1999). The Photograph series of Daily Activities (PHODA). CD-rom version 1.0., Institute for Rehabilitation Research and School for Physiotherapy Heerlen, The Netherlands.

Lang, P.J. (1979). Presidential address, 1978. A bio-informational theory of emotional imagery. *Psychophysiology*, **16**, 495–512.

Lang, P.J., Bradley, M.M., and Cuthbert, B.N. (1998). Emotion and motivation: Measuring affective perception. *Journal of Clinical Neurophysiology*, **15**, 397–408.

Lindstrom, I., Ohlund, C., Eek, C., Wallin, L., Peterson, L.E., Fordyce, W.E., and Nachemson, A.L. (1992). The effect of graded activity on patients with subacute low back pain: A randomized prospective clinical study with an operant-conditioning behavioral approach. *Physical Therapy*, **72**, 279–93.

Linton, S.J. and Hallden, K. (1998). Can we screen for problematic back pain? A screening questionnaire for predicting outcome in acute and subacute back pain. *Clinical Journal of Pain*, **14**, 209–15.

Linton, S.J., Buer, N., Vlaeyen, J.W.S., and Hellsing, A.L. (2000). Are fear-avoidance beliefs related to the inception of an episode of back pain? A prospective study. *Psychology and Health*, **14**, 1051–9.

Linton, S.J., Overmeer, T., Janson, M., Vlaeyen, J.W.S., and de Jong, J.R. (2002). Graded in vivo exposure treatment for fear-avoidant pain patients with functional disability: A case study: *Cognitive Behaviour Therapy*, **31**, 49–58.

Mannion, A.F., Muntener, M., Taimela, S., and Dvorak, J. (1999). A randomized clinical trial of three active therapies for chronic low back pain, *Spine*, **24**, 2435–48.

Mannion, A.F., Junge, A., Taimela, S., Muntener, M., Lorenzo, K., and Dvorak, J. (2001). Active therapy for chronic low back pain: Part 3. Factors influencing self-rated disability and its change following therapy. *Spine*, **26**, 920–9.

McCracken, L.M. and Dhingra, L. (2002). A short version of the pain anxiety symptoms scale (pass-20): Preliminary development and validity. *Pain Research and Management*, **7**, 45–50.

McCracken, L.M. and Gross, R.T. (1993). Does anxiety affect coping with chronic pain? *Clinical Journal of Pain*, **9**, 253–9.

McDonald, I.G., Daly, J., Jelinek, V.M., Panetta, F., and Gutman, J.M. (1996). Opening Pandora's box: The unpredictability of reassurance by a normal test result [see comments], *BMJ*, **313**, 329–32.

Miller, R.P., Kori, S.H., and Todd, D.D. (1991). The Tampa Scale for Kinisophobia. Unpublished Report, Tampa, FL.

Mineka, S., Mystkowski, J.L., Hladek, D., and Rodriguez, B.I. (1999). The effects of changing contexts on return of fear following exposure therapy for spider fear. *Journal of Consulting and Clinical Psychology*, **67**, 599–604.

Moore, J.E., Von Korff, M., Cherkin, D., Saunders, K., and Lorig, K. (2000). A randomized trial of a cognitive-behavioral program for enhancing back pain self care in a primary care setting. *Pain*, **88**, 145–53.

Morley, S., Eccleston, C., and Williams, A. (1999). Systematic review and meta-analysis of randomized controlled trials of cognitive behavior therapy and behavior therapy for chronic pain in adults, excluding headache. *Pain*, **80**, 1–13.

Philips, H.C. (1987). Avoidance behavior and its role in sustaining chronic pain. *Behaviour and Research Therapy*, **25**, 273–9.

Picavet, H.S., Vlaeyen, J.W., and Schouten, J.S. (2002). Pain catastrophizing and kinesio-phobia: predicators of chronic low back pain. *American Journal of Epidemiology*, **156**, 1028–34.

Rachman, S. and Whittal, M. (1989). Fast, slow and sudden reductions in fear. *Behaviour Research and Therapy*, **27**, 613–20.

Rachman, S. (1994). The overprediction of fear: A review. *Behaviour and Research Therapy*, **32**, 683–90.

Rainville, J., Bagnall, D., and Phalen, L. (1995). Health care providers' attitudes and beliefs about functional impairments and chronic back pain: *Clinical Journal of Pain*, **11**, 287–95.

Riley, J.F., Ahern, D.K., and Follick, M.J. (1988). Chronic pain and functional impairment: Assessing beliefs about their relationship. *Archives of Physical Medicine and Rehabilitation*, **69**, 579–82.

Rowe, M.K. and Craske, M.G. (1998a). Effects of an expanding-spaced vs massed exposure schedule on fear reduction and return of fear. *Behaviour and Research Therapy*, **36**, 701–17.

Rowe, M.K. and Craske, M.G. (1998b). Effects of varied-stimulus exposure training on fear reduction and return of fear. *Behaviour and Research Therapy*, **36**, 719–34.

Salkovskis, P.M., Clark, D.M., Hackmann, A., Wells, A., and Gelder, M.G. (1999). An experimental investigation of the role of safety-seeking behaviors in the maintenance of panic disorder with agoraphobia. *Behaviour and Research Therapy*, **37**, 559–74.

Severeijns, R., Vlaeyen, J.W., van den Hout, M.A., and Weber, W.E. (2001). Pain catastrophizing predicts pain intensity, disability, and psychological distress independent of the level of physical impairment. *Clinical Journal of Pain*, **17**, 165–72.

Smeets, G., de Jong, P.J., and Mayer, B. (2000). If you suffer from a headache, then you have a brain tumour: domain-specific reasoning 'bias' and hypochondriasis. *Behaviour and Research Therapy*, **38**, 763–76.

Sullivan, M.J.L., Bishop, S.R., and Pivik, J. (1995). The pain catastrophizing scale: Development and validation. *Psychological Assessment*, **7**, 524–32.

Turk, D.C. and Okifuji (2002). Psychological factors in chronic pain: Evolution and revolution. *Journal of Consulting and Clinical Psychology*, **70**, 678–900.

Van den Hout, J.H.C. (2002). To solve or not to solve. The effects of problem solving therapy and graded activity in non-specific low back pain, Doctoral thesis, University of Maastricht, Maastricht.

Vasey, M.W. and Borkovec, T.D. (1992). A catastrophizing assessment of worrisome thoughts. *Cognitive Therapy Research*, **16**, 505–20.

Vlaeyen, J.W.S. and Linton, S.J. (2000). Fear-avoidance and its consequences in chronic musculoskeletal pain: A state of the art. *Pain*, **85**, 317–32.

Vlaeyen, J.W., Kole-Snijders, A.M., Boeren, R.G., and van Eek, H. (1995*a*). Fear of movement/(re)injury in chronic low back pain and its relation to behavioral performance. *Pain*, **62**, 363–72.

Vlaeyen, J.W.S., Kole Snijders, A.M.J., Rotteveel, A.M., Ruesink, R. *et al.* (1995*b*). The role of fear of movement/(re)injury in pain disability. *Journal of Occupational Rehabilitation*, **5**, 235–52.

Vlaeyen, J.W.S., Nooyen-Haazen, I.W.C.J., Goossens, M.E.J.B., van Breukelen, G., Heuts, P.H.T.G., and Goei The, H. (1997). The role of fear in the cognitive-educational treatment of fibromyalgia. In T.S. Jensen, J.A. Turner, and Z. Wiesenfeld-Hallin (eds.), *Proceedings of the 8th World Congress on Pain*, Vol. 8, pp. 693–704. Seattle, WA: IASP Press.

Vlaeyen, J.W., de Jong, J., Geilen, M., Heuts, P.H., and van Breukelen, G. (2001). Graded exposure *in vivo* in the treatment of pain-related fear: a replicated single-case experimental design in four patients with chronic low back pain. *Behaviour and Research Therapy*, **39**, 151–66.

Vlaeyen, J.W., De Jong, J., Geilen, M., Heuts, P.H., and Van Breukelen, G. (2002*a*). The treatment of fear of movement/(re)injury in chronic low back pain: Further evidence on the effectiveness of exposure *in vivo*. *Clinical Journal of Pain*, **18**, 251–61.

Vlaeyen, J.W., De Jong, J.R., Onghena, P., Kerckhoffs-Hanssen, M., and Kole-Snijders, A.M. (2002*b*). Can pain-related fear be reduced? The application of cognitive-behavioral exposure *in vivo*. *Pain Research & Management*, **7**, 144–53.

Waddell, G., Newton, M., Henderson, I., Somerville, D., and Main, C.J. (1993). A Fear-Avoidance Beliefs Questionnaire (FABQ) and the role of fear-avoidance beliefs in chronic low back pain and disability. *Pain*, **52**, 157–68.

Wolpe, J. (1958). *Psychotherapy by Reciprocal Inhibition*. Stanford, CA: Stanford University Press.

Part IV

Conclusions and future directions

Chapter 15

Future challenges and research directions in fear of pain

Gordon J.G. Asmundson, Michael J. Coons, Johan W.S. Vlaeyen, and Geert Crombez

1 Introduction

The fear of pain construct has received considerable attention in the literature over the past decade or so. As evident in the opening three chapters of this volume, there has been considerable evolution in explanatory models of the association between fear and pain. These models have developed to a point where they now provide a solid foundation from which researchers and treatment providers from a variety of disciplines can conceptualize innovative investigations and approaches to symptom management. This volume comprises a number of contributions that shed significant light on the most important issues and developments in understanding and treating pain-related fear and anxiety. As well, each contribution posits important considerations for future investigation of the fear of pain/(re)injury construct and tenants of the fear-avoidance model. The following is a list of what are, in our opinion, some of the most important issues that remain to be addressed.

1. Why do only a minority of people, albeit significant, experience pain that persists beyond the acute phase? Learning factors have been shown to play a significant role. But, emerging evidence also indicates a role for a general vulnerability factor. What is this factor and how can we best understand its role?

2. How is the fear of pain construct best conceptualized? When is it adaptive versus maladaptive? Is the experience akin to other fears, such as fear of flying or fear of spiders? Should it be considered and classified as a form of psychopathology or can a psychonormal model account for the observed disruptions to cognition, behavior, and physiology. Related to this issue is the question of what the object of the fear is in fear of pain.

3. Are the subtle nuances between pain-related fear and pain-related anxiety important to practical applications, such as assessment and treatment

planning? Are some people more fearful than anxious and does this manifest in different phenomenology and response to treatment? Does avoidance behavior have a fear-inhibiting property and, if so, what mechanisms
are responsible?

4. What are the basic verbal, emotional, environmental (e.g. social learning),
and genetic influences on fear of pain and pain-related anxiety? Which are
most important? What role does culture play in the anxiety-avoidance
cycle as it relates to chronic pain?

5. What are the specific biological mechanisms involved in fear of pain and
pain-related anxiety? Will investigation of autonomic nervous system
responses to pain and other somatic stressors reveal abnormalities in those
patients who respond to pain with fear and anxiety? Will these differences
be observable in only those with chronic pain or do they manifest in
response to acute pain as well? Should functional brain imaging studies be
added to the set of investigative tools in this area?

6. What is the most economical and efficient means of assessing pain-related
fear and anxiety? How is treatment outcome best measured and evaluated?
Which treatment approaches are most effective? What factors predict positive treatment outcome and which predict relapse? How likely is relapse in
these patients?

The purpose of this chapter is to briefly elaborate on some of these questions
and, of particular importance, to outline the directions in which future
research might best be directed. In doing so, we hope to assist in shaping
future efforts at building on our blossoming understanding of fear of pain and
its treatment.

2 Basic issues

Research on many of the issues of critical importance to advancing our understanding of pain-related fear and anxiety are covered in the chapters of Part 1 of
this volume. These issues, stemming from behavioral and cognitive–behavioral
perspectives on pain-related fear and anxiety, span learning of defensive
reflexes, rule-governed behavior, attention, emotion, attitudes, deconditioning,
and the many nuances of these broad categories. In the following section we
highlight some of the key issues that warrant clarification.

2.1 The vulnerability hypothesis

People often experience pain in response to physical injury or other organic
pathology. For most people the pain abates as the physical or organic pathology heals. However, some individuals continue to experience pain that is

either incongruous with the extent of identifiable tissue damage or that persists long after apparent healing of the original pathology. These same people appear to be more likely to also have one or more diagnosable anxiety disorders, most often posttraumatic stress disorder (see Asmundson *et al.* 2000*a*, 2002), that co-occur with their pain. Why? While the answer to this question remains somewhat elusive there are some hints. Information provided in Chapters 1, 4, and 5 suggest that some people may have a vulnerability factor that predisposes them toward the development and maintenance of a chronic pain experience. This vulnerability factor is believed to be shared with certain anxiety disorders (Asmundson *et al.* 2002). Hypervigilance, negative affectivity, catastrophizing, and anxiety sensitivity have been examined as possible factors that influence the development of persistent pain. These factors provide some insight into, and may prove propitious in testing, the vulnerability hypothesis.

Of the constructs that have been implicated as potential contributors in the vulnerability hypothesis, hypervigilance and anxiety sensitivity are perhaps the most fruitful. Hypervigilance refers to a dispositional tendency to attend to and respond to certain classes of stimuli from the external and internal environment. It is a learned phenomenon that is thought to vary with degree of threat associated with a stimulus that, in turn, is affected by individual difference variables (including negative affectivity and catastrophizing). Anxiety sensitivity refers to a dispositional tendency to become fearful of anxiety symptoms (e.g. shortness of breath) based on the belief that they may have harmful consequences. Accumulating research has shown that anxiety sensitivity tends to be elevated in patients who develop persistent headache pain and musculoskeletal pain (for recent review see Asmundson *et al.* 2000*b*). Similar patterns have been observed in nonclinical samples of adults (e.g. McNeil and Rainwater 1998; Keogh and Cochrane 2002) and children (Muris *et al.* 2001*a,b*) who fear pain. In the case of chronic pain, anxiety sensitivity has been found to amplify fear, anxiety, and avoidance behaviors when painful experiences occur. It is conceivable that the likelihood of developing a chronic pain-related condition will be significantly elevated if one has *both* a tendency to be hypervigilant toward internal pain sensations and a tendency to interpret these sensations as dangerous or potentially threatening to their well-being. This notion remains untested.

Perhaps the most convincing evidence to support anxiety sensitivity as a general vulnerability factor comes from the genetic literature. Preliminary studies suggest that anxiety sensitivity is a heritable trait that may be based on dysregulations in serotinergic or GABA-ergic systems (McCarson and Enna 1999). Therefore, unlike negative affectivity and catastrophizing, anxiety sensitivity has been linked to a general predisposition as opposed to a consequence of fear of pain or pain itself. Future research in this area is clearly warranted. While promising, it is too early to say whether anxiety sensitivity, or any other construct for that matter, is a definitive vulnerability factor for the development and maintenance of chronic pain. Indeed, causal relationships between such factors and pain chronicity have not been examined. Further research is required to determine which predisposing factors are the most important in the development of fear of pain or, conversely, if they manifest as consequences of persistent pain. This will involve careful consideration of which potential vulnerability factors are most rudimentary (fundamental) to the development of chronic pain (see Chapters 4 and 5) and what their mechanism of action is. It will also necessarily involve the application of longitudinal designs in which potential vulnerability factors are assessed prior to painful injury or organic pathology and, thereafter, followed in those who do and do not go on to experience pain of a chronic nature.

2.2 Conceptualization

There have been several different conceptualizations of fear of pain presented in the literature. One notion is that it is similar in many ways to other basic fears (or phobias), including fear of spiders, fear of heights, and fear of flying (see Kori *et al.* 1990). This is apparent when comparing the features of specific phobias, as outlined in the *Diagnostic and Statistical Manual of Mental Disorders-IV* (*DSM-IV*) and *DSM-IV* text revision (APA 1994, 2000), with the characteristics of fear of pain. Indeed, both are characterized by (1) marked and persistent fear that is excessive or unreasonable and cued by exposure to or anticipation of a certain object or situation, (2) immediate response upon exposure to the feared object or situation, and (3) avoidance or apprehension in response to the feared object or situation that interferes significantly with activities of daily living and causes marked distress. Vlaeyen *et al.* (2002) have noted that one point on which fear of pain differs from other phobias is the extent to which the fear is *viewed by the patient as* excessive and irrational. Many patients with significant pain-related fear and anxiety do not recognize it as excessive but, rather, see it as useful in protecting them from further pain and (re)injury. A somewhat different view, proposed by Asmundson and colleagues (Asmundson and Norton 1995; Asmundson and Taylor 1996; Asmundson *et al.* 1999), and extended by others (Greenberg and Burns 2003), is that fear of pain is a manifestation of anxiety sensitivity and, as such, is best understood within the context of the more fundamental predilection to be generally fearful of anything that produces symptoms of anxiety.

While of theoretical importance, and with close ties to the vulnerability hypothesis discussed above, the issue of how to best conceptualize pain-related fear and anxiety also holds practical implications. As noted by Greenberg and Burns (2003), the "implicit assumption that fear of pain is a specific phobia, will involve exposure to a range of stimuli too narrow to fully address . . . the more fundamental fear of anxiety symptoms . . . [and] miss the essence of what disturbs the patient" (p. 238). Future research may yield data that will allow a more comprehensive evaluation of this important issue.

2.3 Fear versus anxiety

Fear and anxiety are terms that are commonly used interchangeably (see Chapters 1 and 9). While both manifest in changes in cognitive, physiological, and behavioral reactions to threat, subtle distinctions exist that make these emotional experiences unique and important to distinguish from one another. In order to understand these constructs, especially in the context of pain, it is beneficial to recapitulate their differences.

Fear is a present-oriented state that serves the function of protecting a person from a perceived threat that is immanent. Without fear we would lack motivation to confront or escape from danger. Importantly, fears are not limited to the perceived threat of an object or situation that is external to the self. In addition to fearing *things* (like spiders) or *situations* (like giving a speech to a large audience) people can also fear *internal states* related to somatic arousal or shifting concepts of the self. Thus, the object of fear may involve pain sensations, pain-related activities, potential (re)injury, and threats to self-concept. Anxiety, on the other hand, is a future-oriented state that occurs when a person anticipates threat or danger that is often vague and general. It allows one to prepare (or, in maladaptive cases, to over-prepare) for potential danger. Quite often, as is typically the case for those who fear pain, these anxiety-motivated preparations involve avoidance of things, situations, or internal states that are associated with the experience of pain. Various objects of fear in patients with chronic pain are discussed in detail in Chapters 3 and 8.

Fear and anxiety both influence cognition, physiology, and behavior, albeit in subtly different ways. The main differences arguably lie in the temporal association to the perceived threat (immediate versus sometime in the future) and in the types of behavior motivated (in the case of fear, defensive behaviors such as escape, and, in the case of anxiety, protective behavior such as avoidance). These distinctions are important at the theoretical level and, we believe, warrant careful future consideration in practical applications. While there have been considerable strides in behavioral and cognitive–behavioral approaches to treating pain-related fear and anxiety, there remains much to be learned as we work toward maximizing treatment success. So, if it is the case that some people are more fearful and others more anxious with regard to pain and pain-related objects and situations, then different approaches to treatment may be warranted. Assessment and treatment issues are discussed in more detail below.

2.4 Mechanisms

There is evidence to suggest that certain cognitive factors, including beliefs, attitudes, and attentional focus, play an important role in pain-related fear and anxiety (Chapters 4 and 6). Negative beliefs and attitudes toward daily- and work-related physical activity—both implicit and explicit—are commonly observed in chronic pain patients with high fear of pain. Findings from studies of attention are generally consistent with postulates of the contemporary fear-avoidance models (Chapter 1). They are also consistent with the notion that pain plays an interruptive function (i.e. imposes an overriding priority for attentional engagement and urges escape) that is mediated by the affective characteristics of pain and, in particular, its threat value (Eccleston and Crombez 1999). However, there are findings that, unlike the robust findings characteristic of the anxiety disorders literature, are not consistent with model expectations. For example, findings from research on information processing biases, particularly those using modified Stroop and dot probe paradigms, remain mixed and difficult to replicate. They are also difficult to interpret, with scant evidence, from both clinical and nonclinical samples, that levels of pain-related fear and anxiety may mediate observed attentional biases for pain-related cues. Several key questions remain unanswered.

Are there specific cognitive mechanisms, such as those proposed by Beck (1976) for emotional disorders (e.g. mood and anxiety disorders), that function in those patients with significant pain-related fear and anxiety? Do *general* cognitive mechanisms, like neuroticism (Martin 1985), also play an important role? Future research using clinical and nonclinical samples is needed to clarify the extent to which specific and general cognitive mechanisms are operative in pain-related fear and anxiety and, importantly, to explore their implications for treatment. Indeed, in order to produce notable and enduring reductions in fear of pain and associated functional limitations, treatments need to target all implicated mechanisms.

There is also a need to conduct more research to evaluate the role that biological mechanisms play in pain-related fear and anxiety responses. Fear, regardless of the triggering stimulus, produces physiological arousal. This arousal is characterized, but not limited to, accelerated heart rate, elevated blood pressure, increased respiration, gastrointestinal activity, increased muscle tension, and increased circulation to skeletal muscles along with dermal and cerebral vasoconstriction (Guyton and Hall 1996). This arousal, if prolonged, stresses the body and may have a direct bearing on the physiological processes and anatomical structures implicated in some chronic pain conditions. Some studies (Arntz *et al.* 1991; Flor *et al.* 1992), but not all (Collins *et al.* 1982; Flor *et al.* 1985), have demonstrated lower heart rate reactivity in patients with chronic pain compared to healthy controls when exposed to stress inducing procedures. The mixed results may be the product of method variance, with heart rate reactivity evidenced only under more prolonged or intense stress induction. Regardless, evidence of lower heart rate reactivity in patients with chronic pain suggests an absence of sympathetic outflow (withdrawal) and, perhaps, parasympathetic activation, whereas the pattern in healthy controls suggests the expected sympathetic activation and parasympathetic withdrawal in response to stress. There is also some evidence to suggest that arousal-induced muscular tension plays a significant role in chronic musculoskeletal pain (Flor *et al.* 1992; Merskey 1993; Turk 1996*a,b*). To date, however, there have been no investigations published that specifically address the role of potentially relevant fear-based physiological responses in the context of pain-related fear and anxiety. Studies of this nature are currently underway in the laboratory of the first author of this chapter and will help clarify the role of physiological responsivity in pain-related fear and anxiety and, hopefully, will contribute to efforts to appropriately tailor interventions to the patients comprehensive symptom presentation.

3 Clinical issues

Research on assessment and treatment of fear of pain, particularly the latter, has experienced a dramatic rise in recent years. Much of this emerging research is reviewed in Parts 2 and 3 of this volume and is accompanied by specific practical recommendations. In the following section we provide a brief summary of a number of important points that were raised.

3.1 Assessment

Accurate assessment of pain, and factors that contribute to it, is a necessary component of providing proper and effective pain management services (Asmundson 2002). Given the multidimensional nature of pain, assessment involves not only an evaluation of the sensory aspects of pain (e.g. location, severity, time course) but also its affect on cognition, mood, behavior, and the functions of a multitude of body systems. Both researchers and clinicians have an abundance of targets, strategies, and measures from which to choose when assessing a research participant or patient presenting with pain, whether it be acute or chronic in nature. The same is true with regard to pain-related fear and anxiety. Through the application of semi-structured interviews, behavioral observations, and application of self-report measures, researchers and clinicians can gather pertinent information on core cognitions (i.e. dysfunctional beliefs, catastrophizing, negative expectancies) and behaviors (e.g. avoidance, escape). In particular, it appears important to assess the specific object or objects of the fear, whether they be pain-specific, injury-specific, or more abstract threats to personal well-being (Chapters 3, 8, and 9), and the influence of this fear on cognition, behavior, and physiology (Chapters 7, 9, and 10). This information can be of considerable value in planning treatment and for treatment outcome evaluations. It is generally the case that accurate assessment and maximal therapeutic change are facilitated by a strong therapeutic relationship. Not surprisingly, this appears to be the case when dealing with patients who suffer significant pain-related fear and anxiety (Chapter 11).

Notwithstanding the usefulness of these assessment recommendations, there are a number of important questions pertaining to assessment that remain to be addressed. For example, with regard to behavioral observation and screening methods (as reviewed in Chapters 9 and 10) there is little empirical data available for making a decision on which approach is best at identifying the patient with significant pain-related fear and anxiety. That is, we do not have data to establish whether the *diagnostic* reliability and validity (to the extent that the exercise is one of diagnosis) of one method is any better than another. It will be very difficult to resolve this issue without a *gold standard* for comparison; however, given a lack of consensus on a number of important related issues (e.g. whether fear of pain is best conceptualized as a phobia akin to any other specific phobia or as something else; Greenberg and Burns 2003, Vlaeyen *et al.* 2002), it will remain a considerable challenge for scholars working in the area to identify such a gold standard.

The recent proliferation in the development of self-report measures for assessing fear of pain and related constructs (e.g. pain catastrophizing, kinesiophobia) has given researchers and clinicians a number of psychometrically sound options to choose from. This, on one hand, is an admirable position to be in. On the other hand, when faced with having to select one measure over another in order to minimize the size of self-report packages, there is little empirical information to provide guidance. Which measure of pain-related fear and anxiety provide the maximum unique information with minimal time requirements? Is one measure generally better than others, or are different measures more appropriate to specific applications (e.g. treatment outcome evaluation versus gauging responses to experimental pain induction)?

Is there a need for development and psychometric assessment of new measures of pain-related fear and anxiety? What is the value added by measuring related constructs, such as hypervigilance, pain catastrophizing, and anxiety sensitivity (and what is lost by not doing so)? These questions warrant careful consideration in future investigations of pain-related fear and anxiety. Likewise, practical applications of modified cognitive psychology paradigms (e.g. modified Stroop task, dual task paradigm), physiological assessment (e.g. electromyography, autonomic nervous system responsivity), and overt measures of emotion (e.g. facial action coding) warrant further attention in this context.

3.2 Treatment

Cognitive–behavioral treatments, whether delivered individually or in group sessions, have shown to be generally effective in those with chronic pain (Morely *et al.* 1999). With specific regard to pain-related fear and anxiety there have been recent significant advances in treatment applications. Indeed, strategies for addressing and managing fear of pain in the primary care setting, mainly brief educational and behavioral interventions, appear promising (Chapter 12). General behavioral and cognitive–behavioral treatment approaches for chronic pain can be of benefit to patients with significant pain-related fear and anxiety. This is particularly true when these patients are clearly identified and their specific idiosyncratic issues clearly delineated and addressed (Chapter 13). The application of graded exposure *in vivo* has been shown to have considerable promise in the treatment of patients who have a clearly articulated fear of pain (Chapter 14). Notwithstanding, available support for this latter approach is limited to case controlled designs and, to date, no randomized controlled trials have been published. There remains a need for controlled trials of graded exposure *in vivo* for the treatment of fear of pain. Long-term follow-up assessments with careful evaluation of relapse are also warranted. Such studies are currently underway in our laboratories.

Although recent advances in the assessment and treatment literature have provided some valuable insight into how we can best approach the treatment of pain-related fear and anxiety, numerous questions remain. What is a good treatment outcome? What is an excellent treatment outcome? How is treatment outcome best assessed? Is it a reduction in pain-related fear and anxiety, a reduction of avoidance behavior, an improvement in functional ability, or some combination of these? What parts of the treatment program are ineffective and need to be reviewed and revised? Is the graded exposure *in vivo* strategy appropriate for use with children or the elderly? Are there subtypes of patients, perhaps differing in the object of fear, for whom fear reduction techniques other than graded exposure *in vivo* may be more effective? Are there subtypes who are characterized by more future-oriented worry than immediate fear and, if so, what treatment strategies are best for them?

Williams and McCracken (Chapter 13) assert that an important focal point is in the conceptualization of the patient's problem—recognizing that for many it is not pain but *fear* and *anxiety* that perpetuate suffering and associated functional limitations. Clearly, both patients and clinicians need to recognize this (when it is the case) before they can venture into the territory of appropriately focused treatment strategies. As noted above, this may involve graded exposure *in vivo* for those with clearly defined fears or, in the case of those with significant uncertainty and worry, some other approach. Cognitive–behavioral approaches used to treat those with significant health-related worries that arise from misinterpretation of bodily signs and symptoms (e.g. pain, gastrointestinal distress, cardiorespiratory complaints) warrant consideration in this regard (Furer *et al.* 2001; Taylor and Asmundson 2004). Other approaches that may prove useful, particularly as applied to those patients who live in remote geographic locations or for whom making day time appointments is of extreme difficulty, include self-help programs, community-based psycho-education programs, and telephone or web-based cognitive–behavioral therapy. These have been shown to have general effectiveness in patients with chronic pain (Lefort *et al.* 1998; Sullivan and Stanish 2003) and in a variety of the anxiety disorders (e.g. Walker *et al.* 1999; Lange *et al.* 2003).

4 Future research directions

The above discussion, in combination with the chapters in the volume, suggests numerous directions for future research. The following points highlight what are, in our opinion, some of the most salient avenues for future empirical investigation.

1. Large-scale studies employing a longitudinal design are needed in order to assess the importance of factors—such as hypervigilance, emotional state, and attitudes—that are suggested to influence some presentations of chronic pain. The most important question in the context of these studies is the extent to which these factors contribute to development, maintenance, and exacerbation of chronic pain.

2. Basic mechanism research is needed to clarify the role that dysfunctional behavioral, cognitive, and biological systems play in fear of pain and, importantly, to determine the extent to which these are similar to those observed in other fear and anxiety-related conditions.

3. Clarification of the object or objects of fear in fear of pain is warranted. Understanding the primary object of fear—whether it be continuing pain

sensations, anxiety-provoking somatic perturbations stimulated by pain sensations, or threats to one's sense of identity—would be of great value in clarifying targets for assessment and treatment.

4. Further development of techniques for early identification of those people at risk for developing avoidance-related disability following musculoskeletal injury (and benign somatic perturbation) is needed. This line of investigation would help clarify causal factors and, in doing so, would stimulate work on preventive interventions.

5. Research is needed to improve understanding of what approaches are most effective in treating those with significant pain-related fear and anxiety. Researchers need to establish whether cognitive–behavioral treatments are best applied alone or in combination with other interventions and, in order to increase time-efficiency, what specific components of the cognitive–behavioral approach are most effective. Also, since many patients with debilitating pain-related fear and anxiety live in remote areas where specialty treatment is not available, research is needed to assess the feasibility and efficacy of telephone and web-based treatment protocols.

5 Conclusion

In this volume we have presented contributions from a number of accomplished scholars whose work relates to the fear of pain construct. The chapters provide a comprehensive and state-of-the-art review of current knowledge, key issues and developments, and lingering questions regarding the roles that fear and anxiety play in the development and exacerbation of chronic pain following acute musculoskeletal injury and benign somatic perturbations. Significant advances have been made in understanding the behavioral and cognitive mechanisms involved in fear of pain, its assessment, and approaches to treatment. The weight of the evidence indicates that Waddell (1996, 1998) was on target in stating that fear of pain is more debilitating than pain itself. If this book serves as a useful resource to researchers and clinicians as they prepare their own empirical and treatment protocols for application with those debilitated by fear of pain, we will have met our objective.

References

American Psychiatric Association (APA) (1994). *Diagnostic and Statistical Manual of Mental disorders*, 4th edn. Washington DC: Author.

American Psychiatric Association (APA) (2000). *Diagnostic and Statistical Manual of Mental disorders*, 4th edn. text revision. Washington DC: Author.

Arntz, A., Merckelbach, H., Peters, M.C., and Schmidt, A.J.M. (1991). Chronic low back pain, response specificity and habituation to painful stimuli. *Journal of Psychophysiology*, 5, 177–88.

Asmundson, G.J.G. (2002). Pain assessment: State-of-the-art applications from the cognitive-behavioural perspective. *Behaviour Research and Therapy*, **40**, 547–50.

Asmundson, G.J.G. and Norton, G.R. (1995) Anxiety sensitivity in patients with physically unexplained chronic back pain: A preliminary report. *Behaviour Research and Therapy*, **33**, 771–7.

Asmundson, G.J.G. and Taylor, S. (1996). Role of anxiety sensitivity in pain-related fear and avoidance. *Journal of Behavioural Medicine*, **19**, 577–86.

Asmundson, G.J.G., Norton, P.J., and Norton, G.R. (1999). Beyond pain: The role of fear and avoidance in chronically. *Clinical Psychology Review*, **19**, 97–119.

Asmundson, G.J.G., Bonin, M.F., Frombach, I.K., and Norton, G.R. (2000*a*). Evidence of a disposition toward fearfulness and vulnerability to posttraumatic stress in dysfunctional pain patients. *Behaviour Research and Therapy*, **38**, 801–12.

Asmundson, G.J.G., Wright, K.D., and Hadjistavropoulos, H.D. (2000*b*). Anxiety sensitivity and disabling chronic health conditions: State of the art and future directions. *Scandinavian Journal of Behaviour Therapy*, **29**, 100–17.

Asmundson, G.J.G., Coons, M.J., Taylor, S., and Katz, J. (2002). PTSD and the experience of pain: Research and clinical implications of shared vulnerability and mutual maintenance models. *Canadian Journal of Psychiatry*, **47**, 19–26.

Beck, A.T. (1976). *Cognitive Therapy and Emotional Disorders*. New York: International Universities Press.

Collins, G.A., Cohen, M.J., Naliboff, B.D., and Schanler, S.L. (1982). Comparative analysis of paraspinal and frontalis EMG, heart rate and skin conductance in chronic low back pain patients and normals to various postures and stress. *Scandinavian Journal of Rehabilitation Medicine*, **14**, 39–46.

Eccleston, C. and Crombez, G. (1999). Pain demands attention: A cognitive-affective model on the interruptive function of pain. *Psychological Bulletin*, **125**, 356–66.

Flor, H., Turk, D.C., and Birbaumer, N. (1985). Assessment of stress-related responses in chronic back pain patients. *Journal of Consulting and Clinical Psychology*, **53**, 354–64.

Flor, H., Birbaumer, N., Schugens, M.M., and Lutzenberger, W. (1992). Symptom-specific psychophysiological responses in chronic pain patients. *Pyschophysiology*, **29**, 452–60.

Furer, T., Walker, J.R., and Freeston, M.H. (2001). Approach to integrated cognitive-behavior therapy for intense illness worries. In G.J.G. Asmundson, S. Taylor, and B.J. Cox (eds.), *Health Anxiety: Clinical and Research Perspectives on Hypochondriasis and Related Conditions*, pp. 161–92. Chichester: Wiley.

Greenberg, J. and Burns, J.W. (2003). Pain anxiety among chronic pain patients: Specific phobia or manifestation of anxiety sensitivity? *Behaviour and Research Therapy*, **41**, 223–40.

Guyton, A.C. and Hall, J.E. (1996). *Textbook of Medical Physiology*, 9th edn. Philadelphia: WB Saunders.

Keogh, E. and Cochrane, M. (2002). Anxiety sensitivity, cognitive biases and the experience of pain. *The Journal of Pain*, **3**, 320–9.

Kori, S.H., Miller, R.P., and Todd, D.D. (1990). Kinesiophobia: A new view of chronic pain behavior, *Pain Management*, **Jan/Feb**, 35–43.

Lange, A., van de Ven, J.P., and Schrieken, B. (2003). Interapy, treatment of post-traumatic stress through the internet. *Cognitive Behaviour Therapy*, **32**, 110–24.

Lefort, S.M., Grey-Donald, K., Rowat, K.M., and Jeans, M. (1998). Randomized controlled trial of a community-based psychoeducation program for the self-management of chronic pain. *Pain*, **72**, 27–32.

Martin, M. (1985). Neuroticism as predisposition toward depression: A cognitive mechanism. *Personality and Individual Differences*, **6**, 353–65.

McCarson, K.E. and Enna, S.J. (1999). Nociceptive regulation of GABA-sub(B) receptor gene expression in rat spinal cord. *Neuropharmacology*, **38**, 1767–73.

McNeil, D.W. and Rainwater, A.J. (1998). Development of the Fear of Pain Questionnaire-III. *Journal of Behavioral Medicine*, **21**, 389–409.

Merskey, H. (1993). Chronic muscular pain—a life stress syndrome? *Journal of Musculoskeletal Pain*, **1**, 61–9.

Morley, S., Eccleston, C., and Williams, A. (1999). Systematic review and meta-analysis of randomized controlled trials of cognitive behaviour therapy and behaviour therapy for chronic pain in adults, excluding headache. *Pain*, **80**, 1–13.

Muris, P., Vlaeyen, J.W.S., Meesters, C., and Vertongen, S. (2001*a*). Anxiety sensitivity and fear of pain in children. *Perceptual Motor Skills*, **92**, 456–8.

Muris, P., Vlaeyen, J., and Meesters, C. (2001*b*). The relationship between anxiety sensitivity and fear of pain in healthy adolescents. *Behaviour Research and Therapy*, **39**, 1357–68.

Sullivan, M.J.L. and Stanish, W.D. (2003). Psychologically based occupational rehabilitation: The Pain-Disability Prevention Program. *Clinical Journal of Pain*, **19**, 97–104.

Taylor, S. and Asmundson, G.J.G. (2004). *Treating Health Anxiety: A Cognitive-Behavioral Approach*. New York: Guilford Press.

Turk, D.C. (1996*a*). Psychological aspects of chronic pain and disability. *Journal of Musculoskeletal Pain*, **4**, 145–53.

Turk, D.C. (1996*b*). Cognitive factors in chronic pain and disability. In K.S. Dobson and K.D. Craig (eds.), *Advances in Cognitive Therapy*. Thousand Oaks CA: Sage.

Vlaeyen, J.W.S. and Linton, S.J. (2000). Fear-avoidance and its consequences in musculoskeletal pain: A state of the art. *Pain*, **85**, 317–32.

Vlaeyen, J.W.S., de Jong, J., Sieben, J., and Crombez, G. (2002). Graded exposure *in vivo* for pain-related fear. In D.C. Turk and R.J. Gatchel (eds.), *Psychological Approaches to Pain Management: A Practitioner's Handbook,* 2nd edn, pp. 210–33. New York: Guilford Press.

Waddell, G. (1996). Keynote address for primary care forum. Low back pain: A twentieth century health care enigma. *Spine*, **21**, 2820–5.

Waddell, G. (1998). *The Back Pain Revolution*. Edinburgh: Churchill-Linvingstone.

Walker, J.R., Cox, B.J., Frankel, S., and Torgrud, L. (1999). *Evaluating two cognitive-Behavioral Self-help Approaches for Generalized Social Phobia*. Poster presentation at the Anxiety Disorders Association of America's 19th National Conference, March 1999, San Diego, CA.

Index